FINALLY SOMEHOW HOME

JASON LEE MORRISON

Finally Somehow Home

EDITED BY ELISABETH STUART
Terima kasih banyak, Liz.

Copyright © 2024 Jason Lee Morrison

All Rights Reserved. This book contains material protected under international and federal copyright laws and treaties. Any unauthorized reprint or use of this material is prohibited. No part of this book may be reproduced or transmitted in any form or by any means, electronic or mechanical, including photocopying, recording, or by any information storage and retrieval system without express written permission from the author/publisher.

ISBN: 979-8-337788-56-2 (Hardcover)
ISBN: 979-8-300091-97-2 (Paperback)

Independently Published by Jason Lee Morrison

Finally Somehow Home

FOR MY RECON BROTHERS

Never Above You.

Never Below You.

Always Beside You.

ARUUUUUGAH!

BOOKS BY JASON LEE MORRISON:

The Perfect Fucking Life

Finally Somehow Home

Finally Somehow Home

If offense is herein proffered,
please take only what you need.

Finally Somehow Home

Chapter 1

Have you ever smelled the jungle by the ocean? The very dirt is sweet to smell. And dark. The ocean hasn't made landfall for ten thousand miles. It's wild and dusky and doesn't give a fuck how beautiful you think it is. Its breeze is off at once to drink the jungle mountain mists - unshrouded now - and down to meet on hinterland line. The beach in back and jungle in front. That's where I grew up. On an island of the Celebes. The cottage by the stream where my little brother-swept to sea - almost drowned, but my four-year-old mind rightly surmised the tide was ripping - I could only run harder - it was chest deep - the time stood still and nothing in the world moved except my brother like something I'd never see again soon. But faster. I still remember pale blue cheeks and dad exhausted on the beach. The Indonesian

Finally Somehow Home

tribesmen holding my little brother by the ankles shaking him until the water followed itself out. A cough, a gasp, and he was back. I have some other memories too. But not of leaving. I was too young to remember leaving the only home I've ever had.

The rest were dorms and barracks.

But I'm getting ahead of myself.

I was born in Kellogg, Idaho. When I was two years old, my parents packed up my two brothers and I, and moved us off to Indonesia. Where I grew up. In the jungles of Sulawesi and Borneo. No shit. I can recall being in an airplane before I can ever remember being in a car. It's one of my earliest memories. We lived in a small cottage on the beach. On the island of Sulawesi in a remote fishing village named Bangketa. It was the Indonesian version of a one-horse town. Two motorcycles. One road. The coast road. My dad had one motorcycle, then there was one other one. Remarkably they did manage to get into an accident.

Growing up there was like watching Hemmingway's <u>Old Man and the Sea</u> unfold every day as the natives paddled their outrigger canoes out into the ocean to fish the

Finally Somehow Home

waters teeming with tuna, swordfish, sail fish, dolphins, rays and all kinds of other shit. The water was so clear and calm sometimes that it seemed like if you fell out of your canoe, you'd fall to the ocean floor. It felt like you were flying. I remember that. We lived there until I was five. I don't know what you think about missionaries, but the real ones, the ones that live it day in and day out for their lives for years at a time aren't quite the same as your college kid heading off for two weeks to help build a school. That's all well and good, but it's not the same thing.

I spent 16 years as the child of missionaries in Indonesia, and I spent 16 years as a Special Operations Marine and Paramilitary. Want to know which one requires more courage? It's a wash. I don't know a single Navy SEAL who would travel, at night, with no gun, or weapon of any kind except a machete, in a small, shitty, leaking hand-hewn wooden boat with a 15-horse motor on it, in the dead of night, 200 miles deep in jungle, with only a native tribal person in a loin cloth with a shitty flashlight to call out logs and rocks and sandbars, no one to call to pick you up if you get into trouble, no radio to call them even if you did, five hours up a river with only the gnarliest classes of rapids, an extra prop and a few extra pins for

Finally Somehow Home

it for when you fuck it all up on the rocks and maybe an extra couple of spark plugs and a wrench in case the boat flips, with fucking snakes as fat as FIATs everywhere as well as every other creature in the jungle who'd love to score a human kill out to get you, in order to bullshit with a bunch of people who've never seen a white person before and think you're an evil spirit and believe that you haven't reached manhood if you haven't taken at least one human head, so you can ask them if you can just fucking set up shop in their shitty village for a few years. Like I said... it's a wash.

My dad was more wild Indian fighter than anything, I thought. It just seemed like that's what he'd have been doing if he had been born in another time. He and the missionary pilot used to fly around over the jungle in the little Piper Super Cub, hours by air away from any kind of civilization. They would look for smoke coming up from the jungle below. If and when they spotted smoke, they would mark it on a map, then spend weeks hiking through Sulawesi's mountains and triple canopy rain forest to see if they could make contact with the people groups whose smoke they had spotted from the air. That's why we were in Bangketa. They had made initial contact with a tribe in the mountains and were

Finally Somehow Home

attempting to follow up with them in the hopes of eventually being allowed to live with them in the jungle.

These people were as primitive as time. They had only occasionally met anyone from the coast to trade rattan and rubber for leaf springs to make machetes and spear heads, wire and bicycle inner tubes for their spear guns, salt, and other necessities of war and life. Their whole world since the beginning of the earth had been only them and the jungle with the few other equally primitive tribes with whom they constantly warred. They called themselves the people of Bahasa Madi: the people of the language of "NO". They were all about five feet tall or less, each tribe's trappings were unique, but all wore only a loin cloth, a small pouch for the betel nut they chewed and the tobacco they smoked, and always a razor-sharp machete, its handle adorned with a plume of human hair from the heads they had taken, each in an ornately carved scabbard tied with wicker weaved rope around their waist. Leather would rot in the jungle. Two bamboo tubes about a foot long tied together and filled with blow-gun darts. The poison for the darts there, ready, in the recess of a bamboo lid in the form of a dark tar-like substance, and a pitch made of sap in the other lid to secure the light hand-hewn cones to the back end

Finally Somehow Home

of their darts which caught the sharp burst of breath and stabilized the dart on its deadly perfect path. The blowguns were eight to nine feet long and their spears twelve or more. Some carried short daggers with L-shaped handles and blades treated with poison, the blades intentionally rusted so that the poison intermingled with the powdery rust. They lived in houses that were sometimes twenty to thirty feet above the ground to keep enemies within their own or other tribes from spearing them through the floor as they slept. Constant wars and Baku bunuh – payback murders. Often just an old woman or young child caught alone carrying water from the river. It didn't matter. As long as someone from the other tribe's head was taken.

They did have medicine. From the Dūkūng - the witchdoctor who communed with the demons and ancestors which dominated their daily lives through taboos, curses, and the like. Some of it was very real. My dad once saw a Dūkūng moving a cow skull back and forth across the ground with gestures of his hand from a distance of over thirty feet. There were no strings or mirrors. Others claimed the ability to shape-shift. The taboos were crushing. In some tribes, for instance, it was taboo to cut the grains of rice from the stalk unless done from directly behind it. Any discovered trespass would be punished severely, sometimes by death, lest the tribe bear the ever-present wrath of the spirits they worshiped. The animistic spirits of the trees and mountains and rocks. I saw a look in their eyes I will never forget.

The next time you're tempted to think that those people are happy the way that they are living. Think about this. I'm gonna call you out here, but don't take offense, just think about it... Our entire race. All of humanity, including your very self, are under that ever-present throbbing burden to ease the pain. Whatever pain there is. It is humanity's greatest obsession. And we do it. We do it every day. We are constantly making things easier for ourselves, and thus less painful. We have developed medicines and accomplished great feats of science and innovation in the pursuit of this cause. A parent wants for their children to feel less pain and have a better life than they. We do it. It's a part of cultural evolution. The evolution of humanity.

Those people are us thousands of years ago. They are evolving as well. They aren't making duller knives and spears. They aren't going backwards. Their culture is

Finally Somehow Home

evolving as well. We used to be there. Ironically, the reason they have been trapped there is not because of the desolation of their environment. The reason they have been trapped in that state is because of the abundance thereof. You must be astute and creative, but there is little need to innovate to survive. They are simply continuing what they have always done, but better. They have the food and water that they need, they can make shelter, and the climate is not so intemperate as to make survivability impossible. They are trapped in Eden.

And all the pain that humanity used to feel, all that we have since sluffed off, at the point of our most acute bondage to it, some would wish to keep on them. All that we have done to ease our pain we wish to keep from them because we have some damn fool notion that they are happy that way. What the fuck is that? That's un-thought-out-worldview-horse-shit. Imagine camping for your whole life in the shit-ass jungle with no REI stuff and no medicine, no written language, no electricity, no hope for shit, just scared. Scared of everything, because everything is trying to kill you, including your belief system. It fucking sucks. Think about it. Don't not think.

Finally Somehow Home

Anyway, it was a pretty cool way to grow up. Running around barefoot everywhere. Pet monkeys and the whole nine yards. We had a pet pig too. She was wonderful, but we had to eat her. Sorry Sofie.

I was six when I went off to boarding school where all the other missionary kids went. I was the littlest kid there and the only one in my grade. That was a very difficult and lonely time for me. And formative. We moved from Sulawesi to Kalimantan (old Borneo) about a year after that and lived 15 miles or so outside the city of Pontianak, translated: "Ghost Child". My parents took on the job of dorm parents at the missionary boarding school there called Wajok Hulu. They oversaw the welfare of all the missionary kids who, outside of the school semesters, lived in the interior tribes with their parents. When we first showed up there, the local police stopped by to see my dad. The month before Ramadan was a big month for thieving because all debts had to be paid before it started. "If you catch any penchuris (thieves), just kill them and throw them time the river." They said. Proper guns were illegal in Indonesia because of the attempted Communist Coup in '65-'66 when a shitload of mass killings took place, so my dad made a gun out of a piece of lead pipe and loaded it with big M80 type firecrackers

Finally Somehow Home

and marbles. He did shoot it at a penchuri or two but just over their heads to scare them off as they ran away into the jungle.

The river that the cops had referred to was the Kapuas River adjacent to our property. We called it the "Mighty Ka-poo-poo" because it was shit-gross but we still played in it. It was big and brown and slow and muddy, over 600 miles long and it drained much of Western Kalimantan. We were only ten miles or so from its mouth to the Indian Ocean. The ocean tide would come back up the river. Because the school property was sometimes under two to three feet of water, all the houses were built on stilts to keep out of the high tide. It was a little dicey when the tide would come up, because all the snakes and bugs and other creatures that lived on or in the ground or in the grass had to go somewhere, so they were all swimming around eating each other or climbing up the nearest tree and eating each other. All the while, my brothers and I were frolicking in the water. Of course.

I spent most of my time fishing, hunting with my pellet gun for coconut squirrels, launching firecrackers and bottle rockets into giant ant nests, or – my favorite pastime – throwing knives at the mud crabs. I had a

Finally Somehow Home

parang (machete) when I was 8 years old. I got it for my birthday from my parents... a parang and a Bible. I became pretty good at throwing my knife. I killed a snake with it once. It was a good throw. 12 feet or so. The knife split his head down the middle, just off to one side, so when my buddy and I collected the snake his jaw was hanging off at a wonky angle. We buried the head so no one would step on it and get a dose of the venom, threw the wretched snake corpse into the river, and called the place "Snake's Jaw" after that. But we kept it a secret because only kids nine years or older were allowed to kill snakes without adult supervision. The penalty was confiscation of our parangs and knives for a week. A sentence worse than shoes. So, I guess only he and I called it Snake's Jaw since we were the only ones who knew about it.

We'd go into the tribes sometimes to see our school friends when they were home with their parents. These tribes were up to 2 hours into the jungle by air – a Cessna 185. The missionaries had hacked the little airstrips out of the jungle near their respective tribal villages so the plane could land for monthly resupply or emergency medical evacuations. I always felt jealous of the kids that lived in the tribes. I remember on one of these trips

Finally Somehow Home

interior we decided to go on a hunting trip, so our parents drove us 3 or 4 hours from the village on one of the few red dirt logging roads and dropped us off with nothing but what we could carry. Our parangs, pellet guns, and a cross bow for the "babi hutan" (wild jungle pigs) we were hunting. It was my two brothers and I, along with two brothers of one of the other missionary families. The oldest of us was probably 15 or 16 and my little brother was probably 10. I clearly remember wishing I had brought flip-flops because I kept stepping on thorns with my bare feet. We camped and hunted in the jungle for 3 days, then hitched a ride back on a truck that happened to be going toward the village on the logging road.

We didn't have a TV for a while, so my dad would read books to us every night instead. Dad was and still is an avid reader, historian, and overall lover of knowledge. So, to keep it interesting he read us the classics: <u>The Killer Angels</u> by Michael Shara, <u>Beau Geste</u> by P.C. Wren, C.S. Forester's Horatio Hornblower series, Baroness Orczy's <u>The Scarlet Pimpernel</u>. The goods. We scraped up enough money somewhere along the way to buy a TV. I think it was a 10.5" Black and White jobber. There was only one channel. And it was only on

Finally Somehow Home

for certain hours of the day, but Friday nights at 10:00 or 11:00 the A-Team was usually on and we would be woken up and enjoy our TV show for the week. It was around this time that I started writing poetry for the first time I can remember. I believe this was my first poem, I can remember none before it.

I want to be a pilot,
And fly up in the sky,
Just sitting in my airplane,
And watch the world go by,
It's a nice way of transportation,
And lots of fun to me,
But what I like the most about it,
Is the way I fly so free.

A savant to be sure. I began writing more and more, such as it was.

Finally Somehow Home

Chapter 2

I ended up back in Sulawesi at my old boarding school for alittle while. It was near the city of Palu and it was called Wera Falls. It is still the most beautiful place that I have ever seen. It was up in the mountains, so the air was crisp and cool and the rain was sweet and a river clear and rocky flowed through it and it would flood sometimes. But it was always there, bubbling clear and gently or thundering dark and furious, it was always there like music. Butterflies were everywhere. So many that most kinds we couldn't find the names for. A little brook that shot out from the river was home to most of them where it formed in pools. We would carve our initials in the tree there if we were so bold as to "Like" someone. It was the source of considerable gossip and consternation in the 6th grade. One Saturday, me and

Finally Somehow Home

two buddies decided to hike up the mountain to the big waterfall. I think it took us a couple of hours through the jungle. Zig zagging the river and crossing where we could, back and forth to find the best route up. We climbed up the falls and explored the cavernous hollow in the rock just below its crest over which the torrent thundered, filling the space with cold mist and a constant deafening roar and we put our hands out into the plunging water's ominous weight. When we got too cold we left out on the other side of the falls into the sunlight and laid there on the sun-warmed rocks till we stopped shivering. We went back a different way. Down the other side of the falls to which we had emerged. It was steeper. One of my buddies was using a vine to slide down the side of a rock face and it broke. He fell a good 12 or 15 feet and landed on his back on the point of a rock. The point missed his spine by an inch and left a big bloody gash. He was ok. We washed it the best we could in the river. He still has a scar.

I had a couple of spear guns that I had swapped for from one of the kids from the Lauje' tribe. The Lauje' made good parangs and weapons and spear guns and such, so the missionary kids that lived among them used to make a killing in trades. I have to admit though, that I still have

Finally Somehow Home

a parang from the Wana tribe and it has served me well... And I think Wana made better blow guns. Anyway, we used the spear guns for spear fishing the river and the ocean as well. We'd camp and we'd hunt and we'd ride our bicycles all over that place checking the fruit trees for jambu biji (guava), and other varieties of jambus (water apples). Papaya trees were everywhere. A ripe papaya with the right amount of massaging becomes a perfect papaya grenade. Accurately hurled, or with the big ones, lobbed down a cliff onto the unwary passerby below, would explode in a magnificent splatter of orange goop and black slimy seeds. We thus spent a lot of time at wars. Sneaking around ambushing each other. It was hard being away from my parents. My brothers were there with me, so we all made the best of it and developed very strong friendships with the other kids who were likewise away from their families for four to five months at a time.

We spent a lot of time in that river. When it would rain up higher in the mountains you could see the water get restless and murky. A flash flood was coming. A wall of water five to seven feet high would come hurtling violently down carrying boulders and trees and dirt and whatever else it could find. Then the river would roar

Finally Somehow Home

like a lion. It was fierce. After a few days the flood would subside a bit, though it was still fast and dark and loud. It was then that one of our favorite pastimes ensued: Buttbusting. Tubing the river didn't work. The rocks would literally bust your butt sticking out of the bottom of the hole in the inner tube, so the best way to do it was just lay down, keep your ass out of the way of the rocks, keep your feet pointed down river and try not to die. None of us ever did. Although there were cases of people being caught in the river at the onset of a flash flood only to be found later, miles down-river once the water receded, if ever at all.

I attended Wera for two years, after which, I returned to Wajok Hulu where my parents worked at what had become the 8th - 12th grade high school. There were thirty-some-odd kids there in total. Mostly American kids, but a handful of Aussies and Kiwis as well. My class was the biggest, with eight of us. I was a small kid for my age and always the youngest in my class. But when we took a six-month trip back to the good ole US of A, I had to try out for football in spite of it. I was the smallest kid on the team and my pre-pubescent voice shrieked instead of grunted like the other guys. I had to sit on a pillow in driver's ed. That's how small I was in the 9th

Finally Somehow Home

grade. When I'd wear my football jersey to school on game days it came down past my knees. It sucked, but all the upper classmen on the football team liked me and took care of me. They called me Pee-Wee. One time a sophomore poured a cup full of everyone's piss on me in the locker room shower. The upper classmen got him with some Icy Hot to the bollocks. Anyway, I was a little guy. I don't take much shine to bullies and meanness in general now because of it.

These trips to "The States" happened about every 3 to 4 years that we were on the mission field. We loved it. Apples. Real milk, not the powdered stuff. Cereal. Meat that wasn't full of gristle. It was always wonderful coming back to North Idaho and seeing our family. North Idaho is a beautiful place to come back to. It's like a postcard everywhere you look. The worst part as a kid was that mom and dad had to go visit all the churches that supported them. And we had to go too. Especially when we were younger, it was rough. Going to a different Sunday school every Sunday. All those weird kids oogling at you and asking dumb questions. I spun some wild yarns in some of those Sunday school rooms as a little guy. I eventually quit when one of the Sunday school teachers asked my dad about one of my stories to confirm its veracity. Dammit! Busted. And singing songs in Indonesian in front of a different church every Sunday, then the dinner at the pastor's house... A kid's worst nightmare, but we were stalwart little guys and took it on the chin. It was important to my parents that we were with them. My dad always said that we were all part of the team. So we traveled the United States, a lot of it anyway, in an old LTD Ford. With my little brother asleep up on the car's back window ledge, my older brother asleep on the back seat, and me sleeping on the damned hump on the floor, but those were good days. By the end of six months though, we were always ready to go back. Teachers would look sad and full of pity at me as I handed in my paperwork to get pulled out of school for the flight back. "I'm sorry that you have to go back there." I could only look back at them with incredulity.

High School in Indonesia was fun. I finally started growing and getting picked on less and less until I could bring the hammer down on my bullies and best them or at least give them a run for their money. Sweet relief. I've always made sure to look out for other little guys too, since then. My first motorcycle was a Frankenstein of a creature. It was a Suzuki 185cc. I think

Finally Somehow Home

it was a 1977 or thereabouts. Or at least one or more of the motorcycles that comprised its being was. It was light and quick because it was a two cylinder two-stroke engine. I loved that thing. My brothers and I cobbled it together one summer from spare parts and junked bikes in the garage. My older brother already had a motorcycle and my little brother didn't have a license yet, so "The Beast" went to me. I painted a Flying Tiger's shark mouth on the tank and was the terror of Pontianak on that thing. One time I decided to clean out all the carbon from my mufflers. I got most of it out in the shop with only afew fragments of it left in there. Shortly thereafter a buddy and I decided to take a trip into town. I was driving about 30 yards in front of him and the engine backfired and launched a smoking hot piece of carbon directly between the gaps in his button-up fly. It made for a puzzling spectacle in my rear view mirror. Driving there was dangerous as fuck. That's all there is to it. Even if you survived the accident, if it was your fault, you might get hacked up with a parang alittle bit. The lines on the road were there only as decorations and the only rule was...again: don't die. Just for fun, there were other random factors at play as well. I was coming home from a basketball game late one night and

Finally Somehow Home

suddenly the asphalt in front of me was gone and replaced by 100 yards of pea gravel. All I could do was stay frozen in terror and stay on the gas. I swam the bike all the way through it and came out the other side none the worse for wear except for afew shattered nerves, but that's just the kind of thing you'd expect an Indonesian road crew to do for you. No signs. No asphalt. Pea gravel. Fuckin' pea gravel. I also remember a few times I had to dodge a pissed off cobra on the road. For that you just pin the throttle and lift your feet up as high as you can.

I didn't really care about school and was a dumb kid through most of it. I was always in trouble. I remember back when I was in first or second grade, my teacher asked if anyone had any questions. And, as right at that moment, I happened to be thinking of how, that afternoon, I was going to build an airplane out of blocks of wood from the woodshed. One that could fly. I asked a question about it. About the airplane. The teacher beat on me with the paddle for that one. There was no such thing as attention deficit disorder back then...well, maybe there was, but not out there... so I muddled on through and learned the best I could.

Finally Somehow Home

I had always wanted to be a pilot. I loved it when the mission plane would fly over. Any plane for that matter. Planes didn't fly over very frequently there. I would always stop and look up in the sky with wonder at them. I can't imagine what the Tribal people thought they were. Anyway, the mission plane was great because the pilot would sometimes buzz the school. Especially one of the pilots over in Sulawesi. He would buzz the school low, fast, and loud. First he'd pop out over the ridge with his engine cut and idling so we didn't know he was there, then he'd swoop down on the school building and right above it he would open the throttle all the way and scare the hell out of all of us. Then we'd all bail out of our classrooms and run outside and wave at him as he waggled his wings and flew away. He was great. Funny too. He died in a plane crash in Venezuela a few years later. His son was one of my best friends. He later became an F-15 fighter pilot.

I heard a story about some of the pilots on one of the other mission fields who were trying to do something nice for the kids around Christmas time. They had rigged a dummy to look like Santa into one of the planes. One of the pilots was going to fly over the school and throw the dummy Santa out into the jungle, then the

Finally Somehow Home

other pilot, hidden just inside the jungle, would come strolling out in a Santa costume with gifts and candy for all the kids. Unfortunately, and in view of all the kids, the Santa dummy came hurtling out of the airplane and "shacked" the school roof in a perfect dive-bomb. Direct hit. The kids were distraught, thinking that Santa had just plummeted to his death in their midst, in spite of the most noble efforts of the other pilot who came bounding out of the jungle with his bag full of goodies.

It was around that time that someone burned our house down with us in it. Good thing my dog started barking or my whole family would have been toast. We all made it out. It was about 4:30 in the morning so we only just woke up and ran out of the place before it burned to the ground in front of our eyes. The fire department never showed up. I guess we didn't really expect it to. At the time I didn't know what had happened, I thought it was an electrical fire, but years later I found out the truth about it. When I found out, I thought it over. But I decided not to go back and find the guy and kill him. I know who it was. We lost everything we owned. I don't mind that so much. But ole' boy tried to kill my family and he tried to kill me, and people are always trying to kill me and it pisses me off. But no... Water under the

Finally Somehow Home

bridge and all that. That's kind of the risk you took of living there. It was a truly amazing culture. Directly influenced by people either living in the jungle, or people only just removed within afew generations of living in the jungle. It was a surreal and fascinating glimpse into the ragged evolution of culture happening before our eyes every day just as it does in our present, but to see it thousands of years from what you already know it to become, and see from the tribes still in the jungle to the people living in the city a span of the millennia, really made you think. It is simple. Elegant. They were exceptionally polite and considerate, extremely deferential and gracious to a fault, yet brutally violent and sudden when the time ever came for it. And we were living in it, so it's just one of those things that we had to accept.

As I said, ever since I can remember I had wanted to be a pilot. Well, except Indiana Jones. I remember watching Indiana Jones as a kid and deciding that's what I wanted to be...until I realized that I couldn't, and then I was pissed. But other than Indiana Jones, I'd always wanted to be a pilot. And thanks to Top Gun - the highly edited version with all the swears dubbed out - and a tattered old Naval Academy Admissions guide that I had found

Finally Somehow Home

lying around our library, by the 10th grade I knew I wanted to be a fighter pilot. All of a sudden I started getting A's in everything. Not so dumb after all. My girlfriend was a beautiful Kiwi/Aussie girl. Her parents were one of each. But I never got to see her because her parents worked on an island far away. Over in the Malukus. I got to talk to her on the radio once though. Which was nice. But odd. Since every other missionary within afew hundred miles was listening in on our conversation. My senior year I was the Captain of the Basketball team and the Student Council President. Pee-Wee, the comeback kid! I received Congressional and Senatorial nominations to the US Naval Academy, US Air Force Academy, and the US Military Academy. I went for the Navy. In filling out the admissions packet the Medical equipment that was needed to conduct some of the tests was not available at the hospitals there, so since the Medical portion was incomplete, so was my packet and I was not offered an appointment. I was pretty bummed out. Hell, I was devastated. I had spent the past two years of my young life getting ready for this, and now nothing. I remember running barefoot 3 miles a day on a gravel and dirt road, studying my ass off, and obsessing over it for what had

Finally Somehow Home

seemed an eternity. It's hard to write about this stuff. I don't like remembering all the feelings of disappointment and even shame when I found out that I couldn't go to the Naval Academy. Everyone had very subtly let me know that I shouldn't get my hopes up. It was such a long shot, especially given my situation, that I probably wouldn't make it. Like I didn't already know that. But I wanted so badly to prove them all wrong. And now they were right. All of them. Fuck. I get it now. I understand now. But I still felt slighted and ripped off at the time. I was pissed. I finished up my high school year and came back to the States in June 1995. I turned 18 afew days after getting back. I didn't really have a back up plan for the Naval Academy so I thought I'd just go to the Missionary school that my older brother was going to, to kill time while I figured something out. To my surprise, during that first semester I got a letter from the Naval Academy inviting me to re-apply. So I went through it all again. I got another Congressional nomination and commenced to filling out the paperwork. This time the hospital that I went to for my physical failed to submit the paperwork to the Naval Academy. Yea. That's when I decided: "Fuck it. I'm joining the Marines."

Chapter 3

I dropped out of Bible school at the end of the semester. Everyone there acted like I was Jonah or something. Running away from God. I showed up to Boot Camp in San Diego on February 12, 1996. Guaranteed Infantry. I won't talk much about Boot Camp. You can watch Full Metal Jacket for that. But I will say that the Marine Corps manages to accomplish an awful lot in three months. After that I went to the School of Infantry (SOI) as an 0311 - Rifleman. A few weeks into it we had some guests come in. They were all jacked, and their sleeves were rolled up to just below their elbows - which was out of regulations - and they wore sunglasses on their heads and big watches and a few of them were "dual cool". They wore shiny gold jump wings and a dive bubble on their chests. It was Recon. People always

Finally Somehow Home

talked about Recon but no one really knew much about them. They were taking applications for their selection course. The line to sign up was long. There was still a good chance I could get into the Naval Academy from the Marine Corps, and I had no intention whatsoever of derailing my hopes of it by mucking around with the snake-eater shit that those Recon guys were there to sign us up for, so I stayed in my seat. Until there was only one guy left signing his name. Then I couldn't help it. I went up and signed my name too. I was the very last one. There were well over 200 names on the paper. 12 of us were selected and invited to take the Recon Indoctrination. 3 of us passed and got orders to 1st Recon Company after SOI.

I was at Recon but no way I was a Recon Marine when I first showed up. Not until I went through a lot of shit. They called us "Ropers". We wore a 12 foot sling rope, doubled and tied in a sheet bend in a big loop that went behind the neck, in front of the shoulders and ending at the lower back with the knot. We ran everywhere we went, and at any time any of the Recon Marines, regardless of rank, could stop us and ask us questions pertaining to our knowledge of various subjects we'd been taught, test us on our knot tying, or

Finally Somehow Home

just make us do push-ups or anything else they felt like doing, drunk or sober. I was one of a handful of Ropers floating around waiting for a RIP (Recon Indoctrination Program) class to start up for about a month and a half. It was constant thrashing and studying. There was so much that we had to learn: Radio antenna wave propagation, land navigation, demolitions, patrolling, equipment, calling in air support, calling artillery, calling Naval guns, small craft rigging and handling, nautical navigation, tidal currents, Initial Terminal Guidance, reporting, combat swimming, combat life saving... it was a lot, but all with a very heavy emphasis on patrolling. Patrolling was everything. Patrolling is what makes Recon super-ninja. We do it better than anyone else.

We used to run telephone poles up Margarita Peak all the time. Margarita Peak. Fuck. You didn't exactly run up it. The last 100 yards was more of a crawl on all fours, because the face was so damn steep you could just stick your arms out in front of you and you were crawling. When I went in to see the dentist one time, they asked me why there were bare spots behind my ears where all of the skin had been rubbed off. I said it was from carrying the telephone poles on my shoulders, and

Finally Somehow Home

then I fell asleep while they worked on my teeth. They woke me up after they did their dental work and I left and joined the others to do it again. Another fun game was thrashing in the laundry room. They used to lock us in the laundry room and turn all of the dryers on high heat and we would live in there and thrash and thrash and sweat all night long.

Pre-scuba. Pre-Fucking Scuba. The hardest thing you'll ever do in this life, my Son, is a legit Pre-Scuba. I did 2. Mother – T - Fucker! I did the first one because, like I said, I was a Roper and I was waiting for my RIP class to start and there were not enough new guys at the Company to start up a class yet, so I ended up going to a company Pre Scuba just to pass the time. Holy Shit. They put us in teams in the second week. My dive buddy was a Hispanic dude who they had let into the Marine Corps in spite of the demonic rat tattooed on the side of his head. We called him Chewy. Motherfuckin' Chewy and me tore that shit up. When they'd "hit" you, you just had to make yourself relax in spite of every urge to struggle, and hold on to your dive buddy. Hold on to your dive buddy with one hand and to your tanks with the other. We wore the dive tanks full of air (so they were heavy and negatively buoyant), but no regulator, just a snorkel to breathe through. I tried to breathe shallow so they would hit me on my inhale. It didn't work. The hand comes over the snorkel on the exhale or a knee to the solar plexus. Or both. You have no breath left in your lungs. And down you go in a swirl of violence to the bottom of the 12-foot pool. You can feel the water pressure in your ears. You can only hear dull and flat sounds. It's a flurry of punching and knees and ripping off equipment. Anything that can be ripped off, tanks are stolen if possible, fins come off, masks, everything comes off or is fucked with except for the weight belt that drags you down... and then it's over. It's you and your dive buddy on the bottom of the pool with all your equipment spread across the floor of it. You want to breathe like mad by now. But you know you have to stay calm and conserve your oxygen. If you don't you'll fucking die. Keep your head. Don't panic. Don't shoot to the surface, control the fear and gather up your shit. Help your buddy. Once it's done and you are properly wearing all of your equipment again, you give your buddy the ok and the hand signal to surface, four fingers, and ascend slowly with your hand in a fist above your head. Your mask is still full of water and so is your snorkel. But if you break the surface of the water with

Finally Somehow Home

your face and gasp for air you'll go down again in a flash and without so much as another breath. You break the surface with your snorkel and the top of your head, face still in the water. Use all the air left in your lungs to clear the snorkel of water, then blow the water out of your mask with your nose and continue with the rest of the class to swim slowly in a circle, head and eyes down, waiting patiently for the next hit. Job well done. Me and Chewy were top of the class. He died in a helicopter crash a couple years later. I have scars on my face from when I got drunk that night. One of the best men I've ever known. After that Pre-Scuba my RIP class started.

RIP was where they culled the herd. Attrition was the mission. It was all assholes and elbows the whole time. Constant grinding and classes and ruck runs and paddle drills back and forth through the surf zone for miles along the California coast. We lived on the beach out of old-school shelter halves, or out on patrol under the night sky. We would eat our dinner MRE every night sitting linked together arm in arm in the frigid surf with the waves breaking over us and singing "Leatherneck" till we got it right. This is "Leatherneck" as I was taught it:

Finally Somehow Home

I'm a Recon Ranger,
I live a life of danger,
I run everywhere I go.
I dream about wars,
And slant-eyed whores
At fifteen dollars a throw.

I've had all kinds of kills
and all kinds of thrills,
but the thrill that you'll never know,
Is the thrill that'll get ya when you get your picture on the cover of the Leatherneck.

CHORUS:
Leatherneck,
I'm gonna buy five copies,
Leatherneck,
I'm gonna send them to my Pappie,
Leatherneck,
I'm gonna call the Sergeant Major and tell him I got my picture on the cover of The Leatherneck

I've got an M-16, It's super fuckin mean,
It gets me dozens of kills each day,

Finally Somehow Home

But I don't bitch and I don't moan,
even though I gets no pay,
You see it's all just designed
to fuck with your mind,
but your mind will never know,
the thrill that'll get ya when you get your picture on the cover of The Leatherneck.

We sat in the surf zone in our "deuce gear" to eat. Your deuce gear (short for 782 Gear), no idea what the hell 782 is.... Anyway, your deuce gear was a Y harness and belt and had all of your "go to war" stuff on it. That's why you always wore it, and even slept with it on as something like a pillow, but with arms still through the shoulder straps. Mag pouches enough for at least 12 magazines, grenade pouches, utility and handbook pouch, canteens, sling rope, Med Kit, and an ass-pack that contained a survival kit and usually a survival chow, as well as our only dry things of the night, and if the waterproofing leaked, you slept spooning, shivering under a wet poncho and poncho liner. We got good at waterproofing.

I won't go into all of it. It would take up too much time. I just remember long cold nights swimming all night long

Finally Somehow Home

through that heavy surf zone with El Niño coming down. Doing Confirmatory Beach Reports. Diving for bottom samples 20-30 feet down in the dark. Finning with all your might, and dragging someone's slow ass through that incessant pounding surf. Special Operations is just hard fucking work. It looks cool and all but there is nothing glamorous that is all too important to it. Most of it is just hard fucking shitty work.

Recon was volunteer only, so if at anytime anyone quit they were out. They were immediately separated from the rest of us. The instructors had us construct a cemetery and when someone quit they were made to put a rock in the cemetery as a tombstone. I was instructed to write a eulogy and hold a service with all the students and cadre present. This is what I read that cold, wet, and sandy night on Red Beach:

Dearly beloved,

We are gathered here on this 28th day of August in the year of our Lord 1996 to remember these fallen comrades, and hope in due time, that we can forget all about them and all like them. May we never stoop to the lowness that they did, and never, never in our lives utter the words they did. The words that can disqualify us from our greatest

Finally Somehow Home

hopes and aspirations, and worst of all, disqualify us from being and serving among the best men in God's universe: United States Recon Marines.

May those here among us with a heart like theirs join them soon, and the men who have the heart and mind to drive on, no matter what the obstacles, soon achieve that which we have striven and will continue to strive for: The Title of Recon Marine.

The entire selection and training process never really ended. You could be canned at any time and "sent to the grunts (the Infantry)", and a lot more people quit than passed overall, but within a few months time you had a pretty solid crew of guys that would most likely make it if they didn't get injured, and that was the purpose of RIP. That, and to start things off teaching guys the way it was done in the field before teaching them the way it's done at a school. It was the beginning of the selection process and very ad hoc which made it miserably incessant. There were no rules. The instructors were operators who were in platoons and looking for fresh meat for their own platoons standing up for the deployment cycle, so there was no school mindset. Guys were literally training and screening new guys that they

Finally Somehow Home

would go to war with if they made it through the rest of the training, so the standard was high in both selection and in the quality and care of instruction. Everyone had skin in the game. If you made it through RIP, that meant Recon would give you a chance and send you to the Basic Recon Course or Amphibious Reconnaissance School, West and East Coast respectively. If you could make it through that, you had a shot at a future in Recon. RIP finally ended. A meager and hard ass handful were left and went straight into a Pre-scuba. Round two for me. I used to sing Pearl Jam's "I'm still alive…hey, I'm still alive." Every night on the way home from the pool, crammed into the back of the HMMWV with all the dive tanks and equipment, breathing in exhaust fumes, shivering because you've been in the water for so long that your core temperature has dropped. Haunted by underwater crossovers… over and over and over. Try to come up for air before touching the other side of the pool and shoved down by the back of the head to the bottom of the pool you keep swimming and gulping in your throat because it feels like breathing and the other side is getting closer and one more kick, and you touch it and you have to breathe so bad, and only break the surface of the water with your fist above your head and gasp for air

Finally Somehow Home

and drag yourself up and out, your eyes feel like they're bleeding from the chlorine but you ignore it, and get into the pushup position and hold it. Hold it until your whole body shakes and the sweat drips off your nose and keep your back straight, and keep holding it, then the cadre: "Push...Up", and down and up "One!" you yell, voice shaking. "Push...Up" and "Two!", and on and on... can't catch your breath, "Pays to be a winner" the cadre yells, "crossover!", and gasping for a final breath and splash into the water and down as deep as you can and clear your ears and swim like mad across the bottom, lungs burning, tunnel vision, get there first and you'll get a rest... if you don't, you won't... For hours...

For years after that, I'd sometimes just sit back, relax and be thankful that I could breathe.

Chapter 4

After my second Pre-scuba, I was off to the Basic Recon Course. BRC was by no means easy. I puked my guts out on the Trail of Tears and likewise endorsed many of the physical fitness evolutions. But I was somewhat accustomed to it by then. We would swim and run for miles every day in addition to our class work and field exercises. It never hurt less, I guess I just became used to the pain. And I still hate underwater crossovers, but water became our friend too. It is the ultimate equalizer. The toughest guy in the world can be made into a blubbering pathetic whelp with the introduction of water. Nobody likes to drown. It's a rather unpleasant feeling. I remember a couple of us went on a deep sea fishing charter one weekend and I can clearly recall wondering how anyone could possibly drown if

Finally Somehow Home

they could see the land. In my mind, it was right there. All you had to do was swim afew miles. I had become so accustomed to accomplishing certain things that it actually conditioned my way of thinking. Your mind learns from everything. You can teach it to take the hard shit for granted by doing hard shit all the time. And that's the only way to do the hard stuff: do it anyway. Do it even though it hurts. That's just life. If something hurts, it doesn't mean it's all bad for you. At the top of an athlete's game, he's not sitting around eating donuts all day being comfortable. At the top of your game, in fact, most shit will hurt for you to do. The greatest I've ever been, I felt at that time as if I was just barely keeping my lips above the water. Do the hard stuff anyway. It's supposed to suck. It's ok that it sucks. It's good that it sucks. But it still sucks. It will always suck. Waiting for it to all feel like roses and butterflies isn't going to work. Do the hard shit anyway. There's one caveat to this: there's a difference between difficulty and injury. If you are in a situation that is injuring you, such as an abusive relationship, get the fuck out of it immediately. Don't just stay in it hoping that someone else will change while you get bludgeoned to death. That's not perseverance, it's stupid. Running on a

Finally Somehow Home

leg that's hurt and running on the leg that's broken are two very different things.

I'm not going to try to make it sound all "my class was the hardest" at all. The vetting and the transition from new guy to seasoned operator took years and the first part was a motherfucker. It had to be. If you've ever been a part of a no shit Special Operations selection and indoctrination, you know how much it sucks. And if you haven't, I got nothing to prove to you. Hell, I got nothing to prove to you either way. I learned some important lessons through all of it. I thought the Marine Corps was trying to teach me about war. About how to be proficient in its conduct. But that's not where the real lessons were - the lessons that set us apart from the rest. Not even close. What set us apart from the rest was not what we learned about war, but what we learned about ourselves. Yes, we had to know the technical aspects of operating at an elite level, but what made us elite was the lessons we learned for ourselves about ourselves in those grueling days. I remember when I was at dive school, I asked a friend how he could fin so fast (swimming with fins on). "If you want to be a faster finner, fin faster" was his answer. It's not pain that gives you perseverance. The only way to learn it is to do

Finally Somehow Home

it. Perseverance gives you perseverance. That's it. There is not an easy way. The same is true of life. When it sucks. When you really don't have what you need to keep going. When it really sucks bad deep as fuck and you have only two options: give the fuck up or take one more step...if you take that step, the next feeling you'll have is more and worse pain. It's that feeling where you ran out of the energy to complain a very long time ago. Where there's no more jokes, there's no more bitching about how much it sucks, there's no more of anything but to keep going. At that point it's only pure rage that you're clinging to because that is the only tangible emotion that you can feel toward your tremendous and overwhelming and incessant and un-relieved pain. And you know it will not end soon. That feeling. That is the feeling of you becoming awesome. Becoming elite. That's what it feels like. That's what set us apart. You can only get it that way. That's just how that shit works.

After that I went to Combatant Dive School. This was what all the fuss was about with the Pre-scuba courses. Dive School was so hard, you had to pass another school to go to it. It was in Panama City, Florida. And my class was there during spring

Finally Somehow Home

break. Well I guess it didn't spring that break. Because it was cold as shit. I remember breaking the ice off of my wetsuit to put it on for 3 AM dives. You struggled to get it on. The ice breaks off in little bits as you wriggle into it, shuddering. We had already prepped the boats and pre-dive checked the rigs so all we had to do was just come in and dive. Put on your wet cammies (camouflage utilities) over your wetsuit to further irritate you. Your hood is annoying as fuck hanging off the back of your neck at some wonky angle. Your buddy helps you put your dive rig and buoyancy compensator on. You do so grudgingly; the strap hanging the entire weight of the rig around the back of your neck is another pain in the ass. You waddle over to help your buddy get into his rig. You get your fins, mask, Duece gear, rucksack with a full 5-gallon water can in it, buddy line, buoy line, whoever is "driving" (the lead diver) has the compass board "dummy chorded" and snap linked to his rig. Hanging off. Now put the damned mask around your neck under your chin, and the regulator hanging off your head to the front. Your fucking back hurts. This goddamn weight belt needs to be adjusted and now I gotta piss already, god damn it. Not to mention that we're diving pure oxygen, which makes you irritable

Finally Somehow Home

anyway. Dive Sūp (Supervisor) Checks are starting already. "Dive Sūp. It's my first dive of the day and I feel fine." The Dive Supervisor, supremely comfortable in cammie bottoms (camouflage trousers), Chuck Taylors, and a voluptuous hoodie, inspects each diver and rig in a ritual and thorough inspection. You stand awkwardly and wait your turn.

"Grab all your shit and get to the boats." It's fuckin freezing and there's a wind. The wetsuit begins to prove its worth. You drag and haul your kit to the boats and flop in. The air is thick with the exhaust of the outboard motors. You sit and rest on the rubber gunnel, the weight of the dive rig resting on your lap finally relieving the strain on your sore neck. The wind whips up alittle shit ass spray from the surface of the water, which keeps hitting you in the face, but the surface chop isn't too bad, and there is no swell in the bay, so it's just the vindictive little spitting of mother nature in your face that pisses you off extra. The smell of gasoline and burning oil in blue smoke from the engines hangs in the air. The boats look like chemlight creatures jostling along the choppy surface at a quick clip toward the insert point 2 thousand meters away from the pier, which was the target. It's

Finally Somehow Home

miserable, but you don't bother worrying about it because you know it's about to get even worse.

You had to dive on time and on target. You had to show up exactly when and where you needed to be with only the initial bearing of the compass once you were in the water, then one tactical peak, where 500 or so meters from the target, the driver with the compass board would ease toward the surface while his buddy and other divers below held on to the buddy line that they were all snap linked into. As soon as the diver's head broke the surface he'd be pulled back down by the divers below him. He had just a split second to check his bearing and distance to the target before he was pulled back below the surface. Then it was on to the target to do whatever dastardly deed needed doing.

We learned how to dive SCUBA there as well, but our tool of the trade was a Dräger LAR V closed circuit rebreather. It was a small chest mounted rig and used only pure oxygen while scrubbing the Carbon Dioxide out of the breathing loop with Sofnolime or Sodasorb - the same stuff you use to make lawns nice and green. So essentially you were under water breathing the same air over and over again but it was being supplemented by

Finally Somehow Home

pure O2 and all the CO2 was being scrubbed out of it in a continuous loop. This was handy because there were no bubbles from it to give away the presence of divers to anyone on the surface, as there was with SCUBA. You could only go 20-25 feet deep or you would get O2 toxicity, but it was a great rig for sneaking up on piers, or boats, or fish. I surprised the hell out of something big down there one night on accident. I was 20 feet down skimming the bottom when all of a sudden a shitload of phosphorescence stirred up just below me and scared the ever-living shit out of me. There were Hammer-head sharks in that bay, maybe it was one of those. Sometimes the guys at the dive locker back at the unit would help themselves to any lobster that might be lying around the bottom of the ocean. They were easy as hell to sneak up on with that rig because it was so quiet, and as far as the game warden knew it was just a couple of guys in a rubber dingy out on the water minding their own business. You could stay down for a couple of hours on those things, but they did make you irritable as fuck, and as there were no bubbles, you could yell and cuss at each other through the regulator and hear pretty damn well.

Anyway, back to the story: You had to be OT/OT - On Time and On Target. The engines idle. The boats drift to

Finally Somehow Home

a stop in the wind. The Dive Sūp points to the divers and gives them the command to enter the water. You hold onto your weight belt and back strap with one hand and onto your mask and regulator with the other and roll back in. The icy water shocks the breath out of you and begins to fill your wetsuit. You purge your rig. Your rucks get passed down to you. The driver checks his azimuth. You give the OK. You get a 2 (two fingered hand signal) from the dive Sup, which means to go subsurface, and return it. You let some air out of your buoyancy compensator and sink into the black ocean water. The sound of the idling boat motors is very loud. Everything else is dull. The pressure of the water closes cold and dark around you. Even your sense of touch is tempered by the feel of the wetsuit everywhere, even on your finger tips. You piss yourself finally as you sink, relieving the strain of the past hours. The warmth is delicious in your wetsuit. The driver is ready. It's time to fin. And kick and kick and kick and kick and kick.

Chapter 5

After Dive School, the real training started: Constant, continuous, and intensive patrolling. I learn the hands-on way. And that's how they taught us patrolling. It is a craft and it was taught as such. There's a lot that goes into all that is required of living for days and weeks, surrounded and undetected, in the wilderness, all the while reporting and surveilling, and where possible, ambushing the shit out of bad guys. It was like playing at war again, and I loved it. I paid close attention. We were learning lessons the Vietnam guys had left behind for us. It was like the lessons that the old Samurai had passed along to their following generations. At the end of the day, it was the same thing. The craft's most elite pass along the most essential knowledge, and patrolling

Finally Somehow Home

was something we took very seriously at Recon. Amen and Amen.

Marching and close order drill and spit-shining your boots and not walking on the grass, and all the other stupid bullshit...not so much. I think because, although we could not articulate it, but knew it from our sweat and blood and raw rubbed skin from doing the unthinkable for most other men, that we didn't give a fuck about the appearance of discipline because we knew what the fuck real discipline was. Many in the military pay more attention to the facade of it than to the real thing. I think in the special operations community in general, and definitely in Recon, it seems like the right people just drift into it. It is definitely not the hard-core rule guy or the bean counter, although there were a few of those. But most of the guys I was in Recon with were the dudes that basically said, "I'll do whatever crazy dumb shit you ask of me in combat, if you will just leave me alone and stop with all the marching and yelling and shit." In fact, if anyone ever showed signs of a weak spirit, or of not being able to make it, I hoped for their demise. We all did. In Recon, we never helped each other out by pushing each other along. I didn't want to be dragging someone along who couldn't hang. And I think the rest of us were like that too. If I need to help and encourage you to not give up, then fuck you, limp dick, get the fuck off of my team. You need to motivate yourself to succeed before you ever look to others for it. That's how we helped each other out. By doing whatever we could to not drain the guy next to you. Don't be a life-suck. When everyone was contributing to the team, not taking from it, that's when really good shit would happen and we would challenge each other to excel instead of helping each other to not quit. I'm not necessarily endorsing that as a principle of life. I'm just saying that's how we did it.

The training was incessant and intense. It wasn't just about proficiency, it was about making it second nature, and the only way to get it down like that was to do it right and do it often and do it underwater and do it at night and do it in the snow and do it again and do it again and do it again. Perfect practice that makes perfect. Training is the process of removing excess time and human error from tactical algorithms. I think it becomes a craft when those responses become second nature. It takes thousands of repetitions to make that happen. And what's funny is that I only ever saw it all come together as one, in combat. Where time slows down when the first shots are fired or when something explodes, you have a choice right then. You can panic or you can think. It's exactly the same decision you had to make when they were punching you in the solar plexus under 12 feet of water and every fiber in your body and soul just wanted to breathe. Panic = die. Think = live. Once in combat, I had already been introduced to that decision under duress and I had handled it, I was in familiar territory. This is what I mean about knowing yourself. Damn. Writing this shit out is bringing back a lot. Part of me doesn't really want to write about it because it's a scary time. I've been in afew of them. Those snaps in time where you could live or die. And you walk the fucking tightrope and live. Whew! Makes me want to do a little dance.

I went to good ole Airborne School too. I hated jumping out of airplanes, man. Jumping HAHO (High Altitude High Opening) or HALO (High Altitude Low Opening) is one thing, but dope on a rope - Static Line: filing out of the back of a C-17 in a Mass Attack then smashing into the ground like a bag of smashed assholes? Brother, you're a better man than I. Fuck That. But you had to learn both because there was a lot of merit to the attributes of each insert capability. So, off I went to Army Airborne School and practiced pounding into the ground from all

Finally Somehow Home

different heights and objects, then pound into the ground out of a low flying airplane five times, and you're done. But it takes 3 weeks. It's Hell. And not at all because it is difficult. It's not. At all. The Marines and SEAL students were always in trouble with the Army Cadre. We had the wrong color of t-shirts, we made people cry, any little thing. We, of course, linked up and joined forces immediately, against our shared enemy: the Army. One Marine got in trouble for ripping a soldier's earring out of his ear. The Marine didn't know the Army regulations on that one. Because that might have been OK in the Army, but the Marine was not aware. Just a little misunderstanding about the regs on that one. No harm, no foul.

But they always put Marines in charge of the classes. A couple classes before mine, the class leader had been a lowly Marine E-3 Lance Corporal. But a senior Lance Corporal with a whip to crack is no slouch, so he did a great job.

I was lucky as hell to go to jump school back then too because quotas usually went to more senior guys, but no one was around the Company area when the quota had come in, and my Platoon Sergeant had snatched it up and

Finally Somehow Home

given it to me. Good man. So, when I got back, I was one of the only dual cool Lance Coconuts (Lance Corporals) in the Company. It was cool, but some dudes were pissed. I got lucky.

That's about when I met Troy. He was from Texas. He was shorter than me but stockier and stronger, and one of the smartest people I've ever met. He was also of wrestling and football fame in Texas during his high school years. He had placed second in State in wrestling because he had a broken ankle when he entered the match. He was a tough motherfucker. He is still my best friend. Troy was older than me but he had joined the Marine Corps after a brief stint in college playing football, so he was junior to me and I was to teach him. The first time I took him out to teach him land navigation, we promptly got lost. It was the same day I picked up Corporal. Dumbass. Me and Troy have been on some wild and crazies since. We have fought each other with our fists more than once. We used to go down to Tijuana because I was under 21 and the drinking age in Mexico was 18, if there was one. We'd go down to get steroids and get shitfaced and talk to under-21 SDSU and UCSD chicks.

Finally Somehow Home

Our buddy, Oz, was a big Mexican. He was an LA gangbanger before he joined the Corps, so he knew his way around. Oz used to go with us to keep us out of trouble. On one of these occasions, we were on our way back to the border when I had to take a piss. So, I went into a phone booth and pretended to be talking on the phone and pointing up in the sky with my hands to distract people from the fact that I was actually pissing. Try it, it works. Troy then decided that he had to piss as well, and commenced to pissing on my leg. I would have retaliated at that moment, but I could not help but notice the Federales coming up behind Troy to arrest him, so I did not. Fair is fair. As they were cuffing Troy I was having a good laugh. Oz stepped in to save the day and began to barter for Troy's life in Spanish. I, however, lost interest and stumbled off to look over some trinkets that one of the street vendors had for sale. I chose a nice looking grey poncho and donned and purchased it. After the course of my monetary transaction for the poncho, I turned to find that Oz had talked Troy free from the Federales and that we were headed through the border to the American side once more. Fair is not fair, I guess, Troy. Yes Troy had not gone to jail and must thereby reap the just deserts of his

Finally Somehow Home

pissing on my leg. During extreme cold weather, or in RIP it was considered a favor for someone to piss on your leg if you were standing in the surf zone, because it's so damn warm. But I didn't need the warmth here. We found the car and I let Troy get in first on the right hand rear side. He was a tough son of a bitch so I knew I had to sucker punch him to get him good. I blasted him a good one across the jaw. It took him a second but he got out of the car and started beating on me hard - he pulled that poncho up over my head and was kneeing me in the face over and over again. I eventually fell down. I was bloody and laughing. I put my left hand out so that he could grab a hold and help me up to my feet. He acquiesced. And as he pulled me up toward him, I brought my right hand back and blasted him really good right in the chin. His head snapped back. It was a great shot. But for the grace of God go I. The American police showed up just as he was beginning to retaliate.

About three years after that Oz broke his back in three places in a motorcycle accident. They said he'd never walk again. He now walks fine with a cane, and incidentally, holds a shit load of Olympic gold medals in hand cycling. He is also a well-known public speaker.

Finally Somehow Home

It seems like in life we all want to be go-arounder's instead of over-comers. You'll just wear yourself out trying to go around. Sooner or later you realize that the only way through it is to start climbing. You will then start to feel like you are not strong enough to reach the top. And you'll be right. You aren't. But you only have to be strong enough to take the next step. And you will learn that the only way to get strong enough to climb the mountain is by climbing the mountain. By the time you reach the top you will be strong enough to get there. Oz showed that to all of us.

Chapter 6

In the movies all the Spec Ops dudes are always yoked out and jacked, but in real life the only guys with the beach bods were in Headquarters and never went to the field. I'll also say that I noticed that I only got really good at my job after I quit caring how cool everyone thought that I was. That's when I really became a professional. Anyway, when we were not starving ourselves out on patrol or otherwise brutalizing our bodies and burning up all of our calories in training, we were trying as best we could to stay jacked and fit. We would usually go for a run every morning around 5:30, then hit the pool at lunchtime for a thousand meters or two, then hit the weights in the afternoon, then start drinking. Life at Recon was always busy with some kind of training, so we had to just make do and squeeze in as

Finally Somehow Home

much drinking as we could around the periphery. Most of us were single and lived in the barracks. It was a shit-show. There was a significant rivalry in the company between the platoons. This would manifest itself in spontaneous combat betwixt platoons, called Kumate'. Sometimes the whole company, or all the platoons that weren't out training or deployed would get sucked into it...minus Headquarters, of course. There was no real objective. It was just a massive brawl that usually left the Company area in utter ruin. Usually, the rest of the world left us pretty much to ourselves but sometimes the Officer Of the Day from Headquarters Battalion would come poking around. I remember he was particularly upset once to find the Duty NCO (Non-Commissioned Officer) of our barracks tied to a tree in the front lawn, blindfolded, with Riggers tape (duct tape) over his mouth. That's just the kind of shit that would upset certain kinds of people, so as we never liked to offend, we tried to keep pretty much to ourselves.

Air travel has been kind of a new idea for the Marines. Don't get me wrong, the Marines have been in love with the idea of strafing and bombing people since the miracle of powered flight was first conceived. I think the officers in the higher echelons of the Marine

Finally Somehow Home

Corps have been caught in a conundrum of sorts for years over the issue of powered flight. Although exhilarated at its applications in the tidy destruction of everything from enemy troops to small villages, as well as the benefits of air power in support of troops on the ground, there has always been one application of flight which has haunted Marine officers: the transportation of troops by air.

The reason is actually quite simple. To see the rhyme behind it, however, you must go back to the beginning of the Marine Corps. Philadelphia, November 10th, 1775. The word was passed on the streets that Tun Tavern would be serving free drinks that evening, but only to those who showed up armed. Despite the fact that to some, this may have seemed to be a bad idea, plenty of people showed up armed to the teeth, and proceeded to do what Marines have done since then in such environments: drink until utter failure. The next morning the drunken "volunteers" awoke on the swaying deck of a ship far out at sea and someone yelling at them about something or other. Marines have been in misery ever since.

Finally Somehow Home

By the time they arrived at their first landfall in the Bahamas they were so angry that they destroyed an entire garrison of troops, fortunately the US was then at war with those people. Thus, the Marine Corps doctrine was born, the secret of its success, and it has been viciously adhered to since then. Being on ship is the only proven way to keep Marines pissed off enough to be combat effective. The shit works. At any given time in this world there are at least three Marine Expeditionary Units (MEUs) consisting of airplanes, helicopters, tanks, grunts, and afew other cats and dogs, all loaded on ships and floating around out at sea somewhere waiting for something bad to happen, or on their way to make something bad happen. Back then, we weren't at war with anyone, so we pretty much just sat on the ship for six months and didn't even hurt anyone's feelings. We did training and shit in a lot of different countries and we did manage to make it into some cool ports. We stopped in Waikiki, Hong Kong, Singapore, Malaysia, The Seychelles, were on our way to Kenya when the Embassy there blew up, Bahrain and hung out in the shit ass desert in Kuwait and got to see what the bottom of a beer glass looks like in all of those places except Kuwait. Fuckin Boo, I say. Actually, in Bahrain it was piss warm in cans, not glasses. But back to the Seychelles for a minute. There were some fucking shenanigans in the Seychelles. Damn. Some of it I can't go into, but I'll tell what I can.

So, Troy had hooked up with this gorgeous blonde chick with a British accent whose parents owned an island. And a big yacht. The time was drawing near for Troy and his two buddies from the grunts to get back to the ship because the ship was going to leave the next morning and everyone had to be back on board by midnight. Troy decided that he was not going to return. He chose then and there to live there forever in the Seychelles in the sweet embrace of this hot ass blonde bitch. The two guys from the grunts weren't having it though. They finally talked him out of it but they were still on her parents' private island, and a long way from the ship. So all of them and some other random bitches got into her yacht and put the hammer down because it was getting nigh unto midnight. The ship we were on was an Amphib. An Amphib can drop its rear gate and even flood its well deck with water in order to launch boats and AMTRACS and hovercraft and shit like that out into the ocean. On this particular night that ramp was down and the gang plank from the pier led

Finally Somehow Home

down to the ramp. On the ramp was the duty desk where everyone had to sign in and out of liberty. And, again, everyone had to sign back in by midnight. Just a smidgen before midnight, there are assembled on the ramp the ship's Captain, the Commander of the Battalion Landing Team, and all the other brass that was on board the ship at that time as well as the Command Master Chief and the Sergeant Major, etcetera. Troy made visual of the ship long before anyone on the ramp saw Troy. The USS Cole had not as of yet been attacked and blown up, so fortunately for Troy and the yacht and all the hot bitches and the two grunts, the 20mm blaster didn't open up on them, and they made it all the way up to the ship and beached the yacht on the steel ramp. The bow of the yacht was grinding on the metal as Troy fell off of it onto the ramp and stumbled, falling down twice before reaching the duty desk and signing in just seconds before the stroke of midnight. The yacht revved its engine to get its bow off of the steel ramp and blew smoke throughout the well deck. It pulled back and away from the ship and left into the darkness. There was a moment of stunned silence. The Command Master Chief finally spoke. "I've been in the Navy for 29 years and I ain't never seen no shit like that before."

Finally Somehow Home

Many years later, Troy, now an Intelligence Officer, was sitting around with abunch of guys from 1st Recon during a lull in the second Battle of Fallujah. One of them started regaling his fellow Marines with a legend involving a yacht pulling up onto the stern gate of the ship full of naked chicks committing lewd acts with each other and a Recon Marine humping one of them across the yacht's bow. According to legend, the Marine jumped off the yacht, signed in, then cock blocked the Sergeant Major in front of the naked Sirens before strolling casually away. Troy just laughed along and didn't say anything. He told me he didn't want to ruin it, because: "Their version was much better." Troy had accomplished that for which Achilles had so striven. He had become a legend in his own lifetime. Brings a tear to the eye.

Coming back from deployment is always anti-climactic. There was never anyone waiting or any shit like that. You want to get back to civilization so badly and the process of getting off the ship is such a pain in the ass that by the end of it you're just tired as fuck and glad to be home, such as it was. It was always weird to see that the whole world had just gone on without me and now I

Finally Somehow Home

was back and it just kept on rolling. I figured I might as well just roll along with it.

Finally Somehow Home

Chapter 7

By the time I got back I was getting the itch to go see some more of the world, so I got orders to Okinawa, Japan. Okinawa was a crapshoot. No one wanted to go to Oki, usually people got orders against their will to go there, but I was young and I knew I'd learn a lot there because there was nothing to do but train and deploy and that's what I wanted to do. I was a shit-hot Corporal and picked up Sergeant afew months after. I knew my shit. I was assigned to a Force Recon Unit, which meant more and better toys and missions, in some respects, and more of the same in others. I noticed this with a lot of things in life in general I guess: it seems like there aren't really many "advanced principles", it's just becoming more proficient and fluid with the basic ones that allows you to operate on an advanced level. Any time you

Finally Somehow Home

started trying to make shit fancy, you fuck it up. Same was true for the most part in Force Recon with the addition of the Deep Recon mission. Exactly the same field craft, but now we were a more strategic asset. Our job would be to go in hundreds of miles deep behind enemy lines to blow up bridges, infrastructure, and otherwise just fuck shit up according to whatever the Generals wanted their battlespace to look like by the time they got there with all their guns and grunts. It was called "Battlespace Shaping". We also got the Direct Action Mission which is what everyone liked about Force: Raids. That's the one where we would take down buildings, ships, people's private residences, or anyplace else that had bad guys in it with lots of shooting and explosions. As soon as I got my bearings in Oki, I asked around for the Platoon that did the most deploying and I talked to their platoon sergeant.

Big Duke 6 was a motherfucker. And I mean that in the best possible way. His platoon was always doing the cool shit. Somehow he would wrangle his way into all the best deployments, the most ammo and good schools for his boys. Just not a lot of time off. I wanted in. Fred was the Platoon Commander. He was a motherfucker too. To the other officers. They called him Friendly Fred because

Finally Somehow Home

he didn't dig their dinner parties. We liked him. Fred was an SS Panzer Commander who had been killed in WW2 in 1945 while attacking a column of Russian tanks in his lone Tiger tank. At least I'm pretty sure he was. I wanted leadership that I could learn under, and they needed strong backs and guys who could handle a shitload of responsibility being dumped on them at any given moment with no excuses. They already had a great crew of younger guys that they had molded well into the most deployed Spec Ops platoon in the Pacific Rim. But to go pro, they needed good Team Leaders. Well, hello.

Big Duke and Fred gave me a team. Holy Shit, I was a God Damn Force Recon Team Leader. Even I have to admit that it was pretty early for me to pick up a Force Recon Team. Most of the Force TL's in the Marine Corps were E-7's or E-6's. I had only just picked up Sergeant (E-5) but that's the nice thing about Okinawa. You did get a younger crew of guys out there, and more shenanigans that went along with all that, but somebody had to take responsibility for all of them, so if you were willing to take on a sharp learning curve and a shitload of responsibility for abunch of bad ass dumb asses including yourself, you could find yourself in a position to learn alot fast, but if you couldn't handle it, you'd fail

Finally Somehow Home

like a fuck in front of everyone, then get shit-canned to the grunts, and some people did. So, yeah, it was a crapshoot.

By the way…the grunts. Marine Corps Infantry. Is the best conventional force in the world today when it comes to killing shit. On liberty or in combat, a Marine Infantry Company is a fucking god damn confounding and brutal whirlwind wrought direct from the depths of a cold wet hell. Everyone in the Marine Corps supports the grunts. Everyone. Fucking Everyone. But the grunts had it rough. The roughest of anyone in the Corps. And they got killed the most. So, let's just cover this while we're on the subject, the whole "women in the military" thing. I'm ok with it if that's what everyone wants, and I know afew women who would be great at it, just understand that when you put women in combat roles… well… a lot more of those people die, that's one reason women have been historically left out of those roles, but not the only one. So, why should only the boys get the jobs where everyone gets killed? That's equally sexist against men, you say. Well, when I see an NFL team start and play mostly women throughout the whole Super Bowl against an all male team, and they win, I'll believe that it's just as hard to take a woman's life as it is to take a man's life. And that is the test at the end of the day. Because when you start losing, you lose more. When more infantrymen die, more infantrymen tend to die because of it. It is an exponentially compounding problem. Do whatever you want with women in combat roles. But please understand the facts of why they haven't been there up until now, that's all. I personally don't like that my daughter has an equal chance of being drafted and a compounded lower probability of survival if she is, but I'm sure she'll be fine as long as everyone is happy and we never actually have to kill other humans. Generals aren't sexist, it's killing that's sexist. And it's sexist as fuck.

Some weekends in Okinawa I'd work at a bar on Gate Two Street named Fujiyama's as a bouncer when I wasn't deployed or at schools. It was pretty a fun gig because the bar was upstairs and all you had to do when someone got too rowdy is just push them down the stairs. So, me and this Army Special Forces guy kept an eye on everything for the Japanese owners. The main perk besides the extra cash was that we got free beer while we were working. So, half the time we were just as much in the bag as everyone we were throwing down the stairs.

Finally Somehow Home

This particular night as I recall, after we closed around 2 AM, I made a bet with my SF buddy that I could do seven shots of Jägermeister in a row. He set them up on the bar and I slammed them one after another in short order. Just a light warm up. Then we went out to the afterhours clubs and stayed at it until the sun was coming up.

Driving home was always a little dicey in such a state, but thankfully, there were hibiscus bushes all along the side of the freeway so if you started nodding off they would invariably wake you up by smacking your mirror and the side of your car in a horribly annoying cacophony before you went off the road at a high rate of speed. Nature's rumble strips. Anyway, that morning I was feeling rather guilty for spending my night in such debauchery, and it was a Sunday morning, so I decided to go to church and sluff off some guilt instead of going straight home to my barracks room and bed.

I got to the church on Camp Kinser about an hour and a half before the doors opened for the first service which, was the Protestant service, so I picked a good spot in the parking lot near the front door. It was starting to warm up, so I took my shirt and shoes off and sat down on the hood of my car with a bag of cheesy poofs. I decided I'd

Finally Somehow Home

nod off for a few minutes and wait for the doors to open. I awoke to the blazing Okinawa sun, sweat flowing from every pore, lying sprawled out on the hood of my car, with wind-blown cheesy poofs stuck to the sweat all over my body. The parking lot was completely full. Apparently about four hours had elapsed. The Protestant service had long since ended and the Catholic service was about half way through. Camp Kinser was where all of the family housing for the Marines on Okinawa was located. I have no idea how many innocent Protestant and Catholic children and dependents were scarred for life from witnessing, on their way to the doors of their church service, a half-naked sweaty man with cheezy poofs stuck all over him, but I know it was a lot.

We hit up Korea for alittle skydiving. I had been to Military Free-Fall School by then, so I was jumping HALO and HAHO. One night we were jumping a UH-1 Huey, and I decided to play a joke on my buddies. I'm lactose intolerant and I rip some gnar-gnar farts if I drink milk, so I knew we'd be in close proximity at high altitude with zero cabin pressure which meant a shitload of ass-pressure and very little ambient air pressure, and I knew the damage which would ensue. I

Finally Somehow Home

went with the half gallon of whole milk for dinner. I just remember being up in the god damn Huey. It's a single-prop helicopter and wobbly as fuck at 10,000 feet. It flew like it was barely hanging on. I thought we were getting ready to jump pretty soon so launched my first attack, and I'd been saving up for awhile, so it was a good one. There was about a half-millisecond delay as the cloud instantly permeated the cabin... then it hit like a pestilence from the staff of Moses. I just remember the door gunner exclaiming suddenly: "Oh my GOD!" Then opening the massive sliding doors on both sides of the Huey to expose us to the frigid gusts of the Korean winter. For 15 minutes. While a bunch of F-16s landed on the airfield that we were supposed to parachute in on. It was miserable. Finally, we got out of the damned bird and flopped around in the air alittle bit because the Huey was only doing 80 knots up there, it took awhile to get up to a good stable freefall speed. The next day I met the pilot. It was in the morning, and I still smelled like booze. She was a hammer. Blonde hair, blue eyes. She looked at me as if she knew it was me whose ass had wrought the horror of the night before. God damn it.

We used to go to Guam a lot. I loved going to Guam because the weather reminded me of Indonesia. It was

Finally Somehow Home

warm and humid and had big tall clouds in the sky and when it rained it was thick fat drops and felt like taking a warm shower. We did a lot of skydiving in Guam. But military skydiving is not quite the same as civilian skydiving. The rig and canopy are bigger and heavier because it needs to be able to support the weight of the jumper plus all of his combat equipment and ammo. There was also the added oxygen bottles and O2 mask and flight helmet. Jumping slick – no combat equipment or O2 – was fun. That was a lark. The problem is that if we were going to show up at a nice war, we needed to have a lot of other shit with us. Jumping combat equipment in freefall was always an interesting endeavor because all of your equipment tried its best to kill you the whole time. Once when I was in Australia on a 25,000 foot combat equipment O2 jump I left the aircraft and everything was just fine until I realized I couldn't breathe. One of the valves in my O2 system was stuck closed. Sometimes they would get condensation or saliva on them and then when exposed to the cold air outside of the airplane it would freeze because at 25,000ft that shit is subzero. So, while in freefall, I pulled my hands in to mess with my oxygen mask, which caused my body to rotate to a head down position which

Finally Somehow Home

is not good when you are jumping a front mount rucksack because the wind is blowing it all over the place trying to get it to make you unstable and spin out of control. So anyway, I've been in freefall for a few seconds now and my vision is starting to blur at the edges. I know I'm running out of oxygen and I'm going to pass out pretty soon if I don't do something quick. I could pull high which means that I would deploy the parachute right then and then I'd be stuck under canopy at 22,500 ft with no O2. So, if I pulled high and I still could not get my O2 working I would pass out and either ride the parachute into the dirt face first at 14 knots or maybe wake up once I got down where there was oxygen. I didn't want to do that because mostly I didn't want to be the guy who pulled high. There are a lot of things that you can deal with if you get fucked up, but if you make it through unscathed, you're fucked because now you're the dumbass that pulled his rip cord at 22,500 ft instead of 4000ft with everyone else. I wasn't going to be "that guy". I didn't give a fuck if I died. That's the kind of thought process that dictated most of my decision making at that stage of my life. Sooo, I arched as hard as I could to try and fall faster and get down to where there was some oxygen in the air. Finally, in exasperation I

Finally Somehow Home

just breathed in as hard as I possibly could (nice to fucking know that's all it took after I almost die), and it broke the seal and let oxygen come into my god damn lungs. OK. Problem solved. I got down to 4000 feet with no further drama - other than wrestling with my god damn rucksack the whole way down - and pulled my main chute. I saw the lines go up over my shoulders and I started falling more upright. It used to take a little while for my chute to open the way I packed it because I liked to roll the nose on it which caused it to open slower and not blast you in the balls when it opened all at once, but this time it was taking too long. I looked up and saw the parachute above me still stuffed neatly into its bag instead of in a vast canopy over my head. Aww shit. Bag lock. I reached up and pulled down the risers twice, quick and hard as I could and was getting ready to cut away when the main chute finally opened around 2000 feet. It didn't really occur to me that I had almost died about 12 times in the last few minutes until I landed. It didn't occur to me to be scared. I was just solving problems, doing it by the numbers. As they say in skydiving... you've got the rest of your life to figure it out.

So back to Guam. We were always down there for some reason or another. We had a little place in our hearts for

Finally Somehow Home

this establishment called "The G Spot". All the ladies that worked there were imports from the Vegas strip clubs and were in Guam cleaning up on the Japanese tourists that would come through there wanting to look at a little bit of "round-eye" ass. Those girls were great to us and fun to look at, so we hit it off with them right away. There was a rule in my team that if you got laid the night before you did not have to show up for team PT (Physical Training) in the morning. My ATL (Assistant Team Leader), Pirate, was always skipping out. The ladies loved him.

One fateful night at The G Spot, I decided that I did not need to go back to the barracks with everyone else and that the rules that everyone else had to abide by did not apply to me that day. So, I stayed out. And got ripped. We usually had a very strict eight hours "bottle to throttle" rule which we generally did a pretty good job of adhering to. But not tonight. So, I stayed out till two when the bar closed. Time to think tactical, no shit. No money. No cell phone. Twelve miles from base. And training the next day starts at 0530. What you gonna do hot-shot? I think it would be a great idea to make a Bear Grylls special on how to get out of dicey liberty situations. So, I started running. I ran for several miles

Finally Somehow Home

when a cop pulled over and after I told him what I was up to, asked me if I needed a ride. Right about the time he reaches to open the door and let me in he gets a call and speeds off - lights flashing. So, I ran for a few more miles. A good Samaritan pulled over to see if I needed a ride. Blessed angel of mercy. In the form of a 350-pound Chamorro drag queen. I shit you not. I couldn't be too choosy at that point, so I got in. I kept one hand on the handle as we drove down the road because she was looking at me like I was a 3AM snack. I wisely got out a half a mile from the gate to alleviate myself of the explanation to the gate guards and ran the rest of the way back to the barracks...or thereabouts. The next thing I remember, a couple of Navy Military Police were standing over me poking me with the toe of their boots trying to wake me up. I heard them yell to someone nearby: "Is this one of yours?"

"Yeah, that's my Team Leader."

"Well, he doesn't even know his own name."

"I'll come get him."

Nothing that a quick shower, a couple of IVs and some pure O2 won't fix. Didn't miss a beat. I was back to the

Finally Somehow Home

land of the living by the time we started training that morning.

In order to be in a Force Recon Platoon for Direct Action missions – what we called a "shooting platoon" - you had to pass a six-month shooting course before every deployment. It was called the shooting package. I could shoot a pistol pretty well up until then, but I wasn't great and I wasn't consistent. I had to re-learn a few things, but I started forming good habits and after a few months I was consistently driving tacks with my .45. Some people swear by the 45. Especially the 1911. As a work gun, I'd maybe pick another pistol, they are all just tools anyway. But I'm very glad that I learned on a 1911. It jumps around a lot more than a 9 mm does so it was a good pistol to learn on. For at least a month before we ever fired a round through our pistols we would spend a half an hour to an hour every day doing dry practice. Picking a spot on the wall in front of you, drawing your pistol, step by step, by the numbers, presenting the pistol and pulling the trigger once on target. The pistol is one of those things that there are no real advanced basics to. The more grounded in the basics you are, the more you do every little thing right every single little time. And the more you start doing every single little thing right every single little time, the more professional and fluid you become in the martial art of shooting. It's just like a golf swing. It's all just in the slightest nuance but you have to register those movements and check them and make sure that you don't do anything unless you do it right. And the faster you can link them all together, the better and faster you shoot. However many thousands of repetitions it takes to develop a habit, that's the number we were after. Because when you link them all together fluidly and then you make that function into a habit and it becomes second nature, then you're starting to get somewhere.

I was our Lead Breacher. I had been to Breacher school along with a couple other guys and we started building breaching charges to blow the doors and windows and walls to make points of entry into buildings so we could flood through them and shoot the bad guys. Building breaching charges is like arts and crafts. It's mostly cardboard and scissors and tape and explosives. It's fun. The problem with it is that we always missed lunch because everyone goes to lunch to eat and you have to stay behind and build all the charges. So, it was my job to identify breach points, work with the other breachers to

Finally Somehow Home

build charges for targets and then delegate who was going to be in charge of blowing which breach point.

Direct Action shit looks all glam-glam in the movies. But once again...it ain't. It took a lot of shooting to make it second nature and shooting is hard work. The ballistic plate carrier and all your magazines and your pistol belt and ammo hanging off of you all day in the heat. Your lower back feels like it's going to explode with all the pressure from leaning forward on the firing line ready to raise your rifle or draw your pistol at the sound of the command or the whistle or the buzzer. And then it would happen and there would be a hellacious violence of gunfire and muzzle flashes and the shocks of all the small explosions and hot spent brass casings flying through the air. Sometimes the hot brass would make it down the back of your flight suit and burn the shit out of you. The constant cadence of "Shooters Ready.... Stand by.... UP!" pivoting one way, pivoting another, shooting with only the weak side, that is with the left hand if you're right handed, shooting on the move, shooting with gas masks on, shooting in the rain, at night, shooting in the sun, shooting off the deck of ships at sea, shooting, shooting, shooting, shooting, motherfucking shooting. I broke 3 locking lugs off the bolt of my M4 and I broke

Finally Somehow Home

countless pistols because of all the rounds I put through them. And the whole time learning how to flood into and flow through houses or ships or whatever needed the boots put to it. We were always changing missions. We'd do a "green side" patrol through the jungle and a raid, then the next night be Fast Roping in on another "black side" fully kinetic type mission.

We were always training or doing exercises or flying off somewhere to do it. That platoon was the most combat ready Force Recon Platoon in the world at the time. I have no doubt of that whatsoever and I'm damn proud to have been a part of it. I guess I was doing something to contribute to it, because I was nominated for a quite prestigious award. To this day, I'm still humbled and honored to have received it from the Force Recon Association on behalf of my unit: the Force Recon Team Leader of the Year, 2000. I was 23.

...Then I got fired. Must have been about six months or so after I got the award. We had flown to California to do some training because our range literally had so many bullets packed into the dirt berm behind the targets that rounds were bouncing back and hitting the shooters. They were pretty much spent by the time

Finally Somehow Home

they'd smack you, but we had broken our range and they had to replace the berms. I had been going hard for almost 2 years of constant training and deployment from Oki, and I was starting to fray at the edges. We were finally back in the US for afew weeks and even then we were training through the weekends. The guys needed a rest and it was killing us all to finally be back in the States and not be able to enjoy it. I mentioned something about it, and it wasn't received well. When I showed up 2 hours late for work the next day after a wild night out, they gave me the axe as a TL. It was everything bad. I had failed like a Fuck, and in front my team and of all of my peers. "Hero to Zero" someone told me. Thanks. I know. I languished in that platoon for another 6 months, still operating, but I no longer had my own team. Just tired of being alive, you know. I was very depressed. I was still doing all the cool guy shit, but after awhile it was just the same shit over and over again, which was necessary, but it had all become monotonous and dull to me. I don't know where the mark is that you achieve whatever we were trying to get to as a platoon, and as shooters as a whole, but I think we got damned close to pretty fucking good. I don't think you have to necessarily burn out to get there, but my whole platoon

Finally Somehow Home

did. But we all learned it cold, and I know that none of us will ever forget how to draw and shoot fast and quick and accurate as fuck when your primary weapon goes down, or any of the thousands of other scenarios we lived and breathed through hundreds and thousands of times over. So, overall, in the grand scheme of things it was the experience of a lifetime. I learned, albeit at great expense, how to master an art, then I did it. Maybe for some, the price you pay for it is that you never even want to touch a pistol and rifle again, but you sure as fuck know how to use one. You see, achieving something is usually done at some cost. If you take on something truly great and truly hard as fuck to do well right...then get ready for that thing to try to break you in some way. I didn't know. I wasn't on my guard. And I ate shit.

I was at Military Freefall Jumpmaster School on 9/11. It was surreal knowing that all that we were doing was now going to be put into practice. It was a huge relief in some ways. It's not that I wanted to have a stack of dead bodies to my name. What I really wanted to know was if I was really any good. I just wanted to take all the things that I had learned over the course of the past six years and see if I could do it in combat.

Finally Somehow Home

Maybe this is everyone, or maybe it's just me, but it seems like my life has been marked by some tremendous and wonderful experiences interspersed with flurries of swift and vicious kicks to the nuts. I'm not at all saying that I'm some kind of innocent victim, but that's just how it seems to play out whether I have it coming or not. But I usually do. I got fired AGAIN! I had finished out my time in the Direct Action Platoon and picked up a team in one of the R&S (Reconnaissance and Surveillance) platoons and right out the gate got busted for taking my ATL off base drinking when he was on restriction (he'd gotten in trouble for something and was restricted to base.) We would have gotten away with it, but he got into a fight with a bathroom stall and lost, cutting up his hand in the process, then ending up in the hospital on base to get it taken care of. Of course, I got the axe again as soon as the Platoon Sergeant found out. He didn't like me much and was looking for an excuse, and I gave him one. I stayed on in the platoon as a gear queer (equipment NCO). Overall, it was a good platoon, all really young guys who I was happy to teach. I spent my spare time writing up a new SOP (Standard Operating Procedure) manual as well as a field guide, but my relationship with the Platoon Sergeant continued to deteriorate over the next year

Finally Somehow Home

until I finally got the hell out of Oki and out from under the dark cloud that had been following me around. That was really the biggest problem with Oki. I did 3 years there. The island had a tendency to break people. Even with all the deployments one would tend to get alittle stir crazy, and given enough time, most guys would end up getting in trouble for some stupid shit that had nothing whatsoever to do with training and operating. We often joked that we should build a platoon out of all the guys that got busted down in rank or otherwise in trouble, because it would have been the best platoon in the unit. There was a lot of truth to that. For some reason, most of the guys who were the best in the "J" (jungle), or in the "house" (shooting house) were always in trouble when they were back in the rear with nothing to do.

Anyway, I finally got the fuck out of Dodge. I left there a young Sergeant with a sigh of relief and a smile on my face, and more than my fair share of experience. I was ready to get back to the US. I picked the East Coast and checked into 2^d Force Recon shortly thereafter.

Finally Somehow Home

Chapter 8

2^d Force was a breath of fresh air. It was great not being one of the senior Operators there as I was back in Okinawa. In fact, in my new platoon, I wasn't even senior enough for my own Team, and I was happy with being a very young ATL for 2^d Force. It was great to have so many peers and solid guys I could learn from. In fact, I ended up in the most senior and experienced platoon at 2^d Force. I was among legends. And it looked like we were finally going to war. When I say that I was among legends, I'm not making that shit up. Many in that platoon are now men of lore in the Marine Corps Special Operations community.

Bushhog was a young hearted southern dude. He was the senior TL. He was about medium height and build and very unassuming at first glance. His nonchalance and

Finally Somehow Home

smirky smile belied the fact that he was a complete bad ass. He was stacked with schools and deployments and had won, I think, three or more Recon Team Leader of the Year Awards. He was the most mellow dude I've ever known. It didn't matter what we were doing or what kind of crazy shit was going on around him, he refused to stress out and got pissed off at others when they did. He simply refused to let shit bother him or get inside his cognitive workspace. He was professional as fuck when it came to getting the mission done and he could drink all night long and still run his team into the ground the next morning without sleeping a wink. He used to do that all the time. He was a tough son of a bitch. I learned a lot from just being around him and watching how he handled shit. I got to go on patrol with him once when my team and his joined up in the field. He was a fucking ghost in the woods, like the Recon guys of old. And he knew how to run a team and put all his guys in a position to succeed. One of the greatest men I've ever met. A hell of a family man to boot. One of the best that I saw at making a family work while in the Marines.

Moshpit... Another TL. Moshpit was a monster and a force of nature. Like an earthquake with muscles. He was a lot younger than Bushhog, but he was just fucking

Finally Somehow Home

damn good at everything. He was one of those guys who could go to the field all the time and still looked like a Greek god. He grew up fighting and saw no reason to change anything. He was smart as fuck and a clear thinker under pressure. Moshpit didn't play. He took everything seriously. If you fucked with him and he didn't appreciate it... didn't matter if you were his best friend... you'd get a bottle full of dip spit to the face, or maybe a broken ankle. No shit. Both of those things happened, and more. In spite of that, he was a very thoughtful guy, and cared deeply about his guys. He would fight for his tribe as viciously as he'd fight for himself, if not more.

We were out in Arizona doing some Military Freefall shit and calling in air strikes a month or so after I got to 2^d Force. Moshpit and I were having a beer one night on the outside patio of the bar. We knew war was coming. It was on the back of everyone's mind. I don't know why he told me this because he didn't know me that well yet. I think we just had a healthy mutual respect for each other by then.

"Hey man, promise me something."

"OK"

Finally Somehow Home

"If I ever get burned up real bad or anything, do me a favor, and just take out your .45 and finish it right there for me."

"Ok, man. Me too." I said.

"OK"

Moshpit didn't just say shit. If he said it he meant it. I did too.

In Afghanistan in 2009 Moshpit's gun truck was hit by an IED. The extra fuel cans on the truck ruptured and added to the inferno. He lived through it but was a quad amputee with something like 90% of his body covered in 3rd degree burns. All of the Doctors were amazed that he survived at all. He was just that fucking tough. He was the most injured man in the VA healthcare system until he succumbed to his war wounds and died several years later. I was in Afghanistan at the time he was hit, but I wasn't there when it happened. I don't know what I would have done if I had been. Bushog was killed in Afghanistan within a couple weeks of Moshpit being hit. Before, or after, I forget. I just remember it being a hard couple of weeks. Of the three Team Leaders of that

Finally Somehow Home

platoon, Sammy is still alive, and he is likewise a Recon legend.

Sure enough, 2^d Force Recon Company was going to war. A few platoons were going over on ship and the rest of us were flying over. The guys going on ship were leaving afew weeks before we did so that we could show up in Kuwait around the same time. The company held a massive All-Hands formation the morning the shipboard platoons embarked. It was a somber moment. Every platoon in the company stood at parade rest as families watched in nervous silence from the sidelines. Everyone understood the gravity of the moment. It could very well be the last time all of us were alive together. Dead silence. The company Sergeant Major positioned himself front and center.

"COMPANY, ATTEN -...."

Suddenly, a massive ragged fart erupted from Philthy's ass from the rear of the formation:

"BLAAAAAAPTPTPTPTTTPTPTPP-queeeeeeeePTP!!"

"...-HUT!!!"

Finally Somehow Home

The entire Company and all the civilians burst into laughter for a moment. Then silence again.

"You Motherfuckers." The Sergeant Major muttered, trying in vain not to laugh as he executed a crisp About-Face and reported to the CO. And that's how the war started for 2^d Force Recon.

I hate to admit it, but I actually flew to war on an Air Force bird. I was impressed by the consideration of the Air Force pilots, though. They must have been briefed, because they knew just how to get a guy ready to kill people by the way they flew that thing. It was very impressive. I had strung up a hammock in the back of the bird and was lounging casually until we hit Iraqi airspace. We had plenty of Surface to Air missiles and guns pointed at us, so they took full advantage. Needless to say, their frantic and erratic maneuvers dislodged me from my hammock quite suddenly and fiercely. After a while of dodging fence posts along the desert floor, we landed in Kuwait; I checked my guys and was happy to discover that in spite of the pleasant distractions and soothing alarms ringing every few seconds, we were still in poor enough spirits to be somewhat combat effective.

Finally Somehow Home

So, we were finally going to war. And by the looks of it, it was going to be a big one. Back then we still thought the Iraqis had all kinds of chemical and biological weapons that they planned to use on us. We were expecting very high casualties. The worst possible kinds of deaths and a lot of it. We sat there in the Kuwaiti desert for some time while the world around us filled up with tanks and trucks and guns and bombs, all ready to roll up north and take Iraq. Honestly it was a shit show. We hadn't been at war in so long that not many remembered what it was like or how to do it. It's a pretty standard problem. It takes awhile to get used to anything. The Israelis experienced it against Hezbollah in 2006. It just takes afew months to get the hang of a war and we weren't quite there yet.

Kuwait was a dry country. That did not sit well with us. Not that we could go out or anything anyway. But it did make the acquisition of booze a difficulty aside from having people mail it to you in Listerine bottles. One of the guys in our platoon - Philthy, chose to take matters into his own hands. He got ahold of some yeast and started stealing fruit cocktail from the chow hall and anything else he could get his hands on that he could make into hooch. We had a pretty good grog system

Finally Somehow Home

going. A new batch of booze in a five-gallon water jug was ready for consumption every Wednesday. After a while the operation started growing beyond what we could do to keep it properly concealed. So, we just made a space in the corner of our tent where there were five-gallon water jugs neatly aligned with rubber gloves at different stages of inflation hanging off of their spouts. This was severely annoying to my platoon Commander who walked in one day and left in a huff yelling behind him, "Why can't you guys at least try to hide it!? God Damn it!"

Waiting for the war to start. Just waiting. These sand storms would come ripping through there. It was amazing. The sky and the air all around you glowed orange. There was sand everywhere and it got into everything. On one occasion our sister platoon decided to play Survivor during one of these storms and proceeded to vote several of their members off the island. The poor bastards were made to sleep outside in the blowing sand for the night.

One day me and Slick Kat were on our way to breakfast just walking along as usual when I heard a jet engine flying very low. I thought it was a AV-8B Harrier because

Finally Somehow Home

it was so loud - and Harriers are loud little fuckers. I looked up to see a giant missile flying at about 500 feet above the ground. Right as I saw it the engine cut out. "Oh shit." is all I could say. And me and Slick Kat hit the deck just as it exploded 500 meters outside of the wire. Fuuuuuck. We already had our MOP suits (chemical/biological suits) on, so we put our gas masks on because we didn't know what kind of chemical or biological agents were on board that missile. We got back to our company area about the time the alarm started going off. The missile was a Seersucker anti-ship missile and had come in under the radar skimming the desert floor. It was funny to hear the person on the loudspeaker in panic trying to speak through their gas mask to warn us that missiles were coming in. No shit, Sherlock. We got into the bunker and waited for the cloud of death to come drifting by and kill us all, or the all clear. Dirty Joe showed up in the bunker covered in shit and blue water from the porta-shitters. Apparently he had been in there when the missile came in and somehow managed to get blue shitter juice all over his MOP suit.

That's how the war started. For the next several days it was constant. Fortunately, they didn't seem to have any more of those Seersuckers, or other missiles that could fly under radar. It was all Scuds after that. The Patriot Missile battery was behind us about 10 kilometers and would fire over us as soon as they picked up an incoming Scud. About three Patriots to every Scud, it seemed. You could hear the explosive blast as the Patriots left their tubes, then the crack of them breaking the sound barrier 2.9 seconds later somewhere just over our heads. They'd reach Mach 4.1 as they found and slammed into the incoming missiles. Then the impacts of the Patriots into the Scud overhead and a shitload of warheads and fuel exploding. BOOM-BOOM-BOOM-BOOM. Then you waited. Because all that shit up in the air was falling down to the ground right about then, and you just held your breath and hoped that it wasn't directly above your bunker. Then you heard all that shit slamming into the ground around you. BOOM-BOOM-BOOM-BOOM-BOOM and the ground shook. It was constant and ground your nerves raw, but the Patriot batteries got them all. Kudos, because getting shot at with fucking missiles fucking sucks. Over the next couple days we were just anxious to get the hell out of Kuwait and away from all the Scuds falling all around us. We had a kick ass mission lined up to HALO in and call in airstrikes on an

Finally Somehow Home

Iraqi armored Division until it was all gone, but it got scrubbed at the last minute, so we ended up having to wait around for Headquarters to roll out. Finally, someone pulled their head out of their ass, and we rolled north into Iraq.

It was an awesome sight to behold the full might of the US war machine on the move. At least a big part of it. But what I could see was amazing. Vehicles for miles and miles and miles and miles as far as the eye could see, rolling along the hard ball road with burnt out tanks and armored personnel carriers littering the sides of the road where the lead element had engaged them. Blown up cars and trucks and shit everywhere, especially around An Nasiriya. The Cobras (attack helicopters) had a heyday blasting taxi cabs after the Intelligence boys found out that the bad guys were using them as a logistics and intelligence network. Fuel trucks ran constantly trying to keep the giant beast on the move. Grunts still dug into their fighting positions from last night's battle. Spent brass and expended AT-4 (shoulder fired anti-tank weapon) tubes laying scattered about their fox holes, some on watch, some sleeping in the dirt and others herding the ragged, dirty, and bloody enemy prisoners of war into containment areas. It was a full-on conventional war at first - with of course some guerrilla tactics involved - but either way it was amazing to watch.

My war was shit though. Luck of the draw, I guess. 2^d Force was split up between Task Force Tarawa and 1st Force Recon. My platoon had gotten attached to 1st Force. Really good dudes. I knew a lot of them very well from my days at 1st Recon Company. Some shit-hot operators for sure with a great reputation, but the crew that was running that operation at the time were first class shitheads: AJ Copp and his dipshit Sergeant Major. I don't think there is anyone who was there that would disagree with me, including the operators from 1st Force. We were attachments. So, in spite of our capabilities and experience, all of our best gear and all the good missions went to their own 1st Force Platoons and we were stuck doing all the menial bullshit missions or just rolling around with the damn HQ fucks. I was fucking livid. It may seem like a stupid thing to be pissed about. But I was still fucking pissed. I had learned all this shit, come all this way. Sweated the sweat, bled the blood, and when the chance to do the work came along, the leadership at the top was too incompetent to employ their resources or do anything else but bitch about

Finally Somehow Home

shaving and hair cuts and figure out how many medals they could get without really getting their hands dirty. Unreal. Sure, we ran some missions. Nothing much to speak of though. I was a tourist mostly during the invasion. I remember standing on the hood of my gun truck looking out over the berm of the airfield near Al Kut and watching Cobras do gun and rocket runs on a column of Armored Personnel Carriers that were trying to retake the airfield. The war was all around me and I was immersed in all the emotional turmoil that changes someone in a war, but I wasn't allowed to play. I knew that there were a shitload of people there that didn't want to be there, had signed up to get their college paid for, and that's it, and they were out there fighting. I was there for no other reason than to engage in combat. That's what I had signed up for. But nope. It was shit. Like being in a strip club with no money. Like I said. Luck of the draw, I guess. Maybe it's a good thing though. You never know. Maybe I would have gotten zapped or burnt to toast if it were different because there was definitely a lot of that going around, but I was willing to take that chance without hesitation. And no one would give it to me. I lived and saw and felt it all in spite of the frustration. Enough for it to change me. You

Finally Somehow Home

can't help that. But it changes you in ways that you don't see in yourself until much later and in ways that you just don't see coming. We'll get into that. The biggest contributing factor in that particular conflict, for me, was this: From the earliest age a person begins to build this concept in their mind of a future for them. And what it will be like, and all the hopes and dreams and aspirations that go into that. It is always there and it is always being built upon. It was interesting that during our training operations we would always talk about what we were going to do afterwards. Whether it was go get slam-faced at the bar or go have a big fat juicy steak, or whatever. The misery always inspired us to think of and talk about what we were going to do afterwards that we would enjoy. Moshpit touched on it when he mentioned the favor he asked of me. And when we got over there none of us had any plans at all of anything after. As far as we were concerned it was a one-way trip. It was only about what we were doing right then, because if you are thinking about anything other than what you are doing. If you are thinking about what could happen to you. If you are thinking about going home or anything else regarding your future it could cost you your life, or even worse, your buddy's life. There has to be laser focus on the present. And you can't help it, but when you live like that, you stop developing this concept of your future in your mind. And we lived like that for a long time. The problem is that when you get back no one tells you that you have to start it all up again. You get so used to living in the moment, of focusing on what you're doing right now that you forfeit your future. I saw something that a Marine wrote during the Battle of Fallujah where he talked about living 20 seconds at a time. He nailed it. When you do that for so long under such intense pressure your mind forgets to build your future. I think that's why there is so much hopelessness in some people who have experienced combat or other intense experiences for long periods of time. You have to start it all up again. You have to do it. No one will do it for you. No drugs will do it for you. You have to start hoping again. And you have to start becoming excited about those hopes again. I wrote something awhile back, it goes like this:

Dream big. You would if your dreams were glimpses of your future. Well... They are.

And here's the thing: if you don't dream, if you don't hope, if you have nothing of the fantastic in your mind

Finally Somehow Home

for your own self to accomplish or experience, if there is nothing amazing, no long-shot or hail Mary or long odds to beat, you will, by default, settle for the mediocre. You will never experience anything beyond your expectations because you have none. But don't worry. It's not hard to do. You just have to know that you have to do it. And no one told me that when I came back. It took me many, many years to figure this out. No, I don't have horrific visions of my friends dying in my arms, I was spared from that, but it doesn't matter. I still got it. You may be spared some of the nightmares. But you won't be spared the acquiescence of your future if you don't grab it by the balls again and make it your bitch. Dreams aren't kid's stuff. It's just that that's when you discover them and are best at it. Find your inner kid if you gotta, but you gotta start dreaming again my friend. Unless you're in the shit right now. Then don't think about anything but what you are doing. It's like riding a dirt bike, or anything really. If you are constantly thinking about what bad things could happen, you'll panic, freeze up, or hesitate at the decisive moment and the prophecy will be self-fulfilling. If you're in the shit right now, for God's sake,

Finally Somehow Home

just focus on the now, but when you get back, just remember that you have to start your future up again.

We ended up in Al Hilla. Old timey Babylon. Right at the site of the old ruins. And we made ourselves at home in Saddam's Palace and the surrounding areas there for a little while before we got the order to retrograde back to Kuwait. We had won the war. So it was time to go home. Once we got back to Kuwait, my Platoon Sergeant approached me and asked me a strange question, "Mo, do you have a wife or girlfriend or anyone meeting you when you get back?"

"Nope."

"Good. You're going to stay here with all the vehicles and gear until we find a way to fly it all back."

Great.

So everyone else in my unit flew back home and me and a handful of other poor bastards hung out on the tarmac at the Kuwaiti airport waiting to hitch a ride with all of the unit's shit. Like I said: always anti-climactic. It took us about ten days, but we were finally able to get the hell out of there. We loaded up onto a 747, threw our guns

Finally Somehow Home

into the overhead bin, I took an Ambien and passed the fuck out. I awoke about eight hours later to find that we were still on the tarmac in Kuwait, with the AC barely hanging on. Apparently our plane was broke and they decided to keep us on board while they flew in the new parts from Bahrain. Twelve hours after we got on the airplane we finally left the ground on our way home. We smelled like ass. The whole airplane did. I felt sorry for the poor flight crew they'd chartered to fly us back home. They were great though. We bullshat with them up in the cockpit and told them all about the war.

We landed in America about three in the morning and I was home on my back porch smoking a cigarette when the sun came up. I just remember the colors. So many of them and so bright that it startled the eye. The sky was blue again, not blah and dusty. After living in a world of shit-ass dirt-grey for so long it was fucking beautiful. As soon as the base golf course opened that morning I bought a set of golf clubs and played a horrible and delicious round of golf. I just wanted to be in the lush green I guess. And forget about everything for a while.

My End of Active Service came up in the Fall and I decided to get out of the Marine Corps. I would have stuck around if they had let me try out for Delta Force, but the Marine Corps wasn't having it. Not saying I would have made it. Just saying I wanted to take a crack at it. But nope. Ironically the Marine Corps opened it up the very next year and some good buddies went over there, but for me it wasn't meant to be. I'd had a hell of a good time, the experience in Iraq notwithstanding, but it was time for me to move on. I remember leaving the base for the last time, towing my Jeep with my Uhaul, and realizing that I was no longer Sergeant Morrison. I was just Jason. After almost eight years, it was a lot to deal with.

Chapter 9

The strict adherence to most major ideologies will yield some betterment for you, but I wasn't after betterment. I was after truth. So, I decided to take a year and just study the Bible. I went to school to study the Bible because I'm a cynic. I wanted to see if it held up. I decided to only believe the truth - if I could find it - and that's a hard thing because no matter what you believe about anything, you're at least a little bit wrong about it. That means that when you find truth, you have to give up the lie that you've been believing in its place. I was prepared to do it. It was scary, but I know what I believe. Don't ignore it. Don't minimize it. Don't act like what you believe is unimportant. That's a tremendously popular and insidious lie. It might be hard but it's fucking important. Be ready for it though. As soon as you profess

Finally Somehow Home

to believe anything they'll call you a hypocrite. And they'll be right. You will fail at measuring up to what you profess to believe. Here's the thing: anyone who believes in something is a hypocrite because no one can actually measure up to their own standard. Only those too timid and spineless to believe in anything can claim that they are not hypocrites. And here's something else you have to consider in the quest for truth: there are two types of truth, objective truth, and subjective truth. Subjective truth is the shit that you believe to be true that informs and influences your day-to-day decisions and the way that you live your life. This is what people are referring to when they say, "What's right for you may not be right for me." Many will say that there is no Objective Truth, or that it's too hard to find to be worth the trouble. Kierkegaard said, "All decisiveness inheres in subjectivity. To pursue objectivity is to be in error." The problem with that statement is that if you believe there can be no Objective Truth, well... THAT is your objective truth! That objective belief, then, informs your subjective truth. You don't have a choice in the matter. Everyone has an objective truth, even if their objective truth is that there is no objective truth.

Finally Somehow Home

If there is a God who's the source of all that is, it stands to reason that he is beyond our comprehension because all that is, is. However, if we can't possibly comprehend all of God, that does not mean at all that we cannot comprehend parts of Him. And the parts of Him that we can comprehend are the parts that He shows to us. The same is true with objective truth. If you choose to not seek truth on the grounds that it is in itself totally incomprehensible, you're missing out on the parts of it that are. And that sliver of knowledge that you get if you really do seek the truth, no matter what it turns out to be, that shit is pure fucking gold. And when you find those slivers of truth, I promise you they will point directly at whatever God is. If you do not seek to find objective truth, because you think it can't be found, or for any other reason, you will have nothing upon which to guide your subjective truth. The truths that you know from day to day that define who you are, and how you act within humanity and within this world. If you have no objective truth, you have nothing. Nothing concrete, upon which to guide those nudges of the heart to the really, really good things. The things that are best for you and give you life. It's not about good and bad, right and wrong, it's about life and death. What is it that gives you life, or what

Finally Somehow Home

is it that brings you death? That's what sin is. It's not a rule like in a game: if you break it, you get punished. It's a law like in science: if you do it, it'll fuck up your life.

Nietzsche said, "And those who were seen dancing were thought to be insane by those who could not hear the music." I didn't give a damn about anything else. I wanted to find the music. I wanted to find the Truth.

I remember the first time I drove into Estes Park, Colorado. It was early in the morning. Still dark. The sun in the east behind me wasn't up yet. I crested a rise in the road to see the first fingers of the dawn touch the snowcapped peaks of the Rocky Mountains. It hurt me in the gut it was so God damn beautiful. It was one of the scariest things I've ever done, driving up that hill the first day of Bible School. No possessions to speak of, no identity, and no plans but to seek out the truth. It was a good time in my life. It was a very good time indeed.

I was in Cape Town, South Africa a few months later on a two week break from school when I heard about the Blackwater contractors being killed and hung from the Fallujah bridge. Iraq was getting hot again. I was in South Africa helping a friend of mine build a church. Yep, doing the missionary thing again. College kid style. As soon as I got back to the States, my buddy Potsy contacted me and asked if I wanted to join a company that was hiring former Special Operations guys to do security work in Iraq. Fuck it. "I'm in", I told him. I guess I'm going back to war.

So, I ducked out of Bible school for a few weeks again to attend the selection course. The company was all run and managed by former Delta Force guys. I remember meeting one crusty Delta Sergeant Major and introducing myself. He told me "I've never met a Force Recon Marine who I haven't been totally impressed with." I guess I have some expectations to live up to. The training wasn't really training. It was more of an assessment. The only people there were former Navy SEALs, Army Special Forces, Army Rangers, and Marine Force Recon as well as some Marine Scout Snipers. In spite of the impressive resumes of everyone there, the attrition rate was still through the roof. People were dropping like flies. It was funny because no one else really knew too much about Force Recon before then. I had no idea how we really stacked up against the other special ops guys other than a few operations that I'd done with the SEALs and Army Special Forces guys when I was in the Marines. But I had never worked with

Finally Somehow Home

the Rangers or Delta before at all. Turns out we were trained pretty damn well. Most of the Marines were in the top part of the class. The focus was mostly on shooting and driving with an in-depth medical portion as well. By the end of it about half the class was gone because they couldn't meet the standards, which left us with a very solid contigent of experienced Special Operations dudes who were at the top of their game. I had a good feeling about going to war with them. I went back to Bible school and finished it out, then waited for the call to go to Iraq.

I showed up in Baghdad around the first of July 2004. I was told I was going to be assigned to Team Miami and working out of Ar Ramadi. Ar Ramadi was the provincial capital of Al Anbar province. The triangle between Ramadi, Hilla, and Baghdad was known then as the "Triangle of Death". I knew Ramadi was going to be dicey because every time I told someone that I was going there their eyes got really big and they said, "Shit! You're going to Ramadi?" Team Miami had driven out to Jordan to pick up some of their guys who were flying in, so I waited around Baghdad for them to pick me up. After a week or so they were able to make it out to Baghdad and collect me up and stock up on booze and ammo and spare tires and other such essential bullshit. I found myself in the back seat of an armored Mercedes S500 with a PKM medium machine gun running the "Highway of Death" from Baghdad to Baghdad International Airport (BIAP). (Everything there was dangerous as fuck at the time, so everything was the "_____ of death". There was even a Traffic Circle of Death near Al Asad. It sounded corny as fuck until you realized that people called things that for a reason.) At that time it was a constant gunfight on the BIAP road. And this was back when Chechen mercenaries were still getting paid. Those motherfuckers knew their shit when it came to vehicle ambushes, and they fucked some people up on that road and pulled it off without getting killed. There were some shooters along that road then. There were always burning cars on the side of the road from one side or the other and at any given time a complex ambush could kick off if you made yourself a target, or even if you didn't. Everyone had an itchy trigger finger too, so you had to be careful of everyone, especially the Military who were the main target for Vehicle Borne Improvised Explosive Devices (VBIEDs). Tactical vehicles aren't fast, they had to cruise at 45-55 Mph, and those dudes were getting hit every day, so they didn't give a fuck

Finally Somehow Home

about launching a round into you if you came up on them too fast or aggressively. All we had were American flags and bright orange air panels in 12"x8" ready to display and our smiling American faces behind them. Most of the Personal Security Details (PSDs) would run nut to butt down that road in SUVs. In other words, their high-profile cars were stacked up very close to each other making them an obvious target. We spread our motorcade out and hauled ass in armored sedans. At that time our motorcade consisted of a BMW seven series in the Lead, a Mercedes S600 as the Limo, directly behind the lead, and another BMW 740 as the Follow car. Two Mercedes S500s covered the 6 o'clock and acted as the emergency response, or Crisis Action Team (CAT) and brought up the rear. All of them were factory armored in Germany and they all had big fast engines. We each had our own M4 and Glock as well as a complement of ammo and grenades and in the cars we had PKM medium and RPD light machine guns, a shit load of grenades of all kinds, as well as a few other surprises if anyone wanted to find out what kind of fire power we were packing. Our cruising speed was anywhere between 100 - 120 miles an hour once we got past BIAP and onto Route Tampa. Route Tampa was the

Finally Somehow Home

main artery running west from Baghdad all the way to Jordan and passing through the Triangle of Death.

So, I settled into my new home on Camp Blue Diamond in Ramadi as a member of Team Miami, and was given the nickname "Elvis" which has been my callsign ever since. We were fat with Delta Force and senior Army Green Berets who'd already seen a ton of shit either in Afghanistan or in past secret squirrel shit they were involved in. I was among the young guns there even at 27. A handful of Army Rangers and a few Force Recon Marines rounded out the crew.

Some days it was smooth sailing. In fact, for the first few weeks there wasn't much going on because the first battle of Fallujah had just ended, and the bad guys were regrouping. But we knew they were gunning for us because we were the only PSD in the province, and there had been afew other attempts to take out Miami before I got there. The thing about Ramadi that made it unique is that the Iraqi Special Republican Guard, the Fedayeen, (the most fanatical and well-trained soldiers in the Iraqi Army), were based there before the war. When the Shiite dumb asses, Chalabi and the Governing Council of Iraq, disbanded the Baath Party it left them all without

Finally Somehow Home

jobs, so they were all pissed off, and they all went back to their homes. In Ramadi. Where they had been stationed. Where their families were. Where all of their stockpiles of demolitions and weapons and equipment lay hidden and easily at hand. You see, Iraq was set up for an insurgency war because they were expecting Iran to invade. They already had stashes of guns and ammo and demolitions rat-holed all over the country and had a plan for running an insurgency war in place. All they had to do when we showed up was initiate the plan, ad hoc.

I had just been promoted to Limo driver. It was my second day in that position. It was August 10, 2004. I remember we were out taking pictures of ourselves in all of our cool guy shit before the mission just because there was nothing else to do and we needed pictures to post on hotornot.com. I had a pretty healthy score of 9.5 running for a good long while and I was trying to get it up higher but could never quite maintain a 9.8 threshold. In fact, hotornot.com even contacted me and offered to showcase me as Hotornot Man of the Year. I was honored. I guess a lot of girls out there had a thing for sexy mercenaries. I can't say that. I wasn't really a mercenary. But I was definitely a gun for hire. Close enough. And what's not sexy about that? Anyway, we rolled out that day and took an alternate route in to the Government Center in the middle of Ramadi. It was called River Road. It was usually avoided because it went right through some bad guy land, but we liked to alternate our routes to keep them guessing. Everything was fine on the way there and we didn't even fire a shot on venue. But then suddenly I heard over the radio that the meeting was breaking up and we were getting ready to leave earlier than expected. I didn't think anything of it. I just ran back and got into the Limo and got the god damn AC on and the car into position for pickup. Once we got the Principal safely into the backseat and doors closed, the Shift Leader, Smuggler, came over the radio and said "We just got word that foreign fighters are lining the streets waiting for us on the way back. "

FAAAAK. Here we go.

We were planning on just blasting up route Michigan, which was the primary route through the center of town, but traffic was so bad that we decided to take the route out that we had taken on the way in. It was obvious that something was going on right away because as we turned down toward River Road there were cinderblocks blocking the street. We couldn't stop and bunch up at the intersection, so we cruised along on high fucking alert hoping to push on through as we hadn't yet met any resistance and we didn't want to just be sitting ducks in the middle of the traffic jam. But we knew some shit was about to go down. Suddenly I noticed civilians running and scrambling away, and off to the left I could see masked gunmen with AK-47s and PKM machine guns running to get into ambush positions. And sure as shit everyone else saw it too and everyone got on the radio at the same time and stepped on the Shift Leader's transmission when he gave the command to reverse out. (When more than one person is trying to talk on the radio at the same time on the same frequency, it just garbles everything), so the command never went out over the radio, but the Lead car got the idea and turned, nose in, to the left onto a curb in order to turn around. I queued off of the Lead and backed up onto the same curb getting ready to accelerate out and turn right back down the way we came. As soon as I had backed up, the Principal in the backseat and the Agent in Charge in the right front seat called out: "RPG-RPG!!". There was an RPG gunner standing not 20 feet away from me with his RPG leveled and pointed at my face. "He's going to shoot! He's going to shoot!" All I could do was cringe. I knew this was going to hurt. An RPG-7 can go through 9 inches of armor. Even with the Level-7 armor on our Mercedes S600, the windshield being about 5 inches thick, there was no way that the rocket wouldn't blow us all to smashed and battered dogshit. Remarkably, the RPG misfired, or the gunner forgot to take the safety off. For whatever reason he ducked back away without firing. It's then that I looked up and noticed that there was a very high curb and a telephone pole in the path of my egress on the road median and I had to back up even more. So, I threw the car into reverse again to back up a few feet so I could turn around. This was all taking way too long. We were sitting there stationary on the "X" with AK and PKM fire popping off all around us. The follow car reversed out before I did and caught a tight group of PKM rounds to the right rear window. Sonny was sitting in the back seat and watched the window spiderweb as the rounds slammed into it. The armor held up and only part of one round made it through the crease in the door and lodged in Sonny's seat back headrest as they sped off. It's a good thing that Sonny had his lucky ear plug in that day, and that ain't no shit. I was still reversing. Another RPG gunner then stood up

Finally Somehow Home

about 20 feet to my left and fired. He was expecting me to pull forward. I pulled backwards instead, and the RPG sailed over the hood of my car and slammed into the ground next to the left rear quarter panel of the Follow car. It spread shrapnel all through the gas tank and the right rear side of the BMW. Sonny was taking a serious beating but Bags, the driver, stayed on it and shot down a side road with the CAT team following the crippled BMW as it gushed fuel all over the road. I finally pulled my head out of my ass and got myself turned around and heading back toward Route Michigan. On the way out, my left front tire blew on a rock or someone shot it out but it held up OK. We ran Pirelli P-Zero tires and they performed marvelously in spite of the gaping hole in the sidewall. I was doing about 100 mph by the time I hit Michigan, and I started running cars off the road to make room for myself to get through the traffic and make a hole for the others behind us. The big heavy S600 didn't even notice when it would hit a normal car. It weighed in the ballpark of 17,000 pounds with all the armor on it and the V12 under the hood, and when it ran into something lighter, the lighter thing moved over and out of the way. All along Michigan we saw "broken down" cars blocking the side roads in order to congest the road with traffic. They had been channeling us into their ambush, but we got there just a few minutes before they were ready to kick it off. The Follow got itself turned around and joined back up with us, but not before a sniper put a bullet into the driver's side window four inches to the left of Bags' head. It was an amazing shot at that speed, but again, the armor held up. The Beemer was leaking fuel pretty bad, but it was still mobile. As we made our way back, Johnny Bravo came up on the radio. "Elvis, how's my hair?" I thought he was asking me about MY hair, so I said, "9.5 on Hotornot." The immediate pressure was off, so it was important that we de-escalate and resist the urge to succumb to the adrenaline and stay ramped up. We had to reel it back in again so we could be ready to dial it up instantly if we needed to. "Inflate -Deflate", Rancher, one of the Delta guys, and a personal mentor, used to always say. We managed to get back to base before all the fuel ran out or something caught on fire. All the Marines stared, awestruck at our survival, as we drove back onto Blue Diamond, but we all made it back.

My first big ambush and I had fucked it up big time. Only by the grace of God am I still alive. But it was me screwing up that saved our lives. If I had pulled forward

Finally Somehow Home

instead of backed up it would have been over. You just never know with something like that. We had dash cameras in the cars and somehow a few years after that, the video made it onto LiveLeaks on YouTube. If you search for "RPG machine gun ambush Ramadi", you'll see it. Johnny Cash will be playing in the background. Go ahead. Look it up and watch me screw up in combat and live to tell about it. We managed to get back OK and we didn't lose anyone, but we didn't win. We had gotten very lucky. One thing really burned us all, and that is that we didn't kill a-one of them. After that we decided that if they were going to tangle with us again, they would pay. I think that attitude is what saved our lives in the long run, because after that we didn't take no shit without giving a lot back. And after that it was game on. We knew it and the bad guys knew it, and they would come out to play almost every time we went downtown.

Chapter 10

Our heart and soul were the vehicles we drove, because they were the biggest weapons that we had and because we were so damned mobile. We operated all over Anbar Province, from Baghdad to the Jordanian border. We knew the roads intricately. Every pothole, every mortar round impact, every interruption to the road's surface was memorized by the drivers, as well as called out by the Lead car over the radio en route. I ended up driving Lead car, which to me was a great honor. You had to know where you were going, and you had to know the roads perfect. But I learned to drive Lead car by driving Follow car under the tutelage of Rancher. Rancher and Smuggler were the Shift Leaders and switched off with each other on leave. Rancher taught me to drive. He was a consummate professional and tremendously capable

Finally Somehow Home

across a broad spectrum of skill sets. He could drive, shoot, lead, fucking kick ass as good as anyone I've ever known. He was young too, a couple years older than me. A lot of the Delta guys were older, some of them had been in Delta since the beginning of it. Rancher was the byproduct of what the more senior Delta guys had created with their skill and legacy, and Rancher, like the rest of them, was a very, very, very fucking dangerous man. He always smelled great too. (I have to admit that I adopted his habit of the application of copious amounts of cologne.) After a couple of months driving under Rancher's tutelage I was ready to drive Lead.

I would have to push out in front of everyone else to create a couple miles of dispersion between all the cars, so if the Limo wanted to cruise at 120mph, or even at 100 (when we later added SUVs to the mix), I'd be up to 140mph for a good 10 minutes or so to give everyone behind me enough room. Driving on a blown-up shit ass freeway with dogs and kids and trucks who don't check their mirrors when they change lanes, and bad guys everywhere, and IEDs, and trigger-happy Big Army or the Marines rolling along at 45mph in convoys, is much different than driving on a cambered race track, but for all intents and purposes, we were combat racecar

Finally Somehow Home

drivers. Due to the temperature hitting around at 120*F on some days, the road surface would be hot as hell, and at those speeds on that hot asphalt the tires would sometimes fail at speed, but even with a 17,000 lb armored sedan they would usually hold together long enough with enough rigidity in the sidewall to facilitate safe-ish deceleration provided you stopped immediately to change the tire, because by then it was in ribbons. We did have a BMW spin off the road at about 90 miles an hour due to a flat tire, but that happened because as soon as the tire blew it hit a pothole, which grabbed the rim. Everyone was ok. The weight of the car kept it from flipping over, but in most cases you could get slowed down and stopped safely in time.

We rehearsed tire changing drills. To be a driver you had to, with the help of your right front seater/VC (Vehicle Commander), be able to change a tire in under 2 minutes on a sedan and under 5 minutes on an SUV. You never knew when it was going to happen, or where, so you had to know it cold. The other cars would form as much of a protective cordon as they could, and you just had to get it done with your ass out in the breeze on the side of the road with probably no cover.

Finally Somehow Home

Driving at those speeds and in those conditions takes tremendous focus. You're looking much further out in front of the car because of the high speed, then checking close in, and the sides of the roads, check mirrors, check road far, check road near, check speed, check road far, check road near, check dispersion, check road... it was constant, especially while cutting through traffic at 90-100mph in a city checking rooftops, windows, other cars, scanning everywhere for IEDs and VBIEDs who's suspension would be sagging heavily from all the explosives stuffed into it. Your sense of awareness is totally maxed out, and for very long periods of time. We drank RipIts like mad to stay awake and keyed up. I was on a good healthy diet of Sostenon 250 and Deca Durabolin that I had stocked up on during my layover in Amman, Jordan. I could use the extra energy and aggression. The strength and endurance I derived from it helped as well and of course would come in handy if I ever needed to bust heads with bare muscle. You can't be weak. In my mind it wasn't worth the tradeoff to not be taking that shit. If you weren't aggressive, you were a target. Period. In how you drove and walked and operated overall. Everything. Timidity was the fastest way into a body bag. The bad guys weren't stupid. They

Finally Somehow Home

picked the softest targets and we always made sure that wasn't us, which is why we all made it out of there alive and a lot of others didn't, especially a lot of bad guys who tried to fuck with us. Not that we were out actively seeking engagement per se... well maybe sometimes... but we definitely weren't discouraging the bad guys from mixing it up - on our terms. I was at a job interview afew years ago and I was asked to describe the most highly competitive situation that I had ever been in, and how I had prevailed against the competition: "Well, one time a bunch of people were trying to kill me and my teammates, and we killed all of them instead." Hey... She asked. Plus, what the hell? Am I supposed to lie about my life and dumb it down so it doesn't scare you? I didn't get the job.

The currency of getting things done was booze. The military didn't have access to it, so we found ourselves in a unique position. We always made sure we had plenty on hand both for our own consumption as well as to grease the skids on any favors, such as work done on our cars, issues with the Marines on base, swapping for ammo, or whatever else we needed and also just to hook our buddies up who were in country and still in the military. You always have to remember where you came

Finally Somehow Home

from. There were a few liquor stores in the Baghdad "Green Zone" we could go to and stock up. We would fill a whole Suburban full of booze and then make the run back, or if we had to fly out on a helicopter and load up kit bags full of the stuff we would. However we could get it. It was absolutely essential. Plus, it gave us another way to be popular with the Marines who we relied upon heavily and worked closely with both on base and during our daily operations. Honestly, it did make a few enemies though because some of the female Marines would find their way over to our compound for drinks, which caused considerable jealousy, but all's fair in love and war.

General Mattis was on Blue Diamond as well and used to go to many of the same meetings that we did. Surprisingly, he often showed up late, sweaty, and dusty and I always wondered why until I talked to his PSD crew. He would roll around Al Anbar Province in half a dozen or so LAV 25s (Light Armored Vehicles). The 25 stood for the 25 mm chain-driven autocannon in the turret. Those guys were always getting into some shit. This is just what I heard from talking to the guys on his detail, so I don't know if it's true or not, but they had no reason to bullshit me. Apparently the General's

Finally Somehow Home

standing rules of engagement were, if they took fire, to stop whatever it was that they were doing, locate, close with, and destroy the enemy by fire and maneuver. No matter what. They always had Cobra Gunships and F-18s on call as well, so his crew rolled heavy. They would take fire and just decimate whoever it was that was fucking with them before moving on, which, in turn, made General Mattis late for many of his meetings. One of the Marine armorers told me that every time he would roll out, the General would check out his own M-249 SAW (Squad Automatic Weapon - light machine gun) and an M-16 as well as a full complement of ammo, and would always turn the weapons in filthy and with all the ammo used up. Apparently he didn't leave the shooting to the enlisted guys. Again, that's just what I heard, but it was word-of-mouth.

Ramadi was the backdrop to Fallujah. Zarqawi, the boss of the baddies in Iraq, ran operations out of Ramadi. One day when we were on a route recon I remember seeing a redheaded guy with a beard looking incredulously at us as we brazenly drove through his turf deep into bad guy territory. There were parts of town that the Marines and others just didn't roll through, so we liked to pop in and say hi sometimes. At first they didn't notice us, but then

Finally Somehow Home

they'd do a double take and haul ass back to get their guns and RPGs out, but it was too late, they only ever got afew shots off at us and we made sure they hurt worse than we did by the end of it. I later remember reading a book on Zarqawi and seeing that same red headed guy in the book. It was one of Zarqawi's lieutenants. I wish I'd known it then because there was a nice bounty on his head at the time.

There was a lot of sniper activity in Ramadi. Some of their best snipers were working in that area so we had our own. We had a shitload. But Pappy was a retired Marine Master Sergeant and Scout Sniper instructor extraordinaire. One of the most knowledgeable snipers out of the Marine Corps (read: in the world) at the time, and he was on our team. The bad guys had a habit of launching indirect fire attacks on the base during lunchtime hoping to get a lucky hit on the chow hall or hit people on their way there. It was like running the gauntlet some days just to get lunch. One day I was walking to lunch and a mortar round blew up in the air almost directly over my head but just off to my right. Fortunately for me, there was a large concrete barrier about 15-20 feet tall just to my right and it blew up afew feet on the other side of that. Unfortunately, it killed a

Finally Somehow Home

Marine out on his smoke break, not 5 feet from me on the other side of the wall. I felt bad that I was so lucky, but fucking elated that I was still alive. It was weird hearing indirect fire come in. It's a totally helpless feeling, and as soon as you hear the explosion, you're relieved as fuck because it wasn't you and yet you feel guilty at the same time for being such a selfish bastard. Sounds fucked up. But that's the first thing that went through my mind every time I heard an explosion: "Thank God I'm not hit." It was almost a relief to hear it because you knew that one had missed you... unfortunately it didn't do shit for all the other ones hanging in the air right about that time.

At first, the bad guys were using a lot of RPGs as indirect fire weapons against the base. An RPG will self-detonate 900 meters from launch, so they built contraptions that could launch four RPGs, simultaneously, set to washing machine timers and stashed them within range of the base perimeter, set the timers, and viola! 30 minutes later, once they were well away from the launch sites, the RPGs would come blasting in and blow up over our heads or smack into something and blow up. Eventually the Marines started patrolling the area and found afew of their launchers, so they switched to mortars.

Finally Somehow Home

The mortars were more dangerous because they could sit 2-3 km away in a built-up area (where our counter battery artillery couldn't return fire due to collateral damage), and drop them in on top of us. We really had no way of getting back at them until Pappy set up a Night Force scope on an M2 .50 Cal machine gun in one of the guard towers which allowed us to lob rounds out into the areas where they were launching from. It was always back and forth. We would counter their moves and they would counter ours. But really, all that shit was more of a deadly inconvenience than anything else. Just one more way you could die there. Downtown is where all the magic happened. I wrote this awhile back. You'll get the idea...

What War Feels Like

My mouth is so dry. I can feel my heart beating, especially in my ears against the sweaty radio earpiece that I keep checking to make sure it's in tight, but the sweat won't let it be. I take a quick look around, then take my left glove off and roll a foamy piece of ear protection as tight as I can so it will fill up the ear canal and occlude as much sound as possible. The sweat and dirt on my fingers make it slippery as I roll it. I put it in my right ear and hold it there as it expands and makes the world sound dull and flat. Now I can't hear as well but once the shooting starts I won't hear anything at all if I don't put it in. It's a tradeoff. I put my glove back on then swear to myself and take it back off. I forgot I was going to put a dip in. The tobacco tastes cold and sweet between my gum and lip.

It's so hot you can smell it. Something is about to go down, everyone can feel it. The shops started to close a few minutes ago, the proprietors pulling down the garage doors that open to the dirty street. My back hurts from leaning back to counter the heavy ammo and grenades on the front of my ballistic plate carrier. I have 12 magazines on me and one in the gun totaling 390 rounds, and several types of grenades.

I'm aware that I am scared and it pisses me off. I'm not scared of dying. I'm not scared of pain. I know beyond the shadow of a doubt that nothing will happen to me and I'm terrified of the shock and feeling of incredulity I will feel when it does. And I'm mad that I believe so strongly that nothing will kill me. It makes me feel like I'm not ready for something very big that I have to be ready for. It is insanely irritating. I feel daft. I keep trying to picture myself dead, or imagine the feeling of the explosion or bullet, so I'll be

Finally Somehow Home

ready, but I can't. I'm not ready for death and it is infuriating.

I block it all out. But I'm still livid. I decide to take it for granted that I'm invincible. It's the best I can do. The Marine Explosive Ordinance Disposal (EOD) guys are out on route Michigan getting ready to blow a mortar round that failed to detonate upon impact of the street to my front. I'm in a reviewing stand about 10 feet off the ground and 10 feet from the road. 10 foot concrete Jersey barriers line the street in front of the Government Center compound where we are and continue around its border. Sandbags are stacked two wide and about 3 feet high around the circumference of the 20 X 10 foot reviewing stand floor. It has a tin roof and tin walls on three sides.

The Detail Leader, a former Delta Force guy named Pigpen, is sitting down in a folding metal chair with the PRC-119F radio handset jammed against his ear. "They're going to blow it in 30 seconds." Pigpen says. I take a hard look around before I get down behind the sandbags on a knee.

"CRACK" The explosion is right next to us on the other side of the Jersey Barriers. "Damn bro, that was a lot closer than I thought it was going to be." Pigpen

laughs. The explosion has a catalytic effect on the tension that has been mounting and now it breaks like a dam. We've all been waiting. Thank God, here we go.

Instantly rounds start snapping through the air by us. Sounds like maybe a PKM and some AK fire. The Marine Up-gunner's .50 cal is already answering. Pigpen aims across my front and takes three shots. I see nothing to my front and down the alleyway that I'm covering.

Suddenly it's dead quiet. "Got that motherfucker." Pigpen says smiling. "He was in that one little window we were looking at yesterday." I smile, not taking my eyes off of my sector of fire. I know it's going to kick off again in a second. I feel a lot better now.

Chapter 11

When I was back in Estes Park I'd had my eye on a certain piece of property that was right next my South African friend's house up in the mountains. He was a builder, so I bought the land and started working on plans to build a log house. I was making really good money and the housing boom was on so I thought I would build my dream house and then sell it if I needed to and make a little bit of money. First of all, don't do that. Don't build your dream house for someone else because you end up spending way more money on it than you otherwise would, and the return on investment isn't nearly as high. But I didn't know any better, so I started planning. In November it was my turn to rotate out on leave. I had already been there past the normal three months, and we needed to take frequent breaks to be on

Finally Somehow Home

top of our game, so we usually did 90 days on and 30 days off. Poor bastard Army and Marines were doing 12-18 months with no break. I didn't want to go because I knew that the Battle of Fallujah part two was about to kick off and things were just starting to get really interesting in Anbar Province. Sure enough. The team dropped me off at the airport and headed back for an afternoon run downtown. By the time I got off the plane in Amman, Jordan I had an email in my inbox from Snake telling me vaguely about the gunfight that day. Penlight had zapped a car full of baddies with the PKM and everyone else was busy too. I was pissed. Bad timing. That month, there were a lot of gunfights, and as I suspected, the Marines rolled into Fallujah and cleaned it out. Meanwhile, I was in Australia hanging out with a few Army Ranger buddies and visiting my old girlfriend from the Indonesian days. In spite of missing out on all the fun back in Ramadi, it was good to get away from the war and catch our breath. We were there just after the presidential elections when Bush was reelected and everywhere I went people kept wanting to talk politics with me once they heard my accent. The US wasn't very popular in Australia at that time because of Bush and the war, so neither were we. But we decided - fuck it, we're

Finally Somehow Home

gonna have a good time anyway. It was fun being flush with cash, so we made good use of it because we didn't know if we were going to live through our next deployment. We got the most expensive rental car we could find and blasted up to Surfers Paradise from Sydney. About three o'clock one morning after a wild night of partying we were hungry and decided we were going to get some pizza. The pizza place wasn't really a restaurant, it was more of a place that catered to drunken bastards at 3:00 in the morning and sold pizza by the slice. As we were standing in the very long line we were getting fucked with about being Americans and were getting tired of it. So, much to the chagrin of everyone in line behind us, we bought every god damn slice of pizza they had. As we walked down the street to our hotel with about 10 boxes of pizza. We began handing them out to drunken revelers along the way. One group, after we handed them a box of pizza, yelled "hey you guys are awesome!" I turned back to them and yelled, "Your God damn right, we're fucking Americans." They didn't know what to say. We had a good time, but were happy when the time came to go back. November had been a very busy month and I had missed it. I was bummed but I'd needed the break. Miami met me in

Finally Somehow Home

Amman on the way in and we drove back to Ramadi the next day.

There's so much to say that I am leaving out for various reasons. I ended up hanging around Ramadi until May 2005 doing much the same but with Fallujah taken the enemy activity began to taper off in the area for a few months. In May, Blackwater, our company's main competitor, won most of the security contracts that our company had as they had come up for a re-compete, and we were told to retrograde back to the States, sit tight and wait for future assignments. A few of the guys jumped over onto the Blackwater team to work with them but most of us decided to ride it out. The day that the Blackwater guys came out to Ramadi was a bad, bad day. They were driving Mamba armored cars, rolling slow down route Tampa when an IED blew the shit out of one of them. One guy died almost instantly and there were four more wounded, one of which was my good buddy Fondo, who had jumped over to the Blackwater side from Miami. That same day, Blackwater was sending teams out to the rest of their new sites. We had no sooner linked up with the guys who had gotten hit on the way out to Ramadi, than we heard the news about the Blackwater helicopter being shot down. They lost a lot

Finally Somehow Home

of guys that day and lost another one downtown at the government center about a week later. It was then that I realized how close we had been running the gauntlet. I guess we were just doing some things right, staying ahead of the bad guys, or were just getting lucky, but we all made it out of there alive which I think was a miracle. I came back to the States with mixed feelings, but grateful to be alive and not sure I ever wanted to set foot back in Iraq again.

I went back to Colorado and started working on my house and trying to create a life for myself. Life in the States was good, but I was growing restless. I bought a dirt bike and would spend all my spare time blasting around the woods of Colorado on it or driving out to Moab Utah and exploring all of the single-track riding anyone could ever want.

Right before I left Iraq I had been snooping around on online dating sites and had briefly talked to a pretty little Costa Rican girl who had spent some time in Colorado. We hadn't talked in a few months but one evening I found myself chatting her up online. She dared me to come and visit her, so I bought a plane ticket and flew down to meet her. She showed me Costa Rica in all of its beauty, and we hit it off. A few months later she moved back to Colorado, and we started hanging out more. It was a good summer overall, in spite of a few broken bones in my foot from my dirt bike, but I was still restless and bored and wanted to get back into the mix. My foot healed up and I took a job as an instructor teaching for the same company I had worked with before and was now screening and training their new generation of PSD personnel. I did that for a few months until some positions on the Israel detail opened up, so I jumped on it.

I got to Jerusalem in December 2005 and had my own team shortly thereafter. Israel was a good gig. We lived in apartments around Jerusalem or sometimes in hotel rooms in Tel Aviv and worked for the Consulate in J-town and the Embassy in Tel Aviv moving their people around or whoever else happened to show up. My very first mission as a Shift Leader with my own team was shuttling a young buck Senator around Israel and the Palestinian territory. We were at a restaurant in the West Bank where meetings were often held. It started raining hard and in no time there was 3 inches of water in the street. The armored SUVs had been disbursed around the nearby area so as not to draw too much

Finally Somehow Home

attention, as per our Standard Operating Procedure. Usually when a meeting is breaking up and the Principals are getting ready to leave there is a warning call sent out over the radio by someone in the meeting room so that we on the outside would have time to get the vehicles and personnel in position for a quick and secure pick up and departure. Well, this young Senator just stood up and bolted out of the meeting giving us no chance to get ready. He was ready to go. I got on the radio to get the cars lined up as quickly as possible, but it was too late. It was a cluster fuck. The vehicles came rolling in quickly, but late, leaving this guy standing in 3 inches of water in the middle of the street. Then he got into the wrong vehicle. He was not happy with me. At all. The next stop was the Muquata, which is the equivalent of the Palestinian White House. He was there to meet with Mahmoud Abbas, the Palestinian Prime Minister. No sooner had we pulled up to the Muquata than this guy realized that his tie was in a different car. So, someone had to run back and get it for him and then give him a chance to put it on before exiting the vehicle. It was a complete shit show part 2. After getting my ass chewed by the Department of State Regional

Finally Somehow Home

Security Officer, I went up to the Agent in Charge and asked him: "Who the fuck was that guy anyway?"

"Oh, I don't know. Some new Senator. Name's Obama or some shit."

One of the Palestinian guys who worked for the Consulate in J-town was a young suave cat named Iyad. Iyad was the real deal. If he hadn't been working for the US State Department at the time, no telling what he'd have been up to. Probably running a powerful and thriving mob syndicate. In Palestine, your family name means something, and the culture is very Patriarchal in that, just like in the Italian gangster movies, there's always a family patriarch who runs the family and takes care of everyone. In spite of being only in his late 20s, Iyad was that family patriarch. He never mentioned what fate had befallen his dad, but he did have several uncles, at least a handful of which were doing time in Israeli prisons for their active participation in the Intifadas, so that left the family to Iyad. If you ever needed anything at all, or needed something to happen, Iyad could get it done for you. It didn't matter what it was or whether it was on the Israeli or Pali side of the wall, Iyad was your man.

Finally Somehow Home

A year or so before I arrived there, Hamas was holding a western journalist hostage in Gaza. The State Department was running around in circles with their hair on fire trying to deal with the situation. The Consulate General and the Regional Security Officer crew, who Iyad worked for, had the Hamas fuckers on the phone, and to their exasperated chagrin, were getting nowhere. Iyad walked in. "Hey guys. What's going on?"

The RSOs quietly and quickly briefed Iyad up on the situation as one of them continued vainly on the phone.

"Give me the phone." Iyad said.

Iyad picked up the phone and matter-of-factly told the person on the other end of the line his full name. "Return the journalist immediately," he said.

Afew hours later the State Department picked up the hostage at one of the Gaza checkpoints.

After awhile of mulling it over, I decided to ask the Costa Rican girl to marry me on my next leave back to the States. I toured the diamond stores in Tel Aviv, and got up to speed on what to look for in a diamond, and got a good understanding of the price range and what I could afford. I mentioned it to Iyad one day as we were standing around at a meeting site in the West Bank. "Oh, no bro. Don't get a diamond in Tel Aviv. I have a friend I'll take you to. No problem." That weekend, Iyad and I took a trip to Hebron and met with his friend. I ended up with a stunning fully certified diamond, bigger than what I thought I could afford for about half of what I would have paid in TA. I'm pretty sure it was a blood diamond too, which was a total bonus because, cumon, sentimentally it's worth way more if actual blood has been shed over it. You just can't put a price on some things.

Around that time the Palestinians were holding their general elections and a shit load of politicians showed up from the US to witness them and show their support for the free democratic process, I guess. For whatever reason, they were there, and we were on the hook to show them around. Jimmy Carter and his whole entourage showed up along with a smattering of Senators and Congressmen and other cats and dogs.

A little bit of background for you: Fatah was the party that the US backed and had been in power for quite

Finally Somehow Home

awhile. Hamas (incidentally, started with the help of the US back in the day to counter the then unruly Fatah) was the other major party in the running and had, in the recent past, demonstrated a serious habit of lapsing into terrorist type methods to get attention and gain political leverage. No one really took Hamas seriously as a political entity, and their participation in the elections was looked upon by the west as just token in nature as most of their energies seemed to be focused on just fucking shit up. Well, somehow, right before the elections, there was a huge scandal that broke over Fatah's gross misappropriation of funds that was intended for the Palestinian people and which had instead somehow found its way into the pockets of a select few Fatah officials. This kind of behavior was nothing new, as Yasser Arafat – Fatah's founder - had pocketed a metric shit ton of cash for himself as well over the course of his illustrious career.

Suffice it to say that no one expected Hamas to win the elections, but half-way through election day, with US politicians scattered throughout the West Bank on their tours of various polling stations, and us along to ensure their safety, it started to become apparent that Hamas was winning. This in turn incited the more radical of

Finally Somehow Home

Hamas' supporters to tour the polling stations as well, no doubt to demonstrate their support of the democratic process. About the time this was all going down, me and my team and Senator Joe Biden, all of us totally oblivious to what was going on, showed up at a polling station in East Jerusalem – the Palestinian side of J-town – with all the good intentions that any American politician can muster. We showed up in our big armored SUVs and no sooner had the Senator begun shaking hands and kissing babies, than people started closing in around us and hollering about Guantanamo Bay and a bunch of other remarks and questions equally relevant. Joe started trying to answer the rapid-fire questions, but it soon became obvious that the growing crowd liked his answers even less than our presence at their polling station. The crowd was rapidly growing into a mob, and all indications were that it was not a flash dance. One of the instigators in particular was pressing in trying to get to the Senator, and I stepped in between them, my team creating a barricade around Joe as he continued to shout back answers to the crowd's remarks. "Ok, Sir. It's time to go now." I said. And we got everyone back into the vehicles and got the hell out of there.

Finally Somehow Home

Angry mobs were probably our biggest threat in the West Bank. Personal accountability goes out the window and the mob mentality takes over in situations like that. People in a mob will do what they would never dream to do on their own. It's viscous and scary to watch a mob at work, and in the West Bank they could form in an instant. Frankly, if we would have waited another minute or two the State Department guys would have been seriously pissed at me for letting us all get torn to ragged tattered shit.

Hamas won the elections that day, making the situation over there even more convoluted than it had been before. I used to think that the Israeli/Palestinian situation was pretty straightforward, but after living there for a year and a half, I saw what a quagmire it really is. There's no one thread that can be pulled to unravel the whole knot and there are gross and idiotic injustices on both sides that have left deep scars and continue to do so. I was there during the Israeli-Hezbollah conflict in 2006 and while I didn't participate, of course, I witnessed yet another war, first hand.

And let me just throw my two cents in here. The situation in Israel and Palestine is a massive twisted tanglefuck. It

Finally Somehow Home

will never be unraveled. There is just no way to undo all that has been done. The problem lies in the fact that everyone is approaching it from an aspect of wishful thinking and blame. The Palestinians wish the Israelis had never showed up and displaced them from their land in the late 40s, but they did. The Israelis wish they had never been through all the genocide and other horrible shit that they have been through and many of them probably even wish they would not have had to displace the Palestinians, but that all happened. The point is there's not a god damn thing you can do about what has already happened. No one on either side is focusing on the fact that they are in this situation now. Whoever's fault it is it does not matter, and how the fuck are we going to move on from where we really are in reality at this moment. There is no going back and changing anything. The only question is how the hell can both sides make this work with what they have right now. That's the most salient issue, and the most ignored.

While I was home on one of my breaks in 2006 I married the pretty Costa Rican girl and we moved into my newly built log home in Estes Park. Shortly thereafter, she put the house in bubble wrap and came to Israel to be with me in a nice little apartment overlooking the Old City of

Finally Somehow Home

Jerusalem and the park in the middle of town. It was a very homey and a pleasant time in my life. And after a few months I couldn't stand it anymore.

In March of 2007 I left Israel and got into a classified program working in conflict zones overseas for the next four years. There's very little if anything that I can say about this time or what I was up to, but something very important happened in the midst of it.

I had been kicked out of Afghanistan for a DUI. No shit. A buddy and I were shitfaced and driving to an illegal poker game held by some other civilians on Bagram Air Field around 2 in the morning. We were allowed to have booze because we were civilians, but the Army frowned upon it severely, nonetheless. I was driving in a 15 mile an hour zone - yes the speed limit on BAF was slower than the minimum standard of an Army person to pass a physical fitness test. Anyway, I was in a hurry to get to the poker game but an Army Dragon Wagon (a big ass truck) was ahead of me doing about 10 miles an hour. I changed lanes and accelerated, blasting by him at about 17 miles per hour and suddenly saw in my rearview mirror the red and blue lights of the Army's finest: the Military Police. The speeding alone was a grave offense,

Finally Somehow Home

but when the MP shined his flashlight in the back of the cab of the pickup and saw two cases of beer he immediately called for backup. The situation was tense. My buddy was a Special Forces guy who prided himself on the SF art of negotiation and attempted to talk our way out of the situation. The MP wasn't having any of it though because in spite of my buddy's Special Forces fieldcraft and training kicking in, he was slurring his words so much that no one could really understand what he was saying. I could not believe it myself, but the MPs then went back to their car and produced a breathalyzer test. Yes, a breathalyzer test. In the middle of a fucking war zone. I proceeded to blow into the damn thing and apparently transcended the legal limit for driving in Afghanistan. In spite of their preparedness for such a scenario, they had not yet encountered one such as this, so they called their commanding officer for guidance. They brought us back to their Cop shop and said they were sorry, they knew that we were legally allowed to have booze, but their CO wanted to make an example out of us. So, they threw us in the slammer overnight and confiscated our beer. It wasn't that bad. I even had my own Koran to read. Anyway, I got kicked out of Afghanistan and had to sit on the bench for a few months

Finally Somehow Home

before I could get back to work in a different war. I guess I was too drunk for that one.

It was really good the way it turned out though, because we were expecting my son David to be born in the next few months. In the months and weeks leading up to his birth I was very concerned. Unlike my wife who had a great deal of love and that tender beautiful feeling that a mother has for her yet unborn child, I felt nothing whatsoever. It scared the hell out of me. I thought there's something wrong with me, I'm not going to be a good father because I feel nothing about this and apparently I should. As I watched David's birth in awe of that miracle that only life can produce: the beginning of another life, I still in spite of it all felt nothing. I was horrified with myself. The birth was in Costa Rica and there they do it a bit differently. As they were taking care of my wife they took me and David to an adjacent room where we were by ourselves then they handed him to me. I held him close to my chest to keep him warm as they instructed. And I still felt nothing. Then this little human who had never done anything for me, who did not know me at all, nor I him, reached his little arms out wide and clung to my chest. And in that instant I became a father. In that instant I knew that if anyone or anything ever tried to

Finally Somehow Home

harm him I would lay down my very life in the pursuit of the swift and violent destruction of that thing. I felt a love that didn't come from me. It came from somewhere else and flowed through me like that river in Indonesia in flash flood. It was a raging deluge of love mingled with an intense determination to protect and teach this tiny new human life everything I knew about it. I told David that I would do so to the best of my ability. My face hurt from smiling. And I felt great relief. My life had just changed. There was great beauty in it now.

Again, there's little I can say about what I was doing in those years, but suffice it to say that I worked with some exceptional individuals, and saw a lot more of war in new places and from yet another perspective. I also managed to find time to study in between missions, enough to earn a Bachelor's Degree in International Business from EIEIO Online or some such institution. That part was a hard grind, and somewhat surreal, switching gears mentally from gunslingin' to things like Business Ethics, but I knew that I had to do it if I ever wanted to become proficient at anything other than the conduct of war and I did want that very much. Being a gunfighter is like being a stripper. It's great fun and great money but the longer you're in it, the

Finally Somehow Home

less marketable you are to do anything else and the more difficult it is to effect a transition. There's nothing wrong with doing that kind of thing for your entire professional life, but I wanted to see if I was good at anything else. I've always thought it important to challenge myself in this way, which is why I moved around a lot even in the Marine Corps. This starting over from scratch is hard on you, but the result was that I was always among the best at my job because I always had to be. I had to continually prove myself at an elite level to those who held themselves and their peers to the highest possible standard. And I had to prove the same to myself because I held the same expectation of my peers as well. I wanted to be surrounded by people I could learn from and respect, so I strove to be someone who was the same. To me, this held true in every part of life, and I wanted to see if I could function at an elite level in business as well as in war. I had no idea, at the time, how much of what I had learned would serve me well in my future endeavors. Honestly, I thought I'd hate a "desk job", but I had to try it for myself.

Finally Somehow Home

Chapter 12

This bit might seem alittle dry to you gunslingers out there but pay the fuck attention. The only way you can sling lead forever is if you die doing it. Much like combat, the corporate world is pretty fucking awesome unless you suck at it. It actually is combat. You don't get to shwack the other guy and take his scalp, but you sure as shit get to take all his money if you're smart and quick and agile enough. You already know how to be that. But much like combat, you've got to kinda figure it out and get your groove on with it. We've all dealt with the tunnel vision and audio occlusion in our first few gunfights. These next few bits might help you get beyond that shit quicker if you do one day decide to hang up the gun belt. Either way, here's how I figured it out...

Finally Somehow Home

Back in 2004 when IEDs started blowing the shit out of our troops in Iraq the President allocated a giant wad of cash to the Department of Defense (DOD) to do something about it. The result was the Joint IED Defeat Organization (JIEDDO). JIEDDO had three main lines of effort: they provided equipment such as armored vehicles and counter IED jammers, training to the troops, and an element called Attack the Network (AtN). AtN resided under the purview of the Counter IED Operations/Intelligence Integration Center (COIC). JIEDDO itself was an 800 pound gorilla in the DOD because of its huge annual budget. It could effect a great deal of support to the troops in a very short amount of time and did so regularly as was its mission. The COIC was the technical and intelligence support component. It is, or was anyway, described on their unclassified website as such:

"The Joint IED Defeat Organization's Attack the Network line of operation enables offensive operations against complex networks of financiers, IED makers, trainers and their supporting infrastructure.

Attack the Network is comprised of operations, intelligence, and information fusion and analysis. It

Finally Somehow Home

enhances situational understanding of the global picture. It provides analytic capability and capacity through reachback. It provides training of processes, analytics and software, and enables access to the intelligence community.

JIEDDO provides operational intelligence and analysis on threat networks to commanders by fusing hundreds of national-level data sources. JIEDDO maintains a broad network of partners - more than 30 government and intelligence agencies as well as coalition partners.

JIEDDO supports intelligence operations downrange, via intelligence/operations analysts forward deployed down to the battalion level with reach back capabilities to national-level resources."

My best friend Troy from my old Recon days had gotten himself assigned as the Project Manager of COIC's operation in Afghanistan, and when I reached out to him and mentioned that I was looking for something else to do, he helped wrangle me a job back in the Washington DC area. I don't know what he told them, but they hired me somehow.

Finally Somehow Home

He asked me if I knew anything about computer networks. I said "no", so he told me to get on Wikipedia and look up a few things, so I did. That question should've clued me in, but my understanding was that my job was going to be as a Special Operations liaison of sorts. Someone who, when the guys downrange in Afghanistan or Iraq asked for intelligence reachback support, could translate their request into something intelligible by analysts so that the analysts could give them what they needed. That job did exist at the COIC, but that's not the job I got.

I showed up to the COIC, bright eyed and bushy tailed, in January 2011, two days after flying back from Iraq, and was immediately blindsided by the true nature of my future work there. I found myself in charge of all the Special Operations data centers around the world that the COIC managed. A large part of intelligence analysis is the ability to aggregate and fuse data from all different sources, then be able to derive information from that data. Each of these data centers was called a Federated Node. In other words, they comprised a global network, each of them absorbing and defusing data according to the operational contexts of the units they supported. It was essentially the first functional byproduct of The

Finally Somehow Home

9/11 Commission's report addressing shortfalls in the sharing of intelligence information between government agencies. The result was that new mandates were put on the government to share information and the system that was supposed to make this work was called the Distributed Common Ground System (DCGS), pronounced dee-sigs by everyone in the government. The COIC was the first organization across the entire government that had managed to get a fully federated Distributed Common Ground Integrated Backbone (DIB) up and running. At the time it was the state of the art in data aggregation and, arguably, in data fusion.

My job was to manage and support all the Nodes that had a Special Operations focus. And, at the time, I had no clue what any of this meant. Fortunately for me I had some amazing teachers who, incidentally, didn't know how ignorant I really was. The COIC was rife with intellectual elite, all of whom cared deeply for the mission at hand. My immediate boss was literally a rocket scientist and had worked for NASA building satellites among many other things. It was an amazing environment to work in and I was dumbfounded that I had managed somehow to be a part of it. I started

Finally Somehow Home

learning as fast as I could. It was like going to college undercover because I was terrified that if they found out how little I knew I would get shit-canned immediately, but they were patient with me and if they saw through my façade the first few weeks they didn't let on. One of the other guys, a former F-15 fighter jock named Nico, hooked me up with a list that he had made of all the acronyms that he had to learn when he first got there, and I had it taped to my desk. I remember having conversations with people and stealing glances at the list in order to know what the hell they were talking about. It was literally like drinking from a fire hose but everyone who walked into the COIC experienced the same thing back in those days. There was just so much going on and there was such urgency about it because we really were saving people's lives every single day in one way or another as well as helping to zap baddies in an indirect but very important way. It was here that I learned of the power of a networked organization because that's what we were up against.

It seemed like forever but within several weeks I was able to hold my own and properly manage all the sites that I needed to take care of. Really most of that was personnel management and understanding relationships. True leadership is just clearing the obstacles in the path of those who work for you so that they can run at a dead sprint and don't have to break their stride when they encounter roadblocks. But to clear the obstacles before they reach them, you have to be ahead of them all. So, I endeavored to do that as well as learn the technical aspects of my new job. It was different waking up every day and putting on a suit and tie instead of body armor and pistol belt but to my surprise, I found that I enjoyed it immensely and even began to add value.

It soon dawned on me that my past operational experience was actually a huge benefit. I understood things the way that they actually were in the field whereas an analyst or technician did not. This really helped me craft what we were doing to be able to provide more relevant support to the people who needed it. I found myself becoming the go-to for people who wanted to know what things were really like. Not that I knew everything, because I had been out of the game for a little while as far as military Special Operations, but I still had a keen understanding of their operational context.

Finally Somehow Home

This eventually manifested itself in a concurrent realization for my boss and I that a new type of data architecture was needed for the Special Operations guys unique to what we were providing for the conventional forces. Don't get me wrong, the units like Delta Force and SEAL Team Six and all those dudes in what's called Tier 1 SOF, had some dope ass shit set up for them already, but the rest of the Special Operations Community – the Tier 2 guys, didn't have shit and couldn't share shit with each other. All their data was sitting on a hard drive in a footlocker shoved into a corner of the 2-shop (Intel shop), and the 2's (Intel Officers) at each unit didn't have anywhere to put it, so there it sat. There were SODARS (Special Operations Debrief and Retrieval System) reports that all the SF guys had to write up after a deployment, which were uploaded into a Sharepoint library, and after they were written, never again saw the light of day. There were also the rolled up SOF reports, where a team would send in its daily report which was scrubbed and cherry picked for stuff that went into the Company report, which was scrubbed and cherry picked for shit that went into the Battalion report, that was finally shared, so that by the time another team could access it on our COIC system, all the information

Finally Somehow Home

relevant to another team had been scrubbed out and it was only relevant to Battalion Command and Staff or higher. This is where I learned another important lesson: to get the most critical information to the people who most critically need it within LTOV (Latest Time of Value), a data enterprise must be extended to the most granular and furthest level on the battlefield. Only in this case will the people on the pointy end be able to share, query, and analyze data and information that is relevant to their operational context.

So, under my boss's tutelage, I started learning and planning what this new data enterprise would look like. We came up with a rough sketch of how we could get it done at a low cost and began presenting it to people on up the chain. My boss was very much a part of helping me understand everything that needed to get done in the technical aspects of it, but he let me run with it. There's no better way to learn something than having to teach it or brief it.

The director of the Net-centric Innovation Division, which I fell under, was a Marine Colonel named JJ, so as fellow Marines, we hit it off right away. After I presented the idea to JJ he bought into it and in the months that

Finally Somehow Home

followed the two of us started a whirlwind tour of all the Component and Theater Special Operations Commands we could get to in order to solicit their buy-in for the concept. We traveled all over the US and down to US Special Operations Command (USSOCOM) in Tampa, Florida several times to brief the idea, and soon got a letter from Admiral McRaven, the then commander of USSOCOM asking us to develop and build the new data enterprise. It was very gratifying to go from looking up computer networks on Wikipedia to getting that letter from Admiral McRaven facilitating a much needed revamp in USSOCOM's data sharing plan and system in less than eight months. As far as I know my little idea is still an enduring Program of Record at USSOCOM.

Something happened, however, when we were down at USSOCOM getting final approval to deploy the system. I was speaking with one of Admiral McRaven's action Officers, a Green Beret Colonel named Stu. Stu didn't fuck around. He got shit done. Because of this, he'd been hand-picked to head up one of the new SOF initiatives the Admiral had put in place to transform and modernize USSOCOM. Stu's last assignment had been building NATO SOF Headquarters (NSHQ) in Mons, Belgium, from the ground up, then serving as its Chief of

Staff. He had a keen understanding of the intricacies of SOF as well as its role and impact in the big picture of things. He had good swagger and talked like a surfer, though his speech was somehow incredibly articulate, and from the moment he began to speak, I got the strong impression that I should really shut the fuck up and listen as long as he had something to say. We were sitting down around some picnic tables just outside of a Subway at the massive and perplexing USSOCOM Headquarters building on MacDill AirForce Base. Using some paper slides, I showed him what we wanted to do with SOF data and how we planned to get it done using the new data architecture I had blueprinted. He paused for a moment. "You know what you guys really ought to do? This is good, and I'll approve it and send it up to the Admiral, but you know what would really be valuable for us?" He asked. "What we really need is a system that allows US, Allied, and Partner Nation SOF to all look at the same data around a shared problem in their own language, and conduct collaborative analysis and enrichment on that data. That would be Bad to the Bone." I guess I was looking at him like he had a dick growing out of his forehead, because I'd been after the final approval of this thing for months. Did he just bless off on it? I think he

Finally Somehow Home

did. Holy shit, he did! But then he handed me a problem that I didn't have an answer to. Holy shit, no one did.

The reason that SOF is so important is that SOF is the nation's closest touch to burgeoning enemies as well as future friends. It's a small international community. Invariably, the Colombian Lieutenant that you went to Ranger School with will become a Colonel and maybe a General one day, and those relationships have proven invaluable as they mature over the course of time. Many of our senior military leaders have close relationships across the globe with people who are now leaders of their countries based on shared training experiences when they were younger.

I stayed on at the COIC for another six months or so helping to refine and implement the beginning stages of the new data enterprise and was re-assigned to a position created to maintain relationships with key Special Operations stakeholders. It made sense since I had met them all within the past few months. The majority of the work of my little project was passed on to the technicians and developers who were to build the new system, so I found myself casting around for something new to occupy my time.

Finally Somehow Home

Everyone is always looking for a promotion or something extraordinary to be a part of in the working world. I've found that if you can get your eight-hour-a-day job done in 6 hours or less, then you have 4 or 5 more hours to focus on shit that you would rather be doing but maybe no-one else is, and pretty soon, someone will notice and just make that your eight-hour-a-day job. All you have to do then is repeat the process. And yes, you can't get anything done in only eight hours a day. If you really want to push your career forward, you have to invest more than the bare minimum. That goes without saying.

I had started my work at the COIC as a member of a small company out of Fredericksburg, VA who had won some of the work there as a Subcontractor to the Prime contractor, which was a big DC beltway company. While I was there, another big beltway monster had come in and won the Prime contract, so I found myself having to sign on with them to keep my job. I didn't really like the big corporate feel very much. There was all the work to do at the COIC, then I had to participate in all the "rah-rah, our big company is the best" bullshit after hours that was supposed to motivate people toward business development and

Finally Somehow Home

team spirit - business development being the top priority. I always thought that the best business development model was to kick ass for the client's sake, and the proof would be in the pudding as to why they should maintain or expand their business interest with your organization. Both sides have to have skin in the game in a business relationship. I'm not saying that the big company I was with did a bad job, they actually did a very good job, but so much of the time of the employees was taken up with reporting up to their higher echelons within the corporation that it definitely reduced the amount of attention that could be focused on the client's mission. I found myself reporting to my COIC chain of command as well as two other chains of supervisors within my corporate organization. I spent more time reporting on the work I was doing than I did doing any work. I've noticed this as an Achilles heel in many hierarchical organizations. Especially if there is an emergency of some kind, the people focused on fixing the problem must divert more and more of their time and attention to reporting to their supervisors on how they are fixing the problem the bigger the problem grows because the bigger it gets, the more supervisors become involved and the more they want to know. The result is

Finally Somehow Home

that no one is actually fixing anything, and the only people who are capable of fixing it are spending all of their time trying to explain the problem to people who don't know how to fix it. This is where things can break down and the whole system implodes.

Management and Leadership are two very different things. A manager is an day-to-day administrator of employees. That's about it. A good leader will actually draw fire for their people so that their people can focus on what they need to focus on. If this is done all the way up the chain, it can work, but Managers are seldom taught leadership. They usually think that they are one and the same. This is why so many innovative ideas are squashed in the corporate world. The C-suite is looking everywhere within their organizations for good ideas and bright employees, but the ideas never make it past mid management. Employees are essentially told: "You aren't getting paid to do that, now get back to work." Management without leadership is a sure sign of a dying organization. Or at least a very vulnerable one.

Chapter 13

Within a few months, an opportunity came up for me to venture out on my own as an independent consultant. I jumped at it. I started working at the Combatting Terrorism Technical Support Office (CTTSO) as a Systems Engineering and Technical Assistance (SETA) Subject Matter Expert (SME) in the Advanced Analytics Subgroup. The Technical Support Working Group (TSWG), which CTTSO fell under, was started back in the Reagan days after the bombing of the Marine Barracks in Lebanon. The standard acquisitions process for the government was blueprinted during the Cold War days for things like building tanks and fighter jets and is still wretchedly slow. It takes years to develop and field anything, and in today's world where the timeline to obsolescence of technology is measured in

Finally Somehow Home

weeks and months instead of years, there is a huge need for an avenue to circumvent the arcane acquisitions process to develop and field urgently needed high tech shit. TSWG was created for this purpose. It was unique because it actually fell under Department of State as well as the Department of Defense under the purview of the Assistant Secretary of Defense for Special Operations and Low Intensity Conflicts. The benefit to that is that we could support much more than just the DOD. It was the perfect job. I loved it, because much like the COIC, my job was to help people and organizations in their most pressing needs. You're getting blasted with acronyms here. Sorry, but you might as well get used to it. Anyway, before we get too far into this I want to go off on a rabbit trail really quick.

There is a general sense of distrust in the minds of most Americans when we start talking about Washington D.C. and the government. This is somewhat due to all of the bureaucracy that comes part and parcel with the government and the way that it is managed, but I think most of it stems from a distrust for the elected officials. This makes sense, because, for the most part, none of the skills required to become an elected official have anything to do with the skills required to function

Finally Somehow Home

as one. Most of Washington DC's elected officials are lawyers. Lawyers think very qualitatively as demonstrated by Bill Clinton's famous statement: "it depends upon what the meaning of the word "is" is". When you have an entire portion of government predominantly made up of people who think this way it is going to be frustrating for the rest of us, because they suck at thinking quantitatively. For the rest of us, 1 + 1 is still 2, no matter how much you talk about it. But here's the thing, most of DC is not made up of elected officials, or even of the appointees of elected officials. Most of the people doing the grunt work in the government are just normal everyday Americans from both sides of the aisle. When someone gets elected and places their appointees in position, all the people working on the nuts and bolts are still the same people from one day to the next, and these are the most competent people, for the most part, in the government. These are the people who bear the brunt of government shutdowns, the people most affected by the budget wars and all the other bullshit that comes out of the policy side, but they are, most of them, damn good Americans, just going to work every day.

Finally Somehow Home

Most government contractors don't get to see the money. For the most part, it is only actual government employees who deal with contracts and funding. This is so that companies can't wrangle more contracts from the government by having their own people on the "inside" so to speak. In fact, most of the bureaucracy in DC is meant to prevent fraud, waste, and abuse. They take it very seriously. There's even a fraud, waste, and abuse hotline that you can call if you think something's not on the up and up (ironic for DC, I know). As a SETA contractor I was in a unique position. I could see the money and help build the contracts, but as I had signed a non-disclosure agreement with the government I was not allowed to, and never did, use this information to my advantage. I also had no authority when it came to the selection of vendors or the doling out of money. My boss, who was a government employee, oversaw what contracts were executed and what checks were signed. This put me in a position to learn a lot about how the government works. The reason I had to be privy to all of this information was that my job as a SETA SME was to receive requirements from organizations across the government, then to have whatever they needed built to meet their requirements as fast as possible and get it

Finally Somehow Home

back out to them ASAP. I had to know and understand the state of the art in Advanced Analytics, how the money worked, and, once again, understand the operational context of the end user well enough to be able to do all of this within weeks and months instead of years.

To boil it down, this was my LinkedIn write-up on what I did there:

On paper: find or develop capabilities or concepts to meet user requirements across the DOD and InterAgency, then field these new capabilities in support of efforts which Combat Terrorism. However, the goal, and coincidentally, the commonality in the greatest successes has been much more.

Through constant communication with the edge user, understand and develop within the context, but to the root of the requirement if possible, and get it out to the field ASAP. This inspires the edge user as to the scope of the possible, and usually they then begin to push the capability beyond its breaking point and use it in ways that it was never intended or designed to be used. The next step should be a continuous cycle even after the capability has been transitioned: Instead of blasting the edge user

Finally Somehow Home

when he complains by telling him he's not using it the right way, we improve the capability to meet the newly discovered list of requirements and repeat. The greatest inventors are the edge users themselves. In reality, our goal is not just to improve the tools used to manage the problem, but to improve how the problem is managed.

The P-51 Mustang was designed and built and flown 117 days after the contract was signed and was sent to Theater not meeting all requirements. It performed poorly until an edge user wondered what it could do with a Merlin engine in it. It became the greatest fighter plane of all time. If it had stayed in the R&D shop being refined, we would have never heard of it.

The P-51 didn't only change how Allied pilots shot down airplanes; it changed how the war was fought. It became the lynchpin of daylight bombing because someone had the balls to field an 80% solution then listen to the edge users.

The following has little to do with my work at CTTSO, but it's funny, so I'm putting it in. This was a brief bio that I wrote of myself during that time:

Finally Somehow Home

Adept in the approach of abstruse issues from unique perspectives in order to illuminate often simple courses of action toward resolution or exploitation. Experience-derived expertise in a smattering of disparate fields with a reputation for decisive and creative unconventional solutions and considerations to conventional issues, and concise conventional relevance in unconventional circumstances. Twenty-seven years overseas experience in Indonesia, Iraq, Afghanistan, and Israel, eight years as a Special Operations Forces (SOF) Operator; now facilitating foundational concept and technical capability implementation at the operational vector of future SOF efforts. Specialized in data leveraging concepts and capability development/integration/fielding and socio-cultural stability concept development. University level teaching experience. Sixteen years of industry experience across varying disciplines, but all dedicated to direct participation in, or in persisting the presence, safety, and success of key American people by providing them with an unfair advantage over their adversaries.

I have applied this same great rigor and zeal toward the selfless provision of discomfort for as many of those willing adversarial participants as possible at the behest

Finally Somehow Home

of the US Government with the purpose of facilitating for them even the slightest inconvenience such as the ruin of surprise birthday parties, mockery of arts and crafts, offense of personal feelings, ridicule of hopes and dreams, all toward the increase of their general level of discomfort, including but not limited to the application of high velocity projectiles of various types and sizes including, but not limited to, 5.56mm, 7.62mm, .50cal, the general size and shape of various armored vehicles, items closely resembling JDAMs and other such articles as may be available from time to time in South and SouthWest Asia, so as to diminish those people's ability to influence my access to bacon and freedom.

JDAMs are GPS guided bombs. The rest of the acronyms you'll just have to Google. Anyhoo... My main portfolio when I first showed up there was the fielding of an analytical system for the US Special Operations Forces (SOF) and the Marine Corps. I worked closely with all of the US Special Operations Commands and Headquarters Marine Corps – Intelligence (HQMC-I) at the Pentagon as well as staying in touch with the end users who were putting the system to good use in Afghanistan and Iraq and other far-flung corners of the world. The system was called Palantir. Palantir was a Silicon Valley

Finally Somehow Home

startup that spun off out of PayPal as a fraud detection tool. The nuts and bolts of it were so powerful that it could make sense of a lot of different types of relationships very rapidly. Especially since we were up against a networked enemy, this became a tremendously powerful tool. It is, in fact, the very tool that the CIA used to catch Osama Bin Laden. The CIA got involved with Palantir in its nascent stages by investing in the company through In-Q-Tel, the CIA's venture capital organization that finds and nurtures bad ass new tech startups. After the CIA glommed on to Palantir, afew other government and corporate organizations started looking into them as well. CTTSO had received a Joint Urgent Operational Need for Support (JUONS) from General Mike Flynn - the intelligence chief in Afghanistan at the time - for an analytical system that actually worked. CTTSO had done their due diligence on what was out there and after conducting several evaluations had settled on, and begun to field Palantir. Unfortunately for the Army, the Army's DCGS (remember this from my COIC days?) system, DCGS-A got all riled up and plied their leverage to ensure that they alone supported all the Army units, which meant that the poor Army bastards were stuck with something

Finally Somehow Home

that didn't actually work at the time, while CTTSO offered to support anyone else who wanted Palantir. SOF and the Marine Corps raised their hands. Even after that, Army units were begging us for help and we helped them where we could, but most of the support went to the Marines and the Spec Ops dudes.

DCGS-A, was by then a bureaucratic power house and was vying for all the Government funding they could get their hands on. Back then their budget was something like $30 Billion a year and they weren't going to let some piss ant tech startup out-do them. Just alittle inside baseball for you: the way that takeover wars are fought in the government is that if you have what is considered a redundant capability then you'll probably find yourself getting defunded, so what DCGS-A was trying to do to my little program was nothing more than what they had tried to do to the COIC while I was there the year before, and, although ridiculous, because DCGS-A couldn't hold a candle to COIC's capabilities, nor did they posses the authorities to do so, they had tried to declare that the COIC was a redundant capability to what they were doing, therefore, they wanted to absorb the COIC and horn in on the COIC's funding, or at the very least, try to get the COIC defunded in order to

Finally Somehow Home

solidify their own position. DCGS-A was on a power grab. They were going after everyone's money and when it dawned on them that Palantir was far superior to their shitty capability and far cheaper by orders of magnitude, they went after CTTSO.

Unfortunately for DCGS-A, their system sucked ass and couldn't come close to what Palantir was able to provide for a fraction of the cost. There was a war over the whole thing within the DOD and it got nasty. Then it really blew up and went all the way up to the House Armed Services Committee (HASC) in Congress where Congressman Duncan Hunter from California and General Odierno, Chief of Staff of the Army at the time, were screaming at each other in a HASC session. Guess who was caught in the middle of this shit-storm? Yup. Me. I was writing reports for the HASC and trying to keep my program's ass from getting flamed by DCGS-A while trying to get people what they needed to fight a war and save lives on the battlefield. I was getting Requests for Support (RFS's) from Army units on the down-low hoping to get Palantir for their troops and risking their careers to do it because they were getting the DCGS-A system shoved down their throats instead. It was pretty ridiculous. There are probably still a lot of people who

Finally Somehow Home

have very strong feelings about it. It was a shit-show. I was very popular with some folks who were grateful for CTTSO's support – and simultaneously - viewed as a Palantir stool pigeon by others. It was a pretty uncomfortable place to be, but I just kept on doing my job and tried to keep my ass out of the line of fire as much as I could.

In the end, nobody really won. DCGS-A tried to make their user interface look exactly like Palantir, but the back end never really worked on it, except maybe in a lab somewhere, but I never heard of a deployed DCGS-A capability that actually did all the shit they said it could do. Either way, by the time the dust settled everyone in the Army was too nervous or disgusted to adopt either one in and of itself. Eventually I think the Army ended up using Palantir. I believe as part of DCGS-A, but I'm not sure about that or how it all played out because we eventually transitioned all of those systems over to their new owners and let them hash it out after that.

I built a system for Joint Task Force – North (JTF-N) in El Paso, Texas that was pretty interesting. I called it the CADENA Platform – the Combined Agency Distributed Edge Network Analytics - Platform. CADENA means "chain" or "link" or "network" en Española. It was a fitting name because the idea was to provide a secure system that abunch of different organizations could use together to collaborate toward addressing problems along the Southwest Border of the US. It was pretty slick, if I do say so myself. The idea was that a Cop, or Border Patrol agent, or FBI Agent, or any Agent who had a smartphone with the app on it could, say, take a picture of a license plate or a vehicle or a suspect and get real-time feedback from an intelligence analyst within afew minutes instead of finding out three weeks later that they had just let some MS13 baddie get away. There was a lot more to it than just that, but the idea was to provide a system on which all the Agencies working on the Southwest Border could collaborate together on as one big happy-happy. The only problem was that, to my great surprise, no one wanted to do that. The system worked great and ended up being used to great effect by some agencies for awhile, but overall it didn't take off because of this collaboration issue. I couldn't believe it. Not until I started peeling back the onion a little on what was going on along the Border. There was no scandal or anything like that, but there were a few contributing factors as to why no one wanted to share their information with anyone else who were all supposedly working on the same problem. First of all, the DEA was super sketch about sharing information, because back in the day the Clinton administration had demanded that they declassify and share all of their information, and lo and behold, all of their undercover agents and sources ended up getting whacked. Holy shit! But that wasn't the main reason. The main reason is much simpler. No one owns the "Battlespace". In a war, there is such a thing as a "Battlespace Owner". The Battlespace owner owns the turf they have been assigned, and it doesn't matter who you are, if you want to do anything in someone else's Battlespace, you have to clear it with them, period. Otherwise, you end up stepping all over each other's toes. This was actually a problem in Afghanistan for a while, when some high speed, bad ass, special operations units would come flying in in the dead of night and whack some bad guys, only to find out that the bad guy they had shwacked happened to be an intelligence source that the conventional force guys were working. Issues like that were happening a lot until the Special Ops guys ate crow and realized they were doing more harm than good if they didn't coordinate their operations with whoever

Finally Somehow Home

owned the damn Battlespace. Well, along the Southwest Border, there are no "Battlespace owners" per se. At least there weren't when I was working on the problem. Furthermore, each Agency gets paid to do certain things. The Border Patrol, for instance, gets paid to interdict bad guys at the Border. The FBI gets paid to investigate and indict. So, if they both have access to the same information that Javier of MS13 is coming across the border at a certain checkpoint that night, the Border Patrol is, of course, going to stop that from happening. The FBI on the other hand, is getting paid to track Javier into the US, investigate all the bad shit he is up to and indict a drug ring in St. Louis. See, they are both working on the same problem, but they are working on the same problem differently because they are getting funded by the Government to do different and opposing things and there is no one who owns the Battlespace and says, interdict here, and investigate there. It is a very frustrating problem, but once again, they are mostly all great Americans just trying to do their part. But it's still fucked up.

Finally Somehow Home

Chapter 14

I've only really talked about work until now since I mentioned returning to the US. The main reason for that is because everything else was total shit. When I first came back to the States for the job at COIC, I had found a little house to rent in Herndon, Virginia and got it ready for my wife and David to join me from our place in Colorado that I was desperately trying to sell amidst a housing bubble poppathon. We were pregnant with Danielle at the time. That was the only real spark in it.

I don't know what the reason was. She didn't say why, but even when I had been on the ground in Afghanistan she'd just felt the need from time to time to remind me that she didn't love me anymore. Dani's birth in August was bittersweet. I was amazed at this new little creature in my life. When David was born it was an

Finally Somehow Home

overwhelming sense of ownership and duty: the feeling of fatherhood to a son. But with Dani, it was different. There's something to be said about a daddy/daughter relationship. When I first met Dani, I was again overwhelmed as intensely as with David, and with much the same sentiments but with afew exceptions. It was every bit as strong and intense as what I had felt for David, but it was pink and had purple bows and unicorn stickers on it. I felt for Dani the overwhelming desire to protect and nurture her. Like a delicate chubby little budding flower. I wanted to guard her and help foster the seed within her that would blossom into a strong and courageous and beautiful woman one day. It was a remarkable thing welcoming her into the world. But a heavy and foreboding cloud hung over it all. I hate to admit it, but I didn't make the same promise to Dani that I had made to David. I didn't promise I'd always be there. I promised I'd be there as much as I possibly could. It was the best I could do.

Have you ever noticed that people who have never had kids, later in life it seems like they are missing something? Like they didn't learn some things that the rest of us learned? You can't put your finger on it but there's something different about them. I think that's

Finally Somehow Home

because kids are the University of You. I have learned so much about myself from watching my kids that I would never have otherwise learned. They are little mirrors that reflect the things that you could never otherwise see. I remember watching David contemplate doing something naughty. I knew exactly what was going through his mind. He was weighing the pain of the punishment against the joy of the crime. He knew he was going to get nailed for it and was thinking about whether or not it was worth it to go ahead and do it anyway. I know what he was thinking because I used to think the exact same way about things when I was a little kid. And it brought that back to me in that moment. But then I realized to my amazement that I still do the exact same thing. I will still weigh out the pain of the punishment against the joy of the crime. You don't learn that kind of shit about yourself without loving your kids.

But everything else about home was horrid. When something is off in a relationship, any man worth a shit will pause and objectively consider what he could be doing wrong and what he needs to change to make things better. It was constantly on my mind. I agonized over it 24/7. I looked at it from every angle. But the longer we went on, the worse it got. It was driving me mad. I

Finally Somehow Home

thought that if someone I know thinks I'm a piece of shit, they might well be right. But if the person I'm closest to in this world treats me as such, then they probably are right. I thought maybe I was crazy. There must be something I was doing to make it like this. Something I could change to fix it. I hated looking into the mirror. All I saw was failure. I felt the same disdain that was aimed at me for myself. I didn't want to kill myself, but I really wanted to die. I was living in complete despair. Locked into no hope at all for a happy future.

Rabbit trail : Here's a little pick-me-up factoid for ya - Every single romantic relationship in your life will end in failure except for possibly the last one. (Unless the love of your life dies, and you later find another.)

There's plenty that men need to know about women that I don't know, but there are some things that men AND women need to know about men that I do know. A quick caveat: when speaking definitively about general subjects it is important to delineate that I am addressing not necessarily the 100%, but the large majority. There will always be a ~10% fringe on both ends. I will be referring to that ~80% in between. This applies to all such discussions, not just this one.

Finally Somehow Home

It is often thought that a woman is the only one who thinks ahead of time about marriage. This is not true. The difference is that while a man wonders about it and plans for it, a woman wonders about him and plans it. A man, when he thinks he is close to that time in his life will do his best to prepare for it by "getting his house in order". To carry on with the metaphor, once the man has made all the repairs needed, cleaned, and scrubbed, and gotten his very self in the best possible condition...better than ever before...the best he will ever be, in order to impress and gain the attention of the right woman, he brings her in, and shows her what a magnificent "house" he has. She is impressed. She looks the house over inside and out and is very excited and impressed indeed...and says to herself "This place wouldn't be half bad if we just fixed it up alittle!" It's funny, but unfortunately here's where things start to fall apart. Expectations and intentions are not promises. If they manifest, it's gravy. If they don't it's not a breach of trust.

When a woman says something about something or someone, that is how she feels toward that thing or person at the moment. When a man says something about something or someone, that is a definition of that thing or person's very nature and character. For

Finally Somehow Home

example: if a man sees someone behaving cowardly, he will decide, regardless of what he feels at the time, that the person in question is a coward. Not that he behaved cowardly, or is cowardly, or he felt that the person acted cowardly, but that the person in question IS a coward. Period. He may still act the very same toward that person as he did before, but until that person does something to determine otherwise, that person is, in his mind, a coward. Forever.

So, when a woman feels a certain way toward a man and decides that it is important for the man to know what she is thinking at that moment, the man will take that comment, whether good or bad, uplifting, or debasing, and believe in his heart that she thinks that of his very character. Forever, or until the same person tells him otherwise.

The woman needs to be wanted and desired, and a man wants to be needed and trusted. A man who is not trusted can become a man who is not trustworthy. For a man, suspicion and accusation are the surest and quickest way to undermine a relationship. These are the worst enemy of trust. Unfounded suspicion and accusation invoke bitterness. Bitterness grows into resentment, and resentment into vengefulness. Vengefulness manifests itself in actions that betray trust. The campaign against men has been successful. A man will become what people expect of him. He will be brave, sacrificial, and heroic if that is expected of him. If he is respected, he will be worthy of that respect. If he is dismissed and regarded as a bumbling idiot with no sense or ability, he will deliver.

Similarly, within the context of a marriage or long-term relationship, if a man's best attempts to display his strength and value are met with only negative responses, he will eventually reckon that he is weak and worthless, and he will become so. In other words, if a man is doing all that he can - and he naturally will do so, because men hone in on problems and try to fix them - and it becomes clear to him that in spite of his greatest efforts he is treated with indifference, spurned, or ridiculed, he will shut down. The woman's indifference or rebuke may be, and probably is, simply a ploy to manipulate the man into trying harder to meet her perceived unmet needs, but to the man it is a final judgment of the ineptitude of his character and role. His only way out of this is to prove that he is not. If no chance is given him, or he continues to receive only negative responses to his continued

Finally Somehow Home

efforts, he will either remain weak and worthless perpetually, or he will seek opportunity to validate his strength and worth. At first it will be in other ways, such as at work, but his strength and value must be affirmed in the same context that they were spurned. This is why good men cheat. This will not even be going through his mind when he does, but this is why many men are either emasculated, weak and worthless, or unfaithful.

This is the cost of "managing" a man. Men are not wired to be managed. It simply does not compute. Attempts to help him maximize his "performance" in a relationship will destroy him, and if the relationship survives, it will be devoid of the recklessness, uncertainty, and mystery that give it wonder and adventure. It may include a male and a female, but the man is gone forever. All he really needs, is the occasional assurance that he's doing a good job, and if you want to make him do backflips for you, he will, if he thinks that his woman believes that he could take on any other man alive.

Before I go any further something needs to be said. Spoiler alert: we end up getting divorced. The great temptation here, especially for the sake of the opinions of my children, is to defend myself. But I'm not going to

Finally Somehow Home

do that. First of all, in many cases I have no defense. I really and truly fucked up a lot of shit. Guilty as fuck, as charged. And secondly, everyone has a right to their own opinion. Especially my kids. Regardless of what they've been told. I'm making a concerted effort to communicate the "what I felt" at the time and not the "why I felt it". The "whys" get accusatory very quickly and I won't go there. I will never slander the mother of my children. She has been through enough hell on my account. I have no desire whatsoever to diminish anyone's opinion of her. Furthermore, I am in no way condoning any of what I have done, and I'm not glorifying anything, I'm just telling the story, saying what happened. You can do whatever you want with it. If you think I'm a motherfucker at the other end of it, so be it.

When I was with COIC I was traveling a lot for work, especially down to Tampa where U.S. Special Operations Command is based. I remember one night going back to my hotel room in Ybor City, looking out the window and seeing the purple and pink lights of a strip club across the street. I was very sad and alone. I just wanted someone to be nice to me and to want to talk to me. I just wanted to feel wanted. I didn't give a shit if it was fake. I walked across the street and went inside.

Finally Somehow Home

The club was dimly lit and empty except for a single patron sitting flanked by strippers and gawking at the dancer on stage. I hadn't been in a strip club for a long time so I felt awkward and out of place. I ordered a gin and tonic and looked around. I didn't see any dancers that I liked, so I planned on just finishing my drink in the corner alone then going back to my hotel. But suddenly and somehow in slow motion, out of the dark recesses of the club a beautiful girl materialized in front of me. She had black wavy hair and was part Latina and part black. She didn't say anything at all. She just grabbed me by the hand and walked me into the back. She sat me down in a small room and pushed me back into the couch. "From the second you walked in here I knew you were mine", she said. She took her clothes off in front of me. There's nothing on earth quite so sexy as a beautiful woman taking her clothes off. Her mocha skin gleamed dark between the shadows like moonlit bronze. It was soft and smooth as oil on water to my fingertips. I hadn't been touched by another woman in six years. Hell, I hadn't been touched by anyone at all for over a year. It was sublime. It was exhilarating. It was very wrong. But I embraced it. I embraced her. I felt the warmth of another human for the first time in a long time. I sunk

Finally Somehow Home

into it like an opium high. All the comingled sensations swirled around me. The scintillating touch of naked skin as she twerked and grinded her perfect ass into my lap, the pervasive feeling of extreme guilt like an unbearable weight getting heavier, the elation of being wanted, of being an object of desire instead of one of derision. The musty smell of the shadowy room and the slight taste of sweat on her breasts as she let me break the rules. Her breasts were small and perfect for her. I filled my whole mouth with one, sucking it in while I teased her nipple with my tongue. I remember it all distinctly. "Face down, ass up, that's the way we like to fuck..." was playing over the sound system as she, on her hands and knees now, on the floor, face down, ass up, ground her ass into my crotch while I lightly brushed her naked back with my fingertips. She got up and sat in my lap facing me. She could easily feel all of me through my thin dress pants. She put her hands behind my neck and began to grind her vagina along the length of my shaft. Slowly at first, but quickly working into a frenzy. My hands were around her small waist pushing her down harder and moving her pelvis back and forth in rhythm with her savage gyrations. She didn't stop until I came. She made

Finally Somehow Home

sure of that. She ground out every last drop into my pants.

The song ended. I paid her $20 for the dance and I left. It was strange, I don't know if it was just the lighting in the club or something else, I could easily ascertain that she had a beautiful face, the image of her is still clear as day in my mind's eye. But I still couldn't say exactly what she looked like. Her face seemed somehow strangely obscured. It doesn't surprise me at all to know that demons are angels. She was some kind of angel. That's for sure. On the way back to the hotel I tried to regret it but gave up. Fuck it. I thought. I really needed that. I promised myself I'd never do it again. I promised myself I'd never do it again quite frequently after that. Pretty much every time I traveled, but especially when I went to Tampa. Mons Venus, a club I frequented on my many trips, is still one of my favorite places on earth. Leave it to USSOCOM to build their headquarters in one of the most stripper-heavy demographic areas in the eastern United States.

I still had never cheated on my wife. I know some would call that cheating anyway, and maybe it is, but the point is that I had never slept with anyone else in spite of my -

Finally Somehow Home

what would become a 2-year dry spell. Over the course of our marriage she had made it clear on many occasions that if I ever cheated on her she would leave me. It was very tempting to take her up on the deal. Not only because of the physical aspect of it, of course. But because it would be the perfect out. But that wasn't me. I wasn't that guy. I'd only ever almost cheated once. It was on an all-night layover in Atlanta on my way to Afghanistan. Alot of blow was involved. But I hadn't done it. Chalk it up to a close call. It had terrified me the next day and long after. I didn't want to ever compromise my character like that. Even if I was the only one on earth who knew it. But I was already playing with the fire. And I knew it. And I kept doing it. Maybe I just hadn't felt good in so long that I really didn't give a fuck.

You know, I've never heard a marriage counselor say this. And it's not true in every situation at all, but for me, in hindsight, it would have saved us all so much agony had I just left sooner. My "never quit" attitude from Recon days refused to even consider divorce for the first five years of our marriage. Around year six I finally started contemplating it after a conversation I had with my brother whilst driving all of my shit across country

Finally Somehow Home

from Colorado to Virginia. "I've never seen anyone serve their wife the way you do." He said. It left me dumbfounded. I was living under the impression that I was a complete failure as a husband. Maybe it wasn't just me. Maybe there was hope. Maybe there was a future aside from the prison I was stuck in for the rest of my life.

About a year after the conversation with my brother I finally got up the nerve to tell her that we should get a divorce. I was miserable and she was, according to all of my sensory faculties, not satisfied whatsoever with me on the job I was doing to keep her happy. To my great surprise, she broke down in tears as if something beautiful were dying. I was flabbergasted. I honestly thought she was going to jump for joy. Well, regardless, it looked like mutual agreement was out of the question.

Chapter 15

Once I started working for CTTSO I began to travel even more, and I was making about twice as much money. With all the extra hours I worked I was pulling down +$300K/yr, so not too bad. But unbeknownst to me, the extra money and more travel were the exact ingredients required to conjure a raging level 10 perfect shit-storm. And it was brewing.

The idea of taking the easy out and just cheating on my wife looked more and more appealing as things continued to deteriorate at home. I don't know what it was. Some fucked up and twisted form of chivalry maybe. But I couldn't be the one to walk away from her. I had to give her a reason to walk away from me. Sounds more like chicken shit, but in my mind, I didn't want to shame her. If there was any shame to be carried, I wanted it to be on me. Thus, the idea to cheat, be the bad guy, take the blame, go our separate ways, and be done with it.

The strip clubs in Virginia Beach suck. Or at least they did near where I was staying that night. I had flown in from Monterey California where I'd been meeting with the Naval Postgraduate School and was on my way to Trident Specter on Fort Story near VA Beach. By the time I got to my hotel it was pretty late. I was restless though, and figured I would go find out what kind of trouble I could get myself into. The only strip club I could find was some really seedy joint with busted ass strippers in it. I hung around for a while but lost interest and decided to go back to the hotel. In the past I had, on a couple of occasions, called escorts when I was bored in my room, but I'd mostly either chickened out and not answered the door when they showed up, or I'd just hang out and bullshit with them. I never actually did anything serious. I planned much the same on this occasion as well. Even in the midst of all the stupid shit that I was doing, I still had a great aversion to actually closing the deal with anyone outside of my marriage.

Finally Somehow Home

A very pretty girl just a little on the thick side showed up at my door. We chatted for a few minutes. I offered her some wine. She drank some and I asked her if she could take her top off. She smiled and did so and then removed her bra. Her breasts were enormous and beautiful. Not floppy and saggy but large and full and perky. I couldn't help myself and dove right in. She really began to enjoy it. I could tell by how she was moving and the noises she was making. A few minutes later we were on the bed kissing and playing around. Our clothes were on the floor. I began to massage her clitoris and slid my finger inside her slowly and gently. We continued to kiss and play as her moans and sighs grew in volume and intensity. Her getting so turned on was really turning me on as well. She was very wet. With the tip of my penis I began to massage her clitoris. She was writhing. She squirmed and wiggled and made cute little noises. It was not at all lost on me how close to the line I was. I could feel all of her vagina as I swiped my penis through the soft, wet, warm lips. I was going crazy as well. We were a tangled mess of panting sweat. I could feel the head of my fully erect and throbbing penis pressing against her vaginal opening. All I had to do was shift my weight and I would be inside of her. A million thoughts went through

Finally Somehow Home

my mind in a split second. I paused. Then I drove myself into her. To the hilt. She wasn't expecting it. A gasp of shock and ecstasy erupted through the look of surprise and pain and pleasure frozen for a moment on her flushed face. Her mouth was open and her eyes were wide. Oh... my... God... she whimpered and squeaked between jolting thrusts. I wrapped both arms around her then reached up and grabbed the top of her shoulder blades from behind. My grip loosened as I pulled back, my penis almost entirely outside of her then suddenly I squeezed her tightly and pulled her body down viciously as I drove myself into her. Over and over. All the way out, then slamming back in. Her glorious breasts jumped and quivered like gelatin with every shock and buck of our bodies smashing together. She was so wet it was sloppy and the air I'd driven into her queefed out to make room as I plunged into her again and again and again. She came in a flutter of thrashing and shivers and pants and finger nails down my back. I wrapped my arms all the way around her and squeezed her whole body as I shuddered and quaked gasped and came on the sheets between her legs.

"Wow." She said. "I thought we weren't going to do that."

Finally Somehow Home

"I didn't think we were." I said.

We talked for awhile. Then we fucked again. Then she went home.

It was horrible. Something big had irrevocably changed in me. I was a different person the next day than I was the day before. I tried to tell myself that it had never happened. I would just ignore that the event ever took place. But it didn't work. So, I told myself it was no big deal, it was just a physical act that didn't mean anything. None of it worked. I had just ruined my life. I thought about "the deal" and my new "out" from everything. But the issues in our relationship, for the first time, took a back row seat to the trauma I had just inflicted upon myself. I was stuck in a strange and awful place. I knew deep down that I had only one choice if I ever wanted this new torment to abate: I had to tell her. It seemed strange knowing that this was the reason for me considering it in the first place, but now that I was faced with having to admit to her that I had actually lived up to her low expectation of me, I just couldn't do it. I hoped that with time the sinking feeling in the pit of my stomach would go away or at least subside. I remember sitting in a meeting that day with the Palantir crew and

Finally Somehow Home

just feeling all grey and shitty and dull. Like I had lost something I could never get back. Because I had.

When I got back home, I thought she'd notice the change in me for sure and get suspicious. But between me playing it off the best I could and her not really paying that much attention to me anyway, I was able to get away with it. I prayed like a motherfucker for God to help me and swore over and over to myself that I would never, ever do it again. The first thing I did on my next trip, after getting to my hotel room, was call a hooker.

Hookers and blow. Actually, for me it was hookers, strippers, Adderall, Cialis and Testosterone. And plenty of all of it. I did the best I could to drown out the darkness. I actually needed the Adderall. And badly. Since I was a kid I had undiagnosed ADHD. I only found out and finally got diagnosed afew months after I stopped deploying overseas. Whatever my ADHD had been up to before, it was now off the charts. I was later diagnosed by the VA with Hyper-vigilance. In pretty much any overseas shit hole conflict zone you are always either in the actual shit, or on the edge and ready. Your mind has to be going a million miles a minute all the time to read the environment accurately, process the

Finally Somehow Home

information, and make rapid decisions, all within nanoseconds. But when you get back home and all that stimulus is gone, your mind doesn't know that it's supposed to slow down again, so it just keeps on spinning. That's Hyper-vigilance. It was so bad that I went to a shrink who gave me Adderall to take. And thus begun a beautiful love story. I fucking loved the shit and started taking it by the handful. It mellowed me out. I slept better when I was taking it. And for the first time in recent memory, I could focus. Intensely.

Life is strange. Happiness is elusive. Fun is easy if you have the money. I have always found it interesting that the Spanish word for fun is "divertido". Diversion. That's exactly what it is. Fun is a diversion, a distraction, something to keep you from remembering the present. From acknowledging the sick mess. The ticking timebomb. The countdown to hell. I was Nero. Fiddling while my life burned down around me. I want to make it very clear that I am in no way celebrating or condoning this shit. I'm just telling you what the poison tastes like. Was it fun? Fuck yea it was fun. I won't pretend it wasn't. I will be truthful about it all. One can still smile while bleeding out. Emulate me if you want to. Burn it all down

Finally Somehow Home

grinning like a fool. Yes, it is delicious, but it's still poison. You are only defying yourself.

A lot of the traveling I did was overseas. Bogota, Colombia to observe a training course for the Colombian *Comando de Operaciones Especiales* – National Police Special Operations Command, and bullshit with the Military Attaché at the US Embassy. It was very interesting to me how well-oiled the Embassy was there compared to other Embassies I've worked at/with. And I'll just say it was a fun trip. Holy Cocaina Pura!

I was in Hawaii quite abit talking to Special Operations Command, Pacific (SOCPAC) and Pacific Command (PACOM). They were working the Abu Sayyaf problem in the Philippines, and I was trying to help them bolster their intelligence analysis capabilities among other things. Then, I'd be in Frankfurt or Stuttgart Germany talking to Special Operations Command Europe (SOCEUR) and Special Operations Command Africa (SOCAF) who were working the Boko Haram problem in North Africa. Or I'd be in London and out to the Defense Science and Technology Laboratory (DSTL) near Stonehenge to chat about emerging technologies and our ongoing Bilateral agreement with the UK. Or in Israel,

Finally Somehow Home

meeting with the Israeli Defense Intelligence (IDI), learning from what they were doing and showing them what was working for us in Iraq and Afghanistan. Poland for a Science and Technology Conference in Krakow. And on and on. Not to mention all the traveling throughout the US.

And every place I went, I raged. Science and Technology Subject Matter Expert by day, and World Champion Party Maniac by night. It did interfere with work sometimes, but usually I kept it under wraps. I missed a meeting with Major General Repass, Commander SOCEUR, one morning. At the time of the meeting, I was unconscious in the hospital from fatigue and possibly alcohol poisoning. It had been a wild night starting with a beautiful German brunette and ending with an E&E (Escape & Evade) from the German Coppers. "How do you say, "Fuck Me" in German?" I had asked the brunette. She didn't understand much English, but she knew what I was asking her. She was abit shy, but very pretty and almost sweet. "Ficken Mich", she said. "Yell it out the window I told her." I moved us over to the window in step and waddling alittle so I wouldn't have to pull myself out of her as we moved. I reached in front of her and opened the window. There was a chill as the

-205-

Finally Somehow Home

wind came rushing in, but she didn't care. "Ficken Mich!" she yelled over and over again from the 5th story window, her voice pitching with every thrust. "Ficken Mich!" She was smiling now. Giggling alittle. It's so beautiful to see a woman smiling back at you through her tousled hair as her body sways then lurches almost violently at the apex of every full penetration. Hair waving in the rhythm, head bobbing slightly as if drunk, eyes half closed, biting her lip just alittle. Pushing back hard with each jolting plunge into her. Mouth open now, eyes back, the chin comes up as I pull her hair back. "Ficken Mich!"

I had been in Hawaii only two days prior to this, so my jet lag and internal clock were all kinds of fuct. I had been taking a little extra Adderall to stay ahead of the lack of sleep. The problem with Adderall is that you can drink too much and not realize it because it keeps you awake and somewhat alert...until you crash. I found myself in the backroom of a German strip club with a large Roman style couch and pillows everywhere with curtains hanging down around it. A tall blonde German girl who looked like a toned St. Pauli's Girl had approached me as soon as I came into the place and promptly started making snarky remarks. I loved it and fucked with her

Finally Somehow Home

right back. We hit it off. We ended up just hanging out in the backroom for a few hours talking. That's when I kind of lost track of everything. I vaguely remember throwing my wallet at her and saying, "Fuck it, you can have everything in there." She smiled big as she pulled out twelve $100 bills. The next thing I remember, I was in some kind of outside marketplace. The sun's morning rays cut bright through the scattered early crowd and the sweets and confections and knickknacks and breads of all kinds hanging in front of all the different little shops scattered throughout an open plaza. The morning air was crisp but not too cold. It smelled sweet. Like caramel and fresh baked bread. I noticed the cop about 20 yards away looking at me through the crowd. I wouldn't have given him a second thought except for at that very moment the faculties required for the functions of standing and walking were somehow eluding me. I began to move away smoothly in a nonchalant halting stagger. The cop didn't buy it. He started edging toward me through the crowd. I bolted. Seeing as running is nothing more than falling down over and over again, it was much easier than trying to walk or stand. I took off down an alley running behind some office buildings. I knew the cop was right on my tail. The

Finally Somehow Home

nice thing about being that fucked up is that you really can run fast and not feel the pain. The breathing is the only problem. I knew I had to do something quick or he would have me contained in that alley. I had just a few seconds, I knew, before he rounded the corner and saw me. So, I ducked into the closest office building. It was a corporate building with an industrial interior design motif and enormous windows all around. As I came through the door, an open staircase appeared in front of me going up probably eight stories or so. I began to run up it at a dead sprint. Around the fifth story or so I collapsed on the landing, unconscious. I vaguely remember the excited voices of business people as they discovered and gathered around me, then the jostling feeling of being loaded onto a gurney. When I woke up it was just after dusk. A pretty German doctor and her staff gathered around me. I thought maybe I had been drugged the night before by the stripper and asked the doctor what was wrong with me. She smiled at me the way people smile down at dumbasses and said, "You were exhausted and maybe too much drinking." All of the travel and lack of sleep had finally caught up to me. I managed to make it back to the hotel just in time to get my ass chewed the fuck out. You don't miss meetings with

Finally Somehow Home

General Officers. Thankfully my superiors were merciful, and the ass chewing was the extent of it.

The first night anywhere new, I always wanted to explore and usually did as much as I could on the way to the Strip Club. This is an old Marine Corps Liberty strategy. Invariably before the ship full of Marines would pull into port, the Public Affairs Office released a list of cultural and historic attractions in the area. This was a ruse. An attempt to dissuade Marines from the richest cultural experience afforded the international traveler: the view of the bottom of a beer mug. I've seen the bottom of beer mugs all over the world. Did I go see the Great Wall of China when I was there? Fuck no! I went to the bar. Did I tour Fort Siloso in Singapore, or the WWII battlefields on Okinawa? I would have if I'd had the time, but I was occupied with a much more fulfilling and rewarding ambition: the pursuit of shame and regret.

That's the goal. If you have none, you aren't living hard enough. I'm clowning of course, I don't believe that pursuing your lusts will bring you peace and happiness, but this last part is true. I'm always hearing people say stupid shit like "no regrets". If you live your life with the

Finally Somehow Home

intent of never regretting anything that you do, you really aren't living hard enough. You're being a pussy. And furthermore, if you don't regret anything you've ever done, you probably haven't done a god damn thing. Failure is the only way to find out what you're best at. It sharpens you. It sharpens you because it traps you between the beyond what you thought you could do, and that which you can't yet accomplish. It keeps you right on the knife edge. For most, failure is closer to where they really want to be than where they really are. When you fail, you're reaching just beyond what you can accomplish. You're right next to it. It just takes some tuning to get you there. If you never try hard enough to fail, you'll never understand enough about yourself to learn how to win. And yes, I do find it ironic that I'm putting snippets of wisdom in the middle of a diatribe on my depravity. When you fuck up as much as I have, you learn a lot of shit.

Hookers and I have a long history. Hell, I lost my virginity to one in Hawaii when I was 19. Semper Fi! I had other experiences with hookers when I was overseas as well. Sometimes you take what you can get. Hookers are great because you both have an understanding, and you can literally just take your pick and have a good time and

Finally Somehow Home

be done with it. For some reason that aspect of it was very alluring to me. But this was new and different. This was an obsession. I had no control over it. I was a full-fledged sex addict. You'd think it would be kinda fun. Just letting your dick run amok. But it was a dungeon. It was all shit-mad-hell. One lie upon another. It wasn't only when I traveled. I would ditch work sometimes, go bang a hooker, and be back at my desk shortly thereafter dripping sweat and guilt all over my keyboard.

After afew months, I got to where I'd fuck a hooker a couple times a week. Some were ragged and drug ridden, some beautiful but seemingly dead inside. With very few exceptions a dull look in their tormented eyes. I don't think many of them that I was with were victims of human trafficking, but learning more about it afterwards, I hate to say it, but some probably were. The best ones were pros. Traveling hoes. They'd fly to a city, camp out in a hotel room, make afew grand, then fuck off back to their homes and normal lives. One of my faves, who became a friend, owned a cosmetics company in New York City. She was some kind of Eastern European and had the cutest little voice. Like Bruce Willis' girlfriend in Pulp Fiction – Maria di

Finally Somehow Home

Medieros. She'd come down every month or so for a few days. We actually really enjoyed each other and had a cool energy in bed. Hell, I still owe her a couple hundred bucks from when she spotted me for a fuck-around sesh. The little Jewish girl in Boston who loved to drop acid with MIT students and just couldn't keep my dick out of her mouth. Totally normal 21-year-old girl who just had a secret wild side.

There were other memorable ones, but most were not the Pretty Woman types at all. If you want those, you gotta pay the big bucks – at least a couple grand or so. And even they didn't usually come with the charming personality. The middle-of-the-road hookers were from about $450-$650 for an hour. But most of them were the stuck in their own hell, fueled by drugs, devoid of any spark types. Those were $200-$300 a pop. It was sad as fuck. Even then. It was a dark, dark world from whence few escape, and I was living in it. Whether a hooker or a John, we were all stuck there. We all shared the same shame but we all spared each other the same judgment. That made it somewhat bearable. Even pleasant. Until afterwards sometimes... sitting in the car with my head on the steering wheel. Raked with disgust. Hating every bit of myself. Not just for violating a promise to my wife.

Finally Somehow Home

I was way deeper than that. I hated myself because I was confronted with what a horrible piece of shit I was. And I was disgusted with myself because part of me didn't really give a damn. It was revolting to me that I didn't hate myself more.

I was faced with my seemingly infinite depravity and I couldn't deny it, and I couldn't stop it, and I couldn't run away from it. It was a hell that followed me. I remember excusing myself from the pew, sitting in the bathroom stall at church and scrolling the internet for hookers. It was an obsession that took precedence and authority over everything else. Shipwrecked. Bankrupt. Lost.

Part of it was I don't think I really understood judgment. In a way I was taunting God. I have a bad habit of this in general. First of all, as David had shown me: I was weighing the pain of the judgment against the joy of the crime, and secondly, I like to see how far I can go before the hammer comes down. Well, the thing about that is that if God says you shouldn't do some shit, you're not going to hurt Him at all if you do it anyway. You don't bring a tear to God's eye every time you fuck up. You bring a tear to God's eye every time you get hurt. It just so happens that when you "sin" you hurt yourself. People

Finally Somehow Home

think God hates sinners. No, God hates sin. He hates it as if it were cancer and it were killing his child. He's not mad at you because you're sick. He hates the sickness. He really fucking likes you, so He gets pissed and hates on the shit that fucking kills you. And it was killing me. Make no mistake I was dying. But no matter how much God was hating on the sickness, it still had me. I was under water.

Chapter 16

In hindsight I now realize that post-traumatic stress from all my deployments was taking a huge toll on me as well. Pretty much everyone I know that deployed a lot, after the first year or so permanently back home, their shit started to fall apart in one way or another. And it falls apart big. Everything besides the misery, was bland, and drab, and flat, and dull, and grey, and completely tasteless. I would give anything to taste something again. Anything. Good or bad. And the dirtier and filthier and more wicked, the more I was drawn to it because maybe then I'd feel something. And the deeper I dove into the darkness, the more my tolerance grew and the more numb I became. Until I was completely immersed and still felt nothing at all.

Finally Somehow Home

My life was completely fucked. Nothing about it was functioning except for my professional life, and even in that I was risking it all. You aren't supposed to do the shit that I was doing when you have a Top Secret Clearance. Big no-no. But I didn't know how to get out of it. Needless to say, my finances were in ruin. I suck ass at managing my finances on a good day. But to compound it, I had also spent so much on my little addiction that in spite of the money I was making I was living paycheck to paycheck while trying to get out of the debt that had piled up. Things at home were worse than ever. My wife was rightfully exasperated with our financial situation. More than once humiliated at the grocery store when none of her credit cards worked. I had truly become a piece of shit.

Everything was well and truly fucked and every waking moment I obsessed over how to find my way out of the snarled tanglefuck. I could think of nothing else except when I was working. Work was my only refuge. I knew something had to change. I remember holding my daughter and crying as I rocked her to sleep knowing that I was going to leave them all soon and thinking what a despicable motherfucker am I. But shit was so very fucking wrong. The only thing more oppressive than the

Finally Somehow Home

blatant indifference of the person who professed to love me most was the hell of the addiction it had driven me toward and into which I had, of my own volition, plunged. All of me except for my living flesh was in hell.

There were moments of light sometimes that came though the darkness, like a beacon slicing through the frothing and violence of the abysmal fuckstorm of my soul. I was driving to work one morning. Two hours late because my "offsite meeting" that morning was actually a burnt out hooker in Fairfax with a blank and perfect face. I'd asked her to put her arms around me. "I'm not here for that" was her deadpan response.

I was crying as I drove. Raging at myself. Clenching the wheel of my Mercedes with all the fury and hate and guilt and shame and hopelessness that boiled inside like a pressure chamber with a broken release valve. The radio was on. I wasn't paying any attention to it, but suddenly the words cut through everything straight into my scorched-ass, fucked-up heart.

"Darkness" is a harsh term don't you think?
And yet it dominates the things I see
It seems all my bridges have been burnt
But you say that's exactly how this grace thing works.

Finally Somehow Home

*It's not the long walk home that will change this heart
But the welcome I receive with a restart.*

It was Mumford and Sons' *Roll Away Your Stone*. I was so sick of my own shit. Always "restarting" and promising I'd never do that again, and always, without fail, failing again. The story of my fucking life. I was always starting again from a place of defeat. I never accepted the gift of grace extended to me, the gift of a clean slate. Of truly starting over as justified – just-as-if-I'd never fucked up. That's what justified means. Starting from a place of power instead of a place of desperation. But here's the thing. All those words sound great. But there is nothing behind them if there's no one behind them. Otherwise, it's all in your mind. In my case, all in the same mind that was sabotaging my whole life. I had to be Justified by someone other than myself. To someone with the authority to make it real. To the same person who had just reached down to me through a random song on the radio exactly when I needed it most. To the one who never leaves a fallen man behind. Who will hunt you down and find you in the darkest recesses of your depravity, when even you have given up on yourself. To the one with all the power and dominion, and yet, the

Finally Somehow Home

most gentle spirit of lovingkindness who has ever walked the earth. Yup, that motherfucker: Jesus. If you don't believe he's real, I have a challenge for you. If you have the balls, try it. If you really and sincerely want to know what the fuck the deal is with Jesus, quit fucking asking everyone else, and just ask him. You don't have to get down on your knees or fold your hands or any of that shit. You can speak out loud or say it in your mind, it doesn't matter. Don't you think it's about time you had the sack to see if there's really anything to all this Jesus shit anyway? Just fucking get on with it already and see what all the fuss is about. Just, no shit, sincerely ask Jesus to reveal himself to you. That's all you need to do. And if he doesn't do it, then don't fucking believe in him.

Now stop reading for a minute and think on it. Maybe take a little break. Some of you got some shit you need to take care of.

When he does it you'll know and you'll know it's him... and when he does... you got some decisions to make, by friend. Because you've just found the Truth. And you will have to do something with it.

I had been wild'n out for about 4 months at that time. I quit traveling so much for work. Adjusted my

Finally Somehow Home

environment to help trick-fuck myself into a behavioral change. It's a good strategy to take if you're stuck. Be like a sniper, small adjustments make big changes. But mostly it was a new understanding of grace. That I could start off on a clean slate as far as my addiction was concerned. The only problem was, that I didn't go through with the whole prescription of resolution and treatment for my malady. I still didn't confess it to my wife. I knew I had to if I really wanted to close the door on it, but I also knew that doing so would hand her a huge bag of hand grenades to throw at me on top of everything else, and I just couldn't go through with it.

I made it a good four or five months. I had to start traveling heavily again for work, and the boredom and thirst for flavor of any kind in my life kicked the whole shitshow off once more. And back into the darkness I went.

I was in Denver meeting with Palantir, Naval Postgraduate School, and afew other cats and dogs that would eventually comprise the CADENA Platform that I mentioned previously: The InterAgency Analytics System I'd dreamt up for JTF-North for the SouthWest border problem. I had spent a wild night at the strip club

Finally Somehow Home

which entailed finger banging one of the ladies in the private room until she writhed and squirmed and squeaked and came all over my fingers many times over. I made it back to the hotel about sunrise, my suit all fucked-up and wrinkle-bombed from her frantic clawing and gyrations. I got to my room and flopped onto the bed all askew with my head hanging off the side of it, staring down at the mustard yellow carpet with brown French looking patterns in it. I felt nothing. I felt it so intensely that I could no longer bear it. My soul was completely sensory deprived. I felt imprisoned by it. Trapped in it. And I knew there wasn't a god damn thing I could do about it. And I knew it wasn't temporary.

I got down on the floor next to the bed. On my knees at first, bent forward at the waist like the muslims do when they pray, with my hands clasped in front of me. I didn't feel anything at all but I knew I was crying. "What the FUCK!? God Damn it." I cried. "I know that you can hear me. If there's anyone on this earth that you can hear right now, it's me, because I'm one of the most wretched motherfuckers on this earth right now. And I know you're real... I don't know what to do. Please God, do whatever it takes." "Do whatever it takes." I prayed. I got on my face on the ground, arms outstretched, prostrate,

Finally Somehow Home

the musty carpet grinding my dripping nose and face, mouth wide open. Sobbing. "I don't know what to do. God Damn it. Lord Jesus, PLEASE help me! Do whatever it takes. Do whatever it takes." I cried over and over again into the shitty carpet. I was scared. I know God is real and He doesn't fuck around. I knew when you ask him to do "whatever it takes" that nothing is off the table. I could end up all kinds of fucked up before the "whatever it takes" is over. But I was done. I had nothing else to say to him. I knew he was the only one that could save me, and I knew that he'd only do it if I gave him carte blanche to do so. He doesn't split the credit for shit. And he doesn't half-ass shit. He'll help you, he'll heal you, he'll save you, he'll free you, he'll make you whole again, but he won't do jack shit for you unless you let him do it his way, and do all of it, completely. We think we're going in for a floss and a breath mint, but by the end of it you've got a mouth full of fucking root canals. He don't fuck about. I knew it was coming. I didn't know how or what, or when, but I knew it was coming.

"Who do you love more, Mommy, or Daddy?" The question was addressed to my son, David. Dani was asleep in her car seat. We were in Costa Rica on vacation driving from San Jose to Tamarindo, my favorite place

Finally Somehow Home

in Costa. David looked somewhat confused and alittle panicked. "Mommy or Daddy?", she repeated. "Mommy", she mouthed to him a couple of times, turning in her seat. "Mommy", he said.

"See? You're a failure as a father and a husband and I have no respect for you." I didn't say anything. She then explained that our little family didn't include me. It consisted of her and the kids, and that from here on out, if I wanted to be a part of any of it, I was to shut up and color. I really had nothing to say. Any foundation to stand upon to be a proper father and husband had just been ripped out from under me. That's when I knew. I knew that even if I stayed for my kids, patched everything else up, and kept going, I would never really be allowed access to them. Never be granted the respect or authority to teach them all that I could about life. I felt like I'd just been punched in the solar plexus. I knew that at the end of the day, I was expected to be present, follow orders, and bring home bacon, and that was it.

I slept fitfully that night in the condo we'd rented. The next day I played with the kids in the swimming pool. Dani hadn't really started talking yet. She'd bobbed up and down squeaking and flapping her arms at her sides

Finally Somehow Home

like a chubby little penguin in excitement when I had met up with them in San Jose two days before. I'd picked her up and twirled her in my arms as she gushed with joy to see Daddy. They'd been in Costa Rica for a couple of weeks with family before I was able to meet them. David was sharp as a tack and wise beyond his four years. A fun-loving little stoic who seemed to think deeply about everything. He'd gotten a black eye from a hard hit playing flag football that summer. I told him that if anyone asked him who had given it to him, he was to say: "No one gave it to me, I earned it." That had made him beam with pride for his first shiner.

We went out to dinner downtown. It was a thatched roof bar and restaurant with outside seating on an elevated veranda. The palm fronds of the roof rustled softly in the cool afternoon breeze off the Pacific. It was overcast. Looked like rain. We'd finished our meal. David was acting out over something or other and I addressed it. "He can do that if he wants to! Go ahead, David." She said to him. I pulled the car and condo keys out of my pocket and put them on the table with enough cash for the meal, stood up, and left.

Finally Somehow Home

I felt like I was drowning. The gauntlet had been set. The ultimatum laid down. I was to be either an emasculated indentured servant for the rest of my life, or leave my kids and destroy my family. Those were the only options. That was it and that was all. I snapped. Not in anger. Not in violence. I just departed from my life. The rickety scaffolding propping everything up collapsed under the pressure. Everything melted away into static. Nothing mattered. I no longer felt pain, sorrow, grief, responsibility, or compulsion for anything. Like a rudderless ship with no sails. I was adrift. Everything was completely disconnected. I was suddenly living one second at a time again. Just like Iraq. But with no goal, mission, or desire to be alive. Just one second at a time. Everything else was gone. My entire universe existed only in the space and time that my body occupied as its heart pumped blood through its veins and the air filled and departed its lungs.

I thought I'd have a cigar. I found a tabaqueria and bought a dozen Costa Rican sticks in a yellow wooden box, and a dozen fat Cubans in a woodgrain box, each the size of a notebook. It started to rain. I lit a Costa Rican stick with a thick match I'd gotten from the tabaquieria and felt the heavy delicious smoke roil in my mouth, so

Finally Somehow Home

thick it tasted humid. I found a bar. It was open on all sides and covered with a roof and bare rafters held up by beams around the outside. I ordered tequila. A sweet darkness began to settle on the streets as the lights along it and in the shops and bars grew gradually more brilliant. Everything was a soft blur. My cigar went out, the humidity in the air and the misting of the gathering rain wafting in under the roof choked it out only half smoked. "God Damn it." I chose a Cuban from the hardwood box and lit it with some difficulty in the gusting wet breeze. It didn't have the same earthy heavy feel as the Costa Rican, but its leaves were dryer and it stayed lit at least. I drank more tequila, paid the bartender and drifted out into the cool thick rain, cigar boxes under my arm. Fat drops slapped down lightly onto my head and shoulders and ran in small rivulets down my face. It tasted sweet as it dripped across my lips and its mesmerizing rhythm and drum carried me back to Indonesia. When life seemed delicious. The bars were beginning to fill, almost indiscernibly but steadily, with tourists and Ticos escaping the downpour and embarking with anticipation of whatever adventure the night would soon bring. I didn't even think about it. There was no future. No past. Only now. And just barely.

Finally Somehow Home

I saw a taxi and got in.

"Buenas Tardes, Señor"

"Buenas Tardes. Teine Cocaina?"

"Si, Senior. Cuanto quieres?"

I gave him a US $100 bill.

He produced a baggie of Coke. Probably an eight-ball worth. I didn't care.

"Gracias."

"Pura Vida." He said as I stepped out into the rain.

"Pura fucking Vida", I mumbled to myself as I walked to the closest bar. I grabbed a straw from the bar on the way to the bathroom. I lit a match and burnt the straw in two, three inches from one end and, licking my fingers, tapped the hot plastic, tamping the burnt end flush. It was about as pure coke as you can get. I felt the dry spot building in the back of my throat as my lips began to go numb from the two fat-ass lines I had ripped and hurried to the bar to wash it down. I did whatever came to my mind without hesitation. As if on autopilot. I handed out

Finally Somehow Home

cigars at the bar. Tried to fuck a hooker but couldn't get it up because of the blow, so just rolled around the bed with her. Upon leaving I sent a taxi driver on a mission to find me some Viagra or Cialis. He returned with a couple boxes of 20mg Cialis tablets an hour or so later. I paid him, took two and went back to whatever I was doing at the time. It wasn't fun. It wasn't not fun. It just was.

The sun was starting to come up. I reached into my pocket and realized that the last hooker had stolen my wedding ring. It didn't bother me at all. I guess now's the time to tell her, I thought to myself as I walked up the steps into the condo. I didn't care to hide anything anymore. I just wanted to be done with it all, come what may. She was awake and waiting for me to get back. I put my cigar boxes on the kitchen counter, then I walked into the bedroom and sat down on the bed. I told her everything. Everything I'd been doing on and off for the past year. Everything. I held nothing back. I answered all of her questions. At first she seemed more shocked than anything. I wasn't trying to fix our marriage, that wasn't even part of the equation right then. I really, and truly, and deeply just wanted to make it right with her. As right as it could be. To finally confess all the ways I'd wronged her. I felt terrible for the pain I could see on her pretty

Finally Somehow Home

face as she began to come to grips with the reality of it. In spite of all the problems we had, and regardless of my own pain, she didn't deserve this. I did love her. I loved her a great deal, in fact. So much so that I'd chosen to spend my life with her. I had promised to protect her, and instead had caused her her life's greatest pain. I felt like a fucking urchin and I deserved every god damn bit of it, and more. I know why I did it, but it still didn't make any logical sense. To hurt her so badly, and simultaneously completely expose my fucked-up rotten soul. What she didn't know wouldn't hurt her. But she deserved to know, even though it was excruciating for her. She would have wanted to know, and she deserved to. And even though I could have walked away from our marriage, and she would have been none the wiser, I knew as well that for me to resolve it for myself I had to tell her, so I did. The rest of my life was burning down around me, but for the first time in a year I could breathe again. It was like deep cleaning the cockpit as the plane is about to smash into the fucking mountain, but somehow, I was whole again. My conscience was clear. I was finally clean.

The next day I flew back to Virginia. I'd been dealing with what a fuck-up I was for many months, but she had

Finally Somehow Home

only just found out, and it was horrible for her. What a nuclear clusterfuck I had created for the people closest to me. She didn't rage or lash out at me. She was almost calm about it. Gracious, in fact. I'm very grateful to her for that. I wish I'd not caused her so much pain. I wish I'd dealt with it sooner, before it became an unchecked monster and made me into one. There is no way, and I won't try to make me look or sound any better than I was. I was a god damn fool and a fucking bastard to her. And that's it, and that's all.

Chapter 17

But we were still fucked. I had wronged her gravely. But the resolution of these wrongs did nothing to amend the real problem, and the reason I got tangled up in all that bullshit in the first place. We were still hanging off each other like dead appendages with sharp knives and raw nerves. Is it better to model a severely toxic relationship to your kids, or to remove the toxicity? I knew that the role I was being expected to model to my kids, who would watch it for the rest of their childhood and learn from it, and from it emulate what a man, a father, and a husband should be, would be a watered down, neutered, and emasculated one, if I were to abide there. That was, in fact, the very criteria by which I was to be allowed to participate in my family.

Finally Somehow Home

I sought the counsel of a close friend. The deep lines and wrinkles of Wayne's thoughtful face seemed chiseled into his visage in testimony to his own life's deep anguish past, and through the rich kindness within his eyes and soft, deliberate manner flowed a peaceful assurance that he cared deeply. So much that I could almost discern in his face the wince of an old wound opened as, in spite of it, he allowed my hurt to brush over the painful scars he carried. We sat across from each other at a small table at Wegman's where he liked to work. I had known Wayne for several years. We had coffee together over breakfast once a week as much as our schedules would allow, so he knew the wavetops of my life better than most. I told him of everything else. The deep parts I'd never shared before with anyone. I told him what I'd confessed to my wife a few days before and about the road that had led me to where I was right then. At that very moment. "I feel trapped." I said. "Like I'm in prison and will be for the rest of my fucking life." Till Death do us part.

He paused in his gentle way and looked at me caringly. "Maybe you should leave." He said, peacefully.

Finally Somehow Home

I couldn't quite believe what I had heard. "Really?" I asked, incredulously. "I could do that?"

"Maybe you should."

We both knew what would happen if I did. No one would believe me. It would cost me everything. My reputation would be forfeit. My friends the same. Especially, considering all I had done and confessed to her – that would surely become common knowledge. It meant that I would be the guy who fucked abunch of hookers and abandoned his family. And everyone I knew, not to mention the courts, would hear it and see it that way. Including my kids. I would have nothing. I would be nothing. It would destroy me.

But it was the only real choice I had. It was the only way I could save all that was left of me. As I drove away from Wegman's that day I knew what I had to do. There was some slight relief to have finally come to a decision, but I knew that my life was soon going to suck very, very bad, and probably for a very long time. Then very slowly and subtly something new began to come over me. Something I'd all but forgotten and hadn't experienced in many, many years. It somehow grew into the astounding realization that I had a life ahead and a future again. That

Finally Somehow Home

I was no longer confined inside of a life of disdain and despair until the day I fucking died. It was hope, and it was amazing to feel again. It surged through me like a wildfire. I felt as if suddenly put outside of high prison walls. With nothing. As no one. And I rolled down the windows of my car and screamed for fucking joy at the top of my god damn lungs. And I swore an oath to myself then that I would never, ever, ever in my life again be so imprisoned.

I have no intention or desire to slander anyone, or besmirch anyone's character. None whatsoever. So, I will steer clear of self-justification. That aside, I can't progress past this for myself without acknowledging that whatever she did, and however she did it, and whether she meant to do it or not, she hurt me so badly that I walked away from her and from my kids because of it. That's what fucking happened. You can call me overly sensitive, or weak, or cowardly, or selfish, I am past giving a fuck. Like a battered woman going back for more, I stayed in it until I couldn't stay in it any longer. I wish I had left sooner, but there's no way I could have. The guilt and foreboding and total-fucktness of leaving my kids behind was too much. But I think if I had seen it for what it was, and escaped sooner, I would not have

Finally Somehow Home

compromised my character as I did. Had I understood the situation and got the fuck out while it was salvageable, I'd still be a part of my kids' lives because I wouldn't be so fucked up in my head about it.

For a long time after I left, well-meaning friends would come along and encourage me to go back. I hated them for it. I could only try to control my breathing and heartrate as the anxiety and adrenaline spiked, remind myself that they had no idea what they were asking, and shake my head, painfully acknowledging that in spite of all who they had known me to be in this life, they truly looked at me and saw me as a piece of shit deadbeat who abandoned his kids so he could go be "free" or some such shit. Only a very few people, ironically, mostly people who knew her best, really saw and understood. Look, I've been in three wars. I know god damn well what PTSD is, been diagnosed with it by multiple doctors, I can identify its symptoms, its triggers, and all the shit that goes along with it. Most of my PTSD even after three wars, is from that relationship. Because of all this, it is extremely difficult for me engage with my kids - and this is the most fucked up part about it - my mind has placed them squarely in the center of that whole fucked up situation - in the epicenter of my hell. As if trapped there

Finally Somehow Home

in the eye of the storm, and whenever I spoke with them - when we used to talk - I was forced to go back there to all of it. I don't presently have a relationship with them at all. But now, as the passing of time heals those thick twisted wounds that you can't make sense of when they're fresh, now things are beginning to change. I hope it's not too late, but I understand that it might be. They still don't know who I am. It's been exactly 10 years. From me writing this down, right now, since I left them. I haven't seen them in six years. I haven't spoken to them in four. I tried to visit them a couple years ago. I just got the "That's probably not a good idea." They declined to see me. It's the hardest part of my life, and one that I don't know how to fix. I wrote this book so that maybe someday they would pick it up and read it and understand who their dad really is, despite what they may have been led to believe. The good, the bad, and the ugly, but the god damn truth and nothing but. My writing is all letters to my kids. All the shit that I really thought they need to know about life because I knew I couldn't be there to teach them in person as they grow older. That's why I write as visceral and raw and harsh as the world is on purpose - so they can plug it right in.

Finally Somehow Home

I remember my son David running along next to my car through the neighbors' suburban yards as I was driving away yelling "you're the best daddy in the whole world!" I pulled around the block and stopped the car and wept bitterly. I kept that feeling in my heart in case I should ever need to bludgeon myself with it, in case I had fucked up, in case I deserved to feel it, in case there had been any other way and I had missed it. It's taken many years, but eventually I had to let it rest and stop clinging to my pain. Only now are things starting to come into blurry focus. Only now can I even think about it all without the overwhelming pain and questions and self-loathing followed inevitably by retreat and defeat, yet again – unable to face it. But it's as if that part of my mind, on its own timeline, is slowly coming back to life after a decade of CAUTION tape and "Do Not Cross" lines denoting something like the Exclusion Zone around Chernobyl. That's why it's taken me so long to finish this book. I have not, until now, been capable of it. I had to give it some room.

She's off and good now with a good man who's proven to be a great dad to my kids and I'm mighty glad and grateful for their family and that they are together, but I thank God every day that I'm not in that fucking

Finally Somehow Home

shitshow anymore, while in the same breath I can feel, like a saw cutting slow on bone, the fact that I'm no longer a part of my kids' lives. It's still the worst part of my life and it always will be. I think about it every single fucking day.

Chapter 18

I was a complete mess after I left. I sobbed myself to sleep many nights back then. I had no friends. It was a very lonely time for a while. All of our friends in the area had picked her side, with the exception of a few who would just throw Bible verses at me and tell me what a scumbag I was for wanting a divorce. I definitely knew I was a scumbag for being away from my kids, but I could not physically, mentally, or any other way, bear even the thought of remaining in that relationship another day. We had been living in Leesburg, Virginia, which was almost an hour from work, so I got a one bedroom at Belle Pre Apartments in Alexandria, Virginia just up the road from Old Town and near the Mark Center, where I worked, the Pentagon, and the other places I frequented for my job. Again, it was a friendless and lonely time for

Finally Somehow Home

several months, and nothing but dark despair to keep me company.

I had left pretty much everything except my clothes, guns, tools, books, wine, booze, and cigars when I started over, so that meant I'd had to refurnish from scratch. I cleaned out Bed Bath and Beyond for household shit, Magnolia for AV shit, but still needed basic furniture. I'd noticed a little hole in the wall store across the street that looked more like an abandoned garage, but it had afew unique furniture pieces in the window, so I ambled in. I was greeted by a very kind older Asian lady. She was Malaysian Chinese and as Indonesia and Malaysia are neighbors with very similar languages we bantered and bullshat for awhile about home. It was refreshing to meet someone who knew what the hell Salak Bali was, Langsat, or Nasi Kuning, or Makanan Padang, all foods from Indonesia I still to this day have recurring dreams about. I asked her about the furniture in the window and if she had any more, since I had to fully furnish my apartment right across the street. She motioned for me to follow her outside, and around to the back of the building where she unlocked the padlock on the door and let me in. The building was dark and cold and musty and dust hung languidly there in the only light that cut

Finally Somehow Home

sharply through it from afew narrow slatted windows up near the warehouse ceiling. As my eyes adjusted, mysterious shapes and shadows of all sizes came into form slowly around me. When she finally found the switch she'd been groping for, a dozen or so lamps of all different design and scattered throughout, unveiled the mystery of the central area, the outskirts and corners still shrouded in cold and dust and dark. Some of the forms I'd noticed were covered by sheets and tarps, and some were just covered in the dust that covered everything except for afew pieces in the middle. "Holy shit!" I said, walking toward a nearby table. It was 8 feet long and thick and the center rings of the wood were dark as coffee with a graduating lightness toward the edges of almost a brown mustard which were the natural curvature and grain of the tree's trunk from which it had once been hewn. "Dat manga wood from Indonesia." She said,

"How much?"

"Too atousant", she said. "I give you for Fiteen ahundrut".

Sure as shit, the little white paper tag attached to one of the legs read "$2000".

Finally Somehow Home

"You lika da bed?" She asked pointing to a huge bed with a fucking roof on it and walls around it. It was red and had Chinese shit written on it. Clearly hand carved from hardwood just like everything else in the warehouse. "I have Indonesian one, atoo-hundret years old."

"Uhhhhhh...Fuck yes?" I responded. I had seen these beds in Indonesia, usually whilst touring the old Long houses that some of the different clans like the Dayaks used to live in. The houses and all the furniture hand hewn from the dark hardwoods that grew in trunks over 10 feet across in the dark rich wet tropical dirt of the rain forest. Indonesia, especially Kalimantan, had wood so dense that it fucking sank in water. It was called Belian. I saw someone try to drill a hole through a Belian 4x4 with a 220v electric drill. There was plenty of smoke. First from the Belian, then from the drill. The motor in the drill burnt out before making it halfway through. The fastest way to do it was with a hand drill and a red hot metal rod that you had to keep heating up in the fire as you burned your way through the shit. There was also Kayu Hitam - "black wood", or Ebony, and Mabang – Mahogany, among many others. Somehow that combination of sun and rain and soil right on the equator, and on that particular island especially,

Finally Somehow Home

produced some of the most beautiful and dense woods on this earth. I've seen other hardwoods from all around the world, and while I'm no woodyoligist, I do think there's something unique about Kalimantan's plant ecology.

The bed was awesome. It was about 10 feet from end to end, almost 8 feet tall and 6 feet wide. It was made of Mabang and its assembly was like putting together a puzzle using tongue-in-groove and other unique joining techniques without a single nail or screw to hold it together. The base of it had a secret compartment underneath the mattress, where I eventually put my subwoofer for the surround sound system I rigged into it, and it was walled on three sides with vertical slats an inch or so wide and the same distance apart. An intricately carved lattice work of flowers and hornbills and shit surrounded the entire front and entrance to the bed, atop which sat a roof with carved awnings that reached out a foot on both sides. The wood was still in very good shape, but brittle from age, and unfinished and bare except for a hint of color on some of the flowers and whatnot from whatever paint they'd used on it two hundred fucking years ago. I knew it was the genuine

Finally Somehow Home

article. It looked exactly like the ones I'd seen when I was a kid and was clearly very old indeed.

"I'll take it. How much?"

"Dis afie atousant. But I give you for atirty fie ahundret. Don't atell anybody."

I picked out some dresser drawers made of unfinished re-used Teak from Thailand, a 5'X5' table with large round legs of Mabang and a top 3" thick made, again, of unfinished re-used Teak and treated with a wax that made it smooth to the touch and easy to clean while still exposing the beautiful grains in the old thick planks, ostensibly harvested from an old ship. A bookshelf, some high-backed dark brown Italian leather chairs for the table, a couple of leather sofa chairs, afew lamps, and I had everything I needed. I couldn't pay for it all at once, but the old lady said she trusted me, so I made a down payment and she had all of it delivered to my apartment the next day. It took me some time to pay her for all of it, so every month I'd walk over to her shop and hand her a wad of cash. Then she would pull out her notebook and update the balance and hand me a paper receipt. Sometimes she would have Malaysian food cooked and ready for me when I got there, and we would sit and talk

Finally Somehow Home

about life. I don't know what ever happened to her except that her shop closed about a year later and I never saw her again after that. I still have much of the furniture I bought from her. I've hauled that goddam heavy teak table around with me all these years among other things and am often reminded by it of her kindness to me during a very dark and bitter time in my life.

I had met Steve about a year before when I was working at the COIC. Steve was a former Army Special Forces Officer. He was my age exactly, 6'5" or more, well cultured, and handsome. We had hit it off the previous year over Scotch to discuss business. He called me out of the blue one day and told me he was separating from his wife and wondered if I wanted to go in halvsies on an apartment. In the interest of saving some money I decided, what the hell, why not. That turned out to be a beautiful mistake.

I moved all of my shit to a 6th floor two-bedroom apartment in the same complex and adjacent to the pool and expansive patio area that overlooked North Henry Street and the surrounding projects - #601. The first night in our new apartment we were sitting there looking

Finally Somehow Home

at each other saving money when one of us piped up and said, "Hey, I've got an idea. Let's go to the strip club."

The Crystal City Restaurant, which we affectionately called "The CCR", was just a couple miles up the road in Arlington. I'm pretty sure it was owned by the Russian Mob and/or some Russian Intelligence organization considering its proximity to the Pentagon and the propensity for people with security clearances to run their mouth around alcohol and strippers. Even so, it is still, to this day, my favorite bar in the world. There was a bar and stage in the main area, then a glassed off large room with another bar and small stage wherein one could smoke cigars and cigarettes. That was our favorite spot. Furthermore, the two curtained private rooms were back there where, for a fee, one could get some alone time with one or more of the strippers. The CCR had a full kitchen, and you could get a massive steak and/or lobster dinner there all the way up until closing time. It was a lovely place. I had started frequenting it long before Steve and I got the apartment, and as I had no other friends at all in the area, and was craving any kind of pleasant human interaction, I had become pals with the strippers and staff there. As crazy as it may seem, they became my family and support group of sorts.

Finally Somehow Home

The first time Steve and I walked into the CCR together several strippers came up to us. One of them said, "Holy shit! You guys know each other!?" Apparently, Steve was something of a regular as well. Both of us were well liked because we tipped well and were nice to the strippers. We eventually got to know all of them very well. I still consider them very dear friends of mine. I have a very big place in my heart for strippers. They are mostly great girls who have no choice but to dance for a living. It made me sad that many of them were stuck there. Reminded me of the gunfighter trade. Most of them wished they could get out of it but had nothing else to do and nowhere else to go. Steve and I took good care of them. We made sure no one messed with them, and we also gave them shitloads of money. We had several games we would play. We would usually walk into the glassed off back room and find our favorite table reserved for us. There was a lot that was remarkable about Steve, but by far his most remarkable trait, at least the one that he leveraged the most in such situations, was that his cock was simply enormous. Once, on a low-level, night, combat equipment jump, he exited the aircraft at 800 ft AGL and his chute failed to open. With not enough time to deploy his reserve, he plummeted to the earth. Fortunately,

Finally Somehow Home

Steve's massive cock broke his fall, but it took six hours and the jaws of life to pry it out of the rock it had lodged in. He used one of those beds that rock climbers use when bivouacking on a cliff face to keep it off the ground until the swelling went down. We used to leave our metal cock rings on our table to save our seats when we'd go to the bathroom or were otherwise engaged. As a result, our table reservation sign read: RESERVED FOR THE BIG DICKS. We would take our seats, then give the manager about $500 each and get back 1000 $1 bills. These we would pile up in the middle of our table and pass them out in handfuls, or in some cases, throw them in wads of 100 and watch the dollar bills shower down around the girl dancing on the stage. Sometimes we left afew 50s, 20s, 10s, and 5s in the pile. After a stripper was done with her two dances on stage, she would walk around the restaurant, as was customary, and receive tips from the patrons. The girls always loved stopping by our table, especially when we played this game. When she would arrive at our table we would blindfold her and tell her she could pick three bills out of the pile. I'll just say that the sensory capacity of Strippers has evolved far beyond that of the normal person. Their tactile facilities rival that of the octopus whose brains are in its tentacles.

Finally Somehow Home

Even tightly blindfolded with our hands over her eyes, the experienced stripper could somehow feel out and differentiate those bigger bills from the rest.

A few weeks after Steve and I first rolled into the CCR as a team, we were sitting at our reserved table, as per. I was smoking a cigarette and sipping on a frosty mug of Blue Moon with an orange slice when the silhouette of a woman appeared in the glass door to my front. The door and large glass windows all around separated our back room lair from the main stage and surrounding booths and tables occupied by the proletariat revelers who drifted into the Battlespace over which Steve and I benevolently reigned. There were a shitload of women in there, so I don't know why this silhouettey bietch caught my eye. I could tell she had very short hair. A sign of supreme confidence or equivalent desperation in a woman, but all I could derive from the vague outline of her face is that she was smiling as she spoke to one of the other girls. Huge, like the kind that makes your cheeks hurt. That's all I could deduce from the shadowy figure until the door opened and the smoke dissipated as she came closer and the light from the small stage behind my seat began to illuminate her mysterious visage that walked as though all she really wanted in life was for

Finally Somehow Home

someone to love her unconditionally on her own variable fucking terms, and I have to admit that as the obscurity faded, the closer she came, my resistance to that absurd proposition faded along with it and dissolved into nothing at all when I saw her face. I was smoter than a fucking Philistine.

"Who the fuck are you?" I asked as she floated by.

"Hi Steve... I'm Toni Fix." She said as she paused at our table. You could hear the smile in her voice, with a hint of go fuck yourself. "Who the fuck are you?"

"Jason" I said.

"Hi Jason." she said as she turned, blowing me off on her way to the stage.

"Steve! Who the fuck is that?"

"You don't know Toni!?" he said incredulously.

"No, bro. Never seen her before. Holy fucking shit, man."

...My work phone rang at my desk. It was Toni. "Hey, do you have any Adderall?"

"God damn it, Toni, I'm working."

Finally Somehow Home

"I just got home, and I have shit all over me."

"What the fuck? Why do you have shit all over you?"

"My boyfriend was fucking me in the butt, and I got shit all over us. I'm a mess, I'm going to clean up. Can you bring me some Adderall?"

"God damn it. I'll be there in 20 minutes."

We were more like buddies than anything. It took a minute for her to warm up to me, and I wasn't pursuing her or anyone at all at the time, because I was so head-fucked with other shit. I hated the idea of anyone needing anything at all from me since I had so recently, thoroughly, and clearly fucked that up with everyone else who had so depended on me in my life.

I got to her apartment in Old Town Alexandria 15 minutes later. It was a beautifully quaint little affair. Must have been a shortage space or something at one point. The best Greek restaurant in Alexandria occupied the ground floor, and Toni's apartment was through the patio entrance with tables and tikki torches and shit spread all around, up a flight of steps and into a red-orange door above that reminded me of the doorways to

Finally Somehow Home

homes in Venice. She had a foldout couch that doubled as her bed and occupied the entire living room until restored to its couch form, a small kitchen, a bathroom so small it was hard to turn around in, and a loft area with a ladder where she kept all her extra bullshit. Everything in the place was orange or yellow or aqua or one shade or the other of those colors.

I knocked on the door. She opened it and smiled real big the way I saw her smiling in the shadows when I first saw her. She always smiled like that. It made me happy.

"Tonayyyyy"

"Jayysuuun."

I went inside. She was wearing one of those boot things they put on you at the hospital when you break your foot but don't need a cast. She had broken her foot but didn't need a cast. Stepping off a curb or some silly shit like that. It had ruined her summer. She'd had tickets with her lawyer buddy to Italy or some such shit and the broken foot had put the kibosh on that for sure, not to mention, she couldn't dance.

"You should grow scruffles, Jason."

Finally Somehow Home

"Scruffles?"

"Yes. Let your beard grow out alittle bit. I like it when you don't shave for afew days."

"Ok, fine. I'll grow scruffles."

Aside from a big hug when I saw her, I didn't even touch her for a month or so. She had her shit going on, and our meetings were random and sporadic and usually annoyingly inconvenient, but she was fun as hell to look at, and I liked being around this little ray of happiness in my life, that, in spite of all the darkness she'd been through – she showed me a documentary of the area she'd grown up in, in Kentucky. It was about the Opioid crisis in the US and the title of it was something like "The Poorest Town in America." - and even though she saw all of the shit that was plain and clear and real in the world, she somehow saw through it all as if to unveil the great beauty lying dormant beneath it. She was an incredibly talented photographer, and on her lone random adventures throughout DC at all hours of the day and night, would capture perfect moments in time that gushed with humanity and somehow throbbed with meaning. She could be walking into the shadiest 7/11 in DC at 3 in the morning and Toni would stop and greet

Finally Somehow Home

each of the dirty, smelly, strung-out homeless people lying around the entrance, invariably knowing at least one of them by name, and to those she didn't know, she'd introduce herself. They'd ask for a cigarette, and she'd gladly oblige, and sitting there on the sidewalk next to them would light up one of her own and bullshit and laugh and talk to them as if they were human beings and it was astonishing and enchanting and beautiful the way that word really means, and I found myself beginning to understand something that I never knew before and the more I was around her the seed of this new something began to grow in me and bring into life that which had never been a part of me before, and I learned what it was to love the unlovable and it is a part of me now, and it is a precious beauty in this life that I'd been blind to before, and one I'd never have discovered had she never shown me the way.

The first time we actually went out together, she took me to a gay bar. I laughed and thought it was funny albeit slightly annoying, but we had fun together despite the constant questions as to whether or not I thought this or that dude was hot. Partially, because I can ascertain whether or not a man is handsome or ugly to some slight degree, but "hot" implies actual attraction, and I'm not

Finally Somehow Home

attracted to dudes, but it was always a weird aside to our friendship and I don't know what she was after with it, but it was there.

About that time Steve and I got evicted from our apartment. My room was next to the outside wall and patio area, but the apartment beneath us apparently didn't appreciate the subwoofer in my bed that pulsed directly into their living space at all hours. There were other complaints too. The wall of Steve's bedroom was adjacent to the next apartment which was occupied by a couple of young female business professionals. According to the front desk clerk, a big jacked black dude who was our buddy and let us in on the inside baseball of the whole thing, those neighbors had submitted several official noise complaints against us as well, one of which stated that in the late night to early morning hours there were very loud and incessant noises coming from the next apartment that "sounded like a wild animal dying". Those complaints, coincidentally aligned with the frequent nights wherein female company was present in our apartment and while I and my subwoofer would be delighted to take credit for our eviction, I cannot in good conscience

Finally Somehow Home

usurp the glory from Steve's massive dong and consummate expertise.

Chapter 19

So, we had to find a new place. And since we were both going through a divorce, we adamantly agreed that some low-cost hovel would be just fine and enable us to save money and focus on our jobs, so we settled on a massive suite with 14-foot floor-to-ceiling windows on the top floor of the highest building in Crystal City overlooking Ronald Reagan National Airport afew blocks away from the CCR.

Our apartment at 220 20th St was on the southeast corner of the building and offered a clear view of all the DC monuments and shit as well as line of sight to all the planes on final approach landing at DCA. In the night sky one could see them stacked up, preparing to land and wonder and marvel about all the different people on the unrelenting stream of planes that pummeled the

Finally Somehow Home

runways and imagine who they were and what their lives were like and what had carried them thus to DC, but we didn't. It took about four seconds for a cigarette butt to hit the parking lot from our balcony. We did marvel at that. And during the Marine Corps Marathon you could see all the snipers on the rooftops all around looking down to ensure no fuckery was afoot. That too was marvelous.

After a few months of being separated from my ex I got to see my kids every other weekend. They'd come to my apartment, and we'd build forts out of pillows and blankets and take the mattress off my bed and put a disco ball in there and make a karaoke stage and sing along to Frozen songs, or just walk around down by the Potomac getting ice cream goo all over everything, or ride the Ferris wheel or play in the sand, or play video games. Before they came over, I would always get the apartment ready and make sure everything was childproof and whatnot. I had a pistol I used to keep in my nightstand and one day, before I picked them up, I took it out and cleared it – taking the magazine out - put it in my sock drawer, and put the pistol in my work bag up high in my closet so they couldn't get to it. We had a great weekend, and I went back to work the next week and had

Finally Somehow Home

totally forgotten that the damned thing was in there. I showed up to work and noticed on the way in to the parking lot that they had additional security checkpoints set up and were screening people's bags. Totally forgetting that the pistol was in my bag, I parked my car and took my place in line for afew minutes just trying to get in the building to my office. You can guess what happens next. The security guard's eyes got really big as she pulled the pistol out of my bag. This was only a month or so after the Washington Naval Yard shooting where some government contractor went ape shit and hosed down abunch of his co-workers, so that shit was forefront in everyone's mind. I have to admit that my eyes got really big too. They brought me into the security office and an agent started reading me my Miranda rights. I told them that I waived my rights and then told them what had happened. No dice. The building that I worked in was something of an annex to the Pentagon, so they cuffed me, drove me to the Pentagon, and threw me in the Pentagon jail. I can't imagine who else had been in my cell. A KGB agent or two, maybe. It was really small, almost claustrophobic - about 3' X 3' with a tiny 4" X 6" window to look through if you stood up from the little bench in there. I had been to

Finally Somehow Home

the Pentagon many times before, but I'd never gotten to see this part of it yet. My lucky day. The shitty part of it was that the Pentagon itself has kindof an understanding that things like this can happen from time to time, so their policy was a $50 fine. Well, my building, although annexed to the Pentagon, carried the same penalties that you would get if you carried a gun into any other federal building, which is a misdemeanor, but as everyone was freaked out over the recent shootings, everyone just freaked the fuck out more...even though there was no ammo or magazine in the pistol or in the bag. Someone told me later that they were worried that I would try to smuggle ammunition and magazines in later...are you fucking kidding me!??? Anyway, I had fucked up. And big. So, there wasn't much I could do but ride it out. They suspended my TS/SCI (Top Secret/Sensitive Compartmented Information) security clearance, and I was scheduled to fight it out in court as to whether I had intent to schwack all of my co-workers in a shooting spree. By the next day the Secretary of Defense had been informed of the incident and my boss actually caught a lot of shit for covering my ass and not reporting it up immediately through his chain of command. Thanks for the attempt, Newbs. The suspension of my security

Finally Somehow Home

clearance, though, essentially meant that I had lost my job, because without a clearance I wasn't able to get into the office where I worked. Boom. All done. They told me they'd try to keep the position open for me for as long as they could, but no guarantees because they had to get the work done. Fair enough, I don't blame them for that. I, meanwhile, rotted away fretting for my court date. I lawyered up and waited.

I had been living the high life while providing about $8K a month to keep the ex and the kids afloat in the fancy house we'd been living in, her car payment and all of their bills paid for, then all of my own expenses on top of that. I had to start borrowing money from friends and selling stuff. Even downsizing costs money. All of my guns went among many other things, and I moved out of my high-rise apartment and into a spare room with a good friend. Life was crashing down around me, and I didn't know if I was going to end up in prison after it was all said and done, or not. Finally, the court date came. I had prepared a good defense with the Closed-Circuit Television footage of me driving past the security checkpoint on the way to park in the garage, then standing in line after I had parked and doing nothing to evade the search. The Magistrate threw the case

Finally Somehow Home

out. Thank God. But that was just the first part of everything. The next step was getting my security clearance going again. Well, it turns out that when the Navy Yard shootings went down there was an investigation into it and the findings were that the company who was contracted to do all the security investigations for the Navy had screwed up because they had let this psycho slip through the cracks. So, they were canned. Well, the problem was that those people were the same people that were supposed to reinstate my clearance and there was no one flying the desk upon which my paperwork was languishing.

I waited around DC as long as I could, but I had no income, and in spite of trying to find work, even at restaurants and bars, I couldn't. My resume didn't exactly work for those kinds of positions. I was turned away at every job and without a Security Clearance it is impossible to find corporate work within miles of DC, especially with only three years of corporate work experience. I had been mooching off my friend Dennis, who was a fucking godsend to me, but I had been living in his spare room for too long. He got me an Air B-n-B for afew weeks, and I kept looking for work but couldn't find any and no news was coming through on my

Finally Somehow Home

clearance. And furthermore, I had learned that they had filled my old position, so my old job wasn't available to me even if I did get my clearance back. My life was in ruin.

The only brightness in it at all was Toni. She saved my life. She cared for me when no one else did or could or would. We loved each other easily, as if it were the most natural thing in the world to do, because it was. She offered to let me live with her while I figured my life out, but I knew somehow that I would have just become a horrible burden to her. "Jason, what are we?" She had asked me. I didn't have an answer for her. We were like peas in a pod, for sure, and by that time, spent every free minute together. She was more than a close friend and a lover, but I knew that my life was so fucked up that I would just drag hers down with mine even though she was willing to do it. I didn't know what I wanted, and I had failed to jump at the chance when she'd asked the question of me. I knew that her ex-boyfriend was doing everything he could to get her back as well, and who could blame him. I was too paralyzed to make a move, and it wasn't fair to her for me to keep her in limbo, so she told me she was going to get back together with her ex. At first it didn't bother me. But when it finally hit me that I

Finally Somehow Home

would be losing my Teeny, Tiny, Toni, I almost lost my shit. I almost fucking died. I started fighting for her like a drowning man trying to stay afloat. I knew then that if I ever lost her, part of me would be lost forever as well.

Remember when I said she was always taking me to gay bars and asking me if I liked this guy or that guy? Like I said, I've never been attracted to guys in any way, but I have always, since I was a little kid, imagined I would very much enjoy the sensation of anal sex. And the fact is that it doesn't matter what you believe, when you massage the prostate gland, it feels fucking amazing. Just before I'd met Toni I'd been with my first man. I didn't go in for the kissing and all that shit. Men are amazing creatures, but to me their bodies are still weird and gross and smell bad. Afterward I distinctly remember being amazed at how impersonal it all was. There was no passion, or adoration, or exploration - all the things that make sex with a woman a spiritual experience. It was just straight fucking. As empty as a bank transaction. There is a huge difference. At least for me it felt as if something essential were missing. Almost as if it were something completely different than sex altogether. But I had done it. I had ripped off the bandaid.

Finally Somehow Home

Let's talk about the butthole. That from which boundless poop and debate ensue. Is it wrong or right to put stuff in there? Is it wrong or right to stick your dick in one? Is it ok to stick your pee-pee into a girl's, but not a guy's? The basis of the argument appears ridiculous. It seems as though there shouldn't be any argument at all. Why is it considered a despicable act and an abomination to mash your dong into one hole but not another? It really seems impertinent to any moral debate at all. So, how then is this one of the most contentious squabbles in all of humanity's history? The answer: God hates it. What the fuck? Really!? And yes, believe it or not, this is the only, and most salient position and point against homosexuality that I knew of at the time. It really doesn't seem to make any sense why it should be considered wrong, sinful, immoral, evil, or otherwise very fucking naughty. Except that God said, "Don't do that shit."

So, we've established that God sees this as more than just a preference of penetrable orifices. And it seems odd. Like it shouldn't be made into that big of a thing. But God makes it into a HUGE thing. Seemingly a mountain out of a molehill. Wait a minute, though... God's not the only one who makes this into a big thing. The very proponents of banging other dudes in the butt, or otherwise twaddling

Finally Somehow Home

people of their same sex, make it into a HUGE thing as well. It's such a huge thing that it is a lifestyle and an identity within which adherents take great pride. According to the most ardent of buttfuckers, you don't DO gay. You ARE gay. It IS a big thing. Both sides agree on something at least.

In my experience, gay people are some of the kindest and most courageous people I've ever known. And the gayer, the braver. Yes, the lifestyle seems fabulous, carefree, and marvelous, but it's not all butt-plugs and butterflies. Every person who has ever embraced homosexuality as an identity must endure their own unique onslaught of rejection and pain. People don't do it because it's easy. They do it because they firmly believe that they are being true to themselves in spite of the derision that comes with it. That takes a lot of courage. And it takes courage every single day.

So, what's really the big deal? Is it just because it's gross when you get poopy dick from it? There must be a reason behind why God in the Bible thinks it's an "abomination". It didn't make any sense to me.

But I still hadn't told anyone about this side of me that was drawn to this strange and powerful proclivity. I

Finally Somehow Home

guess I wanted to wait until I understood it for myself. Over the next several months I had a few encounters with other men. I wanted nothing to do with a relationship or even a friendship with any of them, so I'd just order up a male hooker on these occasions. So, when I met Toni, and she would take me to gay bars and shit like that, I couldn't understand it, and it was slightly annoying because that was definitely not my jam, but I just secretly laughed at the irony of it.

I was at Toni's little apartment above the Greek restaurant. She was sitting cross legged on the floor counting and sorting a massive pile of one dollar bills she'd stuffed into her purse from the night before at work. I had walked across the street to a deli that we loved and gotten us both a breakfast bagel or some shit and a 4-pack of Crabbies Ginger Beer. I had been wanting to just tell her and get it off my chest. After all, she was my closest friend. But now I didn't want to be just closest friends. This whole time we had been together we were never officially a couple. She was never mine. I had never gotten the chance to call her "Baby". I wanted her alone, to be mine, and me hers alone. Period. Plus, I figured she'd probably love me even more once she

Finally Somehow Home

learned about the dude stuff since that seemed like a thing for her.

"You know how you're always trying to get me to talk to gay guys and shit, Toni?" I said, breaking the comfortable silence. "Well, I've been with guys before. A couple of times." She stopped what she was doing and looked at me incredulously. Then she flipped the fuck out.

Needless to say, it did not have the desired effect. She was now suspicious of me, and didn't know if she could ever be with me. She called her cousin who was perfectly and happily married, yet who occasionally played around with other girls with her husband. Her cousin assuaged much of her fear, but there was still a very real rift between us suddenly that I had not expected. I had wanted to be closer to her, but she seemed to keep drifting further from my despairing reach.

A few days later, I was sitting in my car drenched in melancholy after yet another job rejection. This one was as a waiter at a nice DC restaurant. One of the managers had been in Long Range Recon in the Pakistani Army many years ago which was the only reason I was asked to come by for a second interview with the General Manager. The GM couldn't quite conceal his irritation at having to talk to me, but I appreciated his feeble attempts at courtesy, nonetheless. He kept it short and sweet and sent me on my way with an apologetic nod on the way out from the Pakistani Recondo who'd been watching the interview and loitering near the kitchen. I nodded back in thanks and respect and stepped out onto the sidewalk toward my car. "Fuck. Goddamn it. Fuck, Fuck, Fuck, Goddamn it, Fuck" I muttered whilst grasping the steering wheel with both hands. "Fuck!" I let all the fucks settle around me and just stared off into space. WRRRRT, WRRRRT, WRRRRT, my cell phone buzzed in the seat next to me where I'd flung it. It was Potsy. Potsy had been at 3rd Recon and 2d Force with me. He and Philthy – the guy who had launched the legendary War Fart at 2d Force, and who'd also been in my platoon at 3rd Recon - had established a pretty prosperous business for themselves doing executive protection, private investigations, and high threat security down in Florida. They knew of my situation and offered me a job. It wouldn't pay much, and I'd have to go through and pass the Florida State Certification process, but it was something, and they were willing to help me with lodging and expenses while I took the week-long

Finally Somehow Home

training course. It wasn't much, but it was a hell of a lot better than nothing.

I told my ex that I could borrow enough money to fly her and the kids back to Costa Rica to stay with her family, but she refused. I could do nothing more for them. I put my remaining belongings in storage and headed to Florida to try to make ends meet as a security guard. I went to see Toni before I left. I stayed the night in her apartment. That morning, I had a waking dream. Toni and I were dancing in a crowded room. Occasionally we'd be separated, then invariably find ourselves dancing back together again. It was an easy feeling. But then suddenly I looked up and she wasn't there. She was gone. I felt utterly alone. My only brightness was gone. I told Toni about it. We clung to each other in silence until we both had to leave, I in my car, and she in hers. We drove alongside each other from King Street down to the merge with the DC Beltway. We were both heading West but were on different and divergent roads. I watched her until I couldn't see her anymore. The metaphor was too real. My Toni was gone.

I drove through the day and reached Boynton Beach, Florida that night. It was great to see Philthy and Potsy

Finally Somehow Home

again and dive into what they were doing with their business and where they wanted to take it. They were doing much more than just giving me a job, they were inviting me in to help them build the future of what they had created.

I stood in my hotel room looking into the mirror and hating what I saw. It wasn't lost on me that no one else in the world liked it either. There was nothing there. Nothing worth a damn to another living soul. It made me crave some kind of connection with someone. Anyone. I didn't care. I just wanted someone to approve of me in any way. I combed through the Craigslist classifieds looking for lonely people and replying to any post I thought might yield some companionship. Finally, I posted my own. It basically said that I was up for anything with anyone. I didn't care. I gave myself away for free. To any takers. There were none.

The next week was full of classes on armed and unarmed security. It was a great little enterprise that Philthy and Potsy had going. The classes were held at their business office with about 20 students in attendance. I paid just enough attention to pass the course by Friday. I knew that if I stayed in my hotel room over the weekend, I

Finally Somehow Home

would very likely go mad. And I had to see Toni. The only person that might give a shit about me in the world. As I left the pistol range, the final qualification event of the course, I saw a coconut tree in the parking lot with young coconuts hanging off it. It wasn't very tall and my tree climbing skills from Indonesia yielded a fresh little orange coconut for Toni. I got back on the ground, brushed the shitty coconut tree bark and residue off my abraised forearms and inner thighs of my True Religion jeans, threw the coconut on the floorboard of the passenger seat, and headed for Alexandria, Virginia. On the way, I googled up a Walmart that was enroute and ordered some small canvas prints of pictures of Toni and me. By the time I got to the Walmart the prints were ready and I likewise stashed them on the passenger seat and kept on truckin'.

I showed up to Toni's apartment early in the morning on Saturday. It was like coming alive again to hold her in my arms and kiss her and know that she was really there next to me. I gave her the coconut and the prints of us and kissed her some more. She was just as frantic to see me again as I was for her. I don't remember what we did that day. I just remember the pure bliss of it. It was like breathing again after spending a week under water. All

Finally Somehow Home

the fear of losing her finally left. And she knew it too. We were meant to be together. Just the two of us against the world. That night she called her ex and told him to pound sand. Finally, after what seemed like forever, she was mine. My love, my girl, my Baby. We made love and I passed into a deep and beautiful sleep.

I woke up early the next morning for the drive back to Florida. I didn't want to leave Toni, but at least I knew that everything was going to be ok. If all I had was her in this life, that was enough for me.

I opened my bleary eyes and sat up in bed. The first thing I saw was Toni's intense gaze upon me and I knew immediately that something was very wrong. "What's the matter?" I asked, racking my brain to figure out what the fuck I could have possibly done in my sleep to piss her off.

"What the fuck is this, Jason?" she said, holding up my phone.

"What the fuck is what?" I asked.

She had been snooping my phone and found the emails from Craigslist confirming the posts from the Florida

Finally Somehow Home

hotel room. A couple clicks and scrolls and she had seen all of it.

It was over. It was over forever. She had been mine for afew hours and now it was all gone. I drove back to Florida. Now I was truly alone.

Finally Somehow Home

Chapter 20

I stayed in Florida for another week. Everything was just grey. I worked a gig for Philthy and Posty's company providing security for some kind of conference full of business executives. I was the Shift Leader, so my job was to interface with the client and ensure that the rest of the team were at their stations over the 48-hour event. One of the more attractive business executives intercepted me on my rounds and dragged me into her hotel room for a little frolic. But even that little incident did nothing to dispel the darkness I was in.

I had no one. I had nothing. I was living on borrowed money. I had no prospects for my future other than being a rent-a-cop, which I already knew would not provide enough to relocate permanently to Florida, let alone pay the bills and provide anything for my kids. I

Finally Somehow Home

thought constantly of I Timothy 5:8 - *But if anyone does not provide for his own, and especially for those of his household, he has denied the faith and is worse than an unbeliever.* But I had nothing to give. I was buried. Under water. I felt like Jonah in the Bible when he said:

For You had cast me into the deep,
Into the heart of the seas,
And the current engulfed me.
All Your breakers and billows passed over me.
So I said, 'I have been expelled from Your sight.
Nevertheless I will look again toward Your holy temple.'
Water encompassed me to the point of death.
The great deep engulfed me,
Weeds were wrapped around my head.
I descended to the roots of the mountains.
The earth with its bars was around me forever...

I couldn't take it anymore. I felt a great longing to go home. Back to Indonesia. But I couldn't. I didn't really have a home to go back to. So, at 39 years old, I did the only thing I could and went to live in my parents' basement in the middle of nowhere, Oregon. From hero to zero, yet again. I was soon after informed that the State of Florida had denied my Armed Security license

Finally Somehow Home

due to the gun incident at the Mark Center anyway, so in hindsight it was the best call to make. It was the only call to make.

Broke and unemployed is a full-time job. I spent every spare moment looking for work. Anything that I could think of I applied for, from corporate positions to waiting tables. All day, every day for months on end, all the while wrestling with the turmoil of my fucked-up mind. My parents were very patient and understanding with me. I still had my car for afew months before the repo people found it. But I could rarely afford gas to go anywhere, so I would sit in my car in front of the house and chain smoke cigarettes and just think, late into the night, trying in vain to make sense of everything. When I could afford some gas, I'd go fishing.

Eastern Oregon is high desert country. At first glance it appears desolate and ugly and dry and dead. But when you look more closely you learn a new kind of beauty that you haven't seen before. The air is clean and the sun's light cuts through it sharp in pastel hues against the sage and rocks and knobby mountains bowed down like so many dead giants, afew cut through with jagged wounds like the Owyhee River running down, clear and

Finally Somehow Home

cold and full of big German brown trout, then slowing like it got old and tired where it meets the high desert plain and waters the onions, corn and wheat and hay in fields spread out as far as there is water and then the purple sage again.

One day I was fishing from the bank at Unity Reservoir and agonizing in continuous and fruitless analysis the condition of my fucked-up life. And looking at the desolate beauty around me and the water which had yet to yield any trout that day, I thought of Jacob in the Bible when he wrestled with God on the bank of the Jabbok and how it must have looked something like the place that I was. It hit me like a freight train. I was mad at God. No, I was furious with God. I had never realized it until now. I stopped fishing, set my pole on the bank and broke down in tears. Angry tears. And I started praying. Angry Prayers. I was pissed off at God for not getting into the Naval Academy. I was pissed off at God for not saving my marriage when I had spent years and years tormented, praying for him to do something, and it all went to shit in a giant fucking fireball. I was pissed off at him for a lot of things and I started letting him know it: "What the fuck, God!?"

Finally Somehow Home

There's this idea out there that you're not supposed to do this with God. Here's the thing about God or anyone, really. You never really know them until you've fought with them. Until you've disagreed with them and had it out with them. In a business, in a marriage, with your parents, with your kids, with your best friends, it's the same. It's the people that you don't really care about that you just go along with, because to you it's not worth the effort to disagree. Well, God ain't like that with you. Once you start getting to know him, you're going to have some run-ins with Him, just like Jacob did at the Jabbok. And in that little story in the Bible, it wasn't until after this fight with God that Jacob really began to prosper in his life. That's when God named him "Israel".

Then Jacob was left alone, and a man wrestled with him until daybreak. When he saw that he had not prevailed against him, he touched the socket of his thigh; so the socket of Jacob's thigh was dislocated while he wrestled with him. Then he said, "Let me go, for the dawn is breaking." But he said, "I will not let you go unless you bless me." So he said to him, "What is your name?" And he said, "Jacob." He said, "Your name shall no longer be Jacob, but Israel; for you have striven with God and with men and have prevailed."

Finally Somehow Home

It was a turning point for him, and my duking it out with God on the shore that day was a turning point for me. I let him have it. I poured out my anger and my frustration with Him. Stuff I'd been holding in for years and years came gushing out, stuff I didn't even know was there, and it wasn't until then that I realized, because I had been holding all of this in, I had been shaking my fist at God my whole life, saying: "You haven't helped me, but look at what I have accomplished!" And I realized both the absurdity and the beauty of it when I understood that in spite of my attitude toward him, he had helped me all along the way to great successes, and while I stood on the mountain tops that I thought were my own creation, even while I shook my fist at him and claimed all of the credit, I realized then that he had been applauding me. Every time. All along the way. At every mountain top. Holy Shit. That's how God humbles people. Through realizing shit like that. The Bible says that it is the kindness of God that leads people to change their ways of thinking.

Furthermore, I realized that because I hadn't gotten in to the Naval Academy all those years ago that I had been believing a big lie: that because my life hadn't taken that path, I had been living a second-best life ever since. I'd

Finally Somehow Home

always felt like I was on the "B" team, or "if people really knew..." even when I had been at the top of my game. That lie vanished before an onslaught of truth and all the things that I'd accomplished in my life suddenly became legitimate to me and I could take pride in them. The truth does set you free. Suddenly all the things that I was so pissed off at God about began to unravel one by one as I saw them in the light of truth.

Here's the thing about PTSD, it not only brings its own lovely set of dysfunctions to the party, but it exacerbates all of the other shit that you're carrying around with you as well. For that reason, this was a huge turning point for me in my battle with it. I had many more battles to come before I got it to the manageable level that it is now, but this was really the beginning of my recovery.

That summer was like being in a pressure cooker. The pain and despair were tremendous in spite of these little victories. But here's the thing about victories: they only come at the end of the battles. Everyone wants to win, but few are willing to show up, and even fewer are willing to fight for it. That's just how that shit works.

Still, if it wasn't one thing, it was another, and I had plenty of miserable circumstances to keep it going and

Finally Somehow Home

the fire was constantly being fueled as those circumstances grew worse over time. I couldn't find a job, I was in debt to the IRS, I was in debt to many of my friends, I couldn't support my kids, and the list went on. They were not easy problems. The day I went in to pick up my food stamps card was like a kick in the nuts. I had gone from making $147 an hour to this in six months. I was in utter misery, and worse yet, I had it all coming.

On the way back I was raging. "What do you want from me, God?!" I plunged once again into the despair that was there waiting for me, with open arms, as it always is. I got home and told my parents that I had bankrupt my life and over leveraged my future and there was nothing left, then told them I was going to bed. I went to bed and heard a knock on my door. I knew it was my dad. I brought him the pistol that I had in the room and handed it to him. Neither of us said a word. Before I went to sleep that night I told God that I needed him to help me. Like really show me something real. Not a Bible verse or a cute quote but really come through for me because otherwise I didn't know if I could make it till the next day. I woke up around 2 am and went outside for a smoke. Thrown across the night sky like handfuls of

Finally Somehow Home

brilliance, the stars shone down so bright that you didn't need moonlight to see the fields of wheat and the cows sleeping in pastures all around. Dead silence. A thought came into my head as I took a drag off my cigarette. If I jumped around on one leg, would that change how much I owed the IRS? No. What if I did jumping jacks, or stood on my head, or ran around yelling? Nope. Well, then moping around isn't going to change a god damn thing either, for anything. In fact... Holy Shit, I can actually be happy right now because nothing I feel can change any of my circumstances anyway, so, Fuck it! I'm gonna be happy. And that's how I learned that happiness is a decision, not a destination. I went back to bed with a smile on my face for the first time in a very long time.

You know those moments where you learn something that you know is a game changer for you? Throughout that summer I had a lot of those. They are all amazing experiences, but they are mostly uncomfortable. God's desire for your life isn't that you'll be comfortable. People don't go to Beverly Hills in search of wisdom and fulfillment. His greatest desire for your life is that you will have life itself and have it more abundantly.

Finally Somehow Home

Chapter 21

Finally in September -10 months after the incident - I got word that the hold had been lifted on my security clearance, so I went back to DC in late September with a couple of six-month consulting contracts lined up. It was just enough to get by, but at least I was near my kids again. In January my clearance came up for its five-year review where you have to fill out all the paperwork and go through the whole process again to renew it. That was fine except that I was head over heels in debt and that didn't sit well with whoever was doing the review so it ended up taking longer than it normally does. The reason that having a lot of debt makes you a security risk is that you are more susceptible to bribery, extortion, and blackmail and shit like that, which is totally understandable. Frankly, I didn't expect that it would get renewed, but I never had the chance to find out because the work I was doing that was keeping me afloat dried up in March and I was left scrambling and looking for something to do, once again. It was a very contemplative time, and I was very depressed. The meds that the VA gave me weren't keeping the PTSD at bay either. It was there with a vengeance, on top of everything else. Meds are fine to treat PTSD to some degree and with the right approach. The problem with them is that they make you feel like everything is ok. But everything is not ok. So, a lot of the other problems that come along with PTSD continue on, un-addressed as long as you are on the meds. I was on anti-depressants, anti-anxiety, a hormone imbalance drug, drugs for hypervigilance – ADHD drugs, and all of it by the handful, but it all just made the world dull and bland and sank me deeper into depression. I felt like I was being crushed. As if everything was just too heavy and I was too weak to hold up under it anymore. One night it was so much that the thought of blowing my brains out occurred to me as a viable option. As soon as it did, I stood up and said out loud "I ain't doin' that shit", and I picked up my phone and called the Veteran's Crisis Hotline. The Cops came. Them showing up the way they

Finally Somehow Home

did, all tactical and shit, shocked me back to reality. I volunteered to go to the hospital where they watched me for a while then released me. I'm so glad I didn't go any further down that road in my head or I might not be here today.

On that note... I struggled with these ideas popping into my head quite frequently. I think all of us combat vets do. When you're around death so much, it makes it an easier option. What freaked me out then is that I was actually considering it. What ultimately helped me overcome these ideations for good was this question: "Am I OK with dying if I died today? Is my house in order? Am I as good as I can possibly be on all accounts with those I love and with those to whom I am otherwise indebted? Do they all know that I love them?"

If not, fix it now. Immediately.

And if so, or once that's settled, I guess I'd actually be OK with it right now. I'd be kind of bummed, but I'd be at peace with it. It's been a good run.

So, if I'm happy with the way the important things are, I guess that all things considered, I'm doing pretty well right now.

Finally Somehow Home

Well, shit! If that's the case. Fuck it, might as well keep it going.

That line of reasoning saved my life.

But I was at 0. I once again had no job, no career, and no prospects for my future at all. Then the thought occurred to me as if it were a gift: If I'm at 0, I can do whatever the fuck I want. I have to do something with my life, and I have nothing now, so I might as well choose to become whatever the fuck I've always wanted to be. The only question was: Well, what the fuck do I really want? I thought about it for awhile. I had always loved writing. It was almost annoying, I loved it so much. When I was younger, I used to write a lot more, but it always bothered me that when I would sit down to write, hours would fly by and I would waste all my time at it. Then I realized what a stupid way of thinking this was. The hours flew by because writing captivated my mind. It is also hard fucking work, but it was something that I could pour all of myself into, and at the end of the day, that's what I really wanted most: something that would use up all of whatever all of my strengths are. But once I realized that what I really wanted most was to be a writer I was almost afraid to want it. As if it were too

Finally Somehow Home

wonderful a thing to desire. So, in that moment I courageously decided to become a writer and I got down on my knees and begged God to make me one. It's funny how some of the greatest gifts that I have been given, I've always already had. The real gift is the true desire. I think God waits for you to know what you're asking for so that you know what you're getting. That day I wrote in my notebook. "God, let me be a great writer that I may write well." And that's still why I want to be a writer: so that I can write amazing shit. And that's it. And I've found that whenever I get sidetracked onto any reason for writing other than just to write well, I get lost. I always have to come back to that to keep me on track as a writer.

So, I started writing. Mostly just a few little ideas in a couple of sentences each. And most of them had nothing to do with hardship but were instead little beacons of light for me. Ideas that I could hold on to, like:

Now is the most important moment of your life.
It is the only time in your entire life that you can change it.

Or

Finally Somehow Home

Prayers are the little clouds that form beneath your feet when you are walking on nothing at all.

I went on social media and told all my friends that I had decided to be a writer. Troy reached out to me immediately. After running JIEDDO-COIC's operations in Afghanistan, he had taken up a few other jobs here and there over the years and had landed in Entebbe, Uganda as the Managing Director of a Nonprofit Aviation company. He had a big house on the shores of Lake Victoria and invited me to stay there and write. I told him I would think about it. I blew it off at first, but he kept after me, so I decided to give it some real thought. The idea seemed absurd. My first thought was: "I have bills to pay." Then it dawned on me. "I have BILLs to pay?! I have FUCKING BILLS to pay?! Is that what life is about, then? So I can pay FUCKING BILLS!? Fuck paying bills. The only reason I have the bills is that I live here, dumbass. If I don't live here, I won't have the bills. Fuck it, I'm going to Uganda."

And that's how that shit happened. It was then that I learned the importance of making decisions from my courage, instead of from my fear. The decision to write and to pull chocks and go to Uganda saved my life. Both of them took a tremendous amount of courage, but I

Finally Somehow Home

would have rotted and died had I stayed in DC. And I mean it. Those two decisions changed everything.

> *When you dare to take that step.*
> *When you leap into nothing.*
> *And plummet from the heights.*
> *If you are an eagle, then you will fly.*
> *And if you are not, then you won't.*
> *But there is no other way to find out.*
> *And there is no other way to learn how to fly.*

I had no idea how I was going to afford any of it other than Troy offering to buy me a plane ticket, but I decided to go for it and see what happened. When I got out of the military, I hadn't claimed any disability compensation because like most of us, I was still under the impression that I was bullet proof, and frankly was just busy with all the bullshit bureaucracy of out processing, so claiming my aches and pains and other ailments just took a back seat to getting through it. Plus, PTSD didn't really hit me until after I stopped deploying to combat zones, so I really didn't think I had any of it when I got out of the Marines because it hadn't manifested itself yet. When I had been staying with my parents out in Oregon, I spoke with a local Veterans Affairs advocate and they helped

Finally Somehow Home

me submit for disability compensation based on documented incidents from my medical record and my combat experience. I had all but forgotten about it until I checked my bank account one day and saw a shit ton of money in there. They had approved my claim and given me afew months of back pay on top. Not only that, I was to receive a little bit every month as well, which certainly helped. Hell, it was a life saver. Miraculous. Perfect.

I put everything I had in storage, gave a big wad of cash to the ex for the kids, got some essential supplies for the trip, and afew days later, on April 27, 2016, I leapt into nothing and got onto a plane with a one-way ticket to Entebbe, Uganda. To write.

Uganda is wild and beautiful. Entebbe sits on the equator at over 3,800 feet above sea level and touches the shores of Lake Victoria, which covers over 26,000 square miles of Africa making it the largest lake on the continent. The headwaters of the Nile flow from Lake Victoria for over 4,000 miles and empty into the Mediterranean Sea. The air is full and fresh and pushes the laden clouds thick with rain off the lake in stern grey billows where they dump fat sweet morning rain into the

Finally Somehow Home

lush greenness and the rich orange-red dirt below them. The sun is bright and big and mixes with the young lake breeze in a cocktail of airy warmth, hovering between 70 to 75 degrees Fahrenheit all the year round. Troy's house was a colonial style home on the lake and the whitewashed walls and columns set off the brilliance of the garden flowers and trees around it and birds of all kinds would come there to rest and sing or squawk at each other. I would awake whenever I pleased and sit at the table on the covered garden patio and take in the morning. The housemaids would bring me fresh coffee while I waited for breakfast to come of eggs and fruit or whatever I desired that morning. I would stumble back to my room after breakfast and get ready for the day.

As with everything in life, there seems to never be a time where you can have your cake and eat it too. In spite of the heavenliness of my situation, my decision to go there was not a popular one among most of my friends back in the US. I could tell by talking to them that they were extremely skeptical of it and of my reasons for it, and it hurt me in a very hard way. I wrote this the first few days I was there.

Finally Somehow Home

The Heavy Kind of Pain

It is a heavy kind of Pain.

That look of doubt from a good friend.
To bear the ire of the good men.
Kindly pitied as if a fool
By those who once believed in you.

And note the disappointment from
Your last and greatest champions.
To see those pleading eyes that say:
"Oh, Please don't throw your life away.

Be strong and brave to what is true.
Be what you'd want your children to."
Conceding to your errant way,
As long as you return one day.

It is a heavy kind of Pain.

For when at last I chased my dream,
They said I'd run from everything.
I left the lie for truth in trade.
They said I'd thrown my life away.

Finally Somehow Home

The bravest deed in life I've done,
They say it was a cowardly one.
For my children I became a man.
They're told that I've abandoned them.

When Nineveh I finally found,
They said that I was Joppa bound.
When I my greatest calling win,
They'll say it is my greatest sin.

It is a heavy kind of Pain.

I carry it with no offense,
With love's sole indifference.
For they are most, dearest of friends,
And wish for me the best of ends.

To do great things they know I can.
And be sought out from other men.
Just as those who know the gods' true voice
Seek men to build their dreams of choice.

Finally Somehow Home

They seek only the best of men.
And I will not be one of them.
For theirs I'll not put mine a-shelf,
For I can hear the gods myself.

I had my favorite writing haunts. There were afew bars and restaurants near Troy's house that looked over the water, and as soon as they would open in the late morning I would show up at one and enjoy a gin and tonic whilst scribbling down my thoughts. One of the plants in Troy's garden was a ghost pepper plant that the locals called Peele-Peele. I started experimenting with the fiery little fuckers and found that when muddled ever so slightly into a gin and tonic, they made the gin sweet to the taste and provided a little kick to the drink as well. They were also amazing in chocolate flavored vodka. Just let afew soak in it for a day or so and it was delicious. You could drink it straight from the bottle it was so good.

Some weekends we'd go to Jinja, the red dirt city at the Nile headwaters. The Kakira Nile Polo Club was there, and Troy and his wife would play Polo, and I would drink Gin and tonic and Pimm's Cup cocktails and watch from the open-air thatched roof covered lounge above

Finally Somehow Home

the field with the big clouds billowing over it and the sun shining down in spite of them. It was all magnificent and it breathed its thick fresh air into my life.

While I was there, I battled with the idea of what or who God is and kicked furiously at mankind's propensity to be comfortable with things that didn't add up. To tolerate lies.

Pick whichever God you would prefer to beat you.
All of us are dogs owned by animals that eat you.
Come believe in me, I won't hesitate to beat you.
I will be your God and you will let me defeat you.
You will praise my name because I did not delete you.
Even though the battle's lost, I will not retreat you.
But you may die for me, and I will consecrate you.
And kill for me so that I may fully dominate you.
Give all to me unselfishly and I will tolerate you.
Slander my conspiracy and I will intimidate you.
Go and sin and fail again so I may liberate you.
And owe to me eternally, otherwise I'll hate you.
And cast your damn-ed soul to hell and fully violate you.
Until the end when I descend to obliterate you.
So, get on your knee and worship me and I'll claim to create you.

Finally Somehow Home

Now feel the shame to think again. See how I manipulate you?

The first title of the poem above was "Make me your God". It was not received well by many, but it was really a riddle of sorts. Because it reflected something else I'd realized some time before. I later published it in The Perfect Fucking Life under the title: "the way you are", because here's what the poem reveals to each person who reads it: You don't see things the way they are. You see things the way you are.

Chapter 22

Before I left for Uganda, I had applied for an internship program in New York City. The program was specifically for former Special Operations types as the corporate nerds recognized the value of attributes that tended to prevail among our ilk that could be leveraged in the corporate world. I had all but forgotten about it when I received an invitation to participate in a review board in NYC in late May. I wrote back and let them know that I was in Uganda and asked if they would still consider footing the bill for me to fly back to the States, and they said they would do it. So, after a month of living like a king, I boarded a plane and headed to The Big Apple.

I had been to New York City before, but only on very brief trips for work back when I was at CTTSO. I had never really seen the city. I was in awe. They put me up in a hotel in Midtown, right across the street from Rockefeller Plaza. I walked around the night before the interview and explored a little. I was in love. All of the candidates for the board met up the night before and we had dinner together. It was going to be a challenge. There were eight of us. All Navy SEALs, Army Green Berets, or Marine Corps Special Operations dudes. It was a great crew of people and by the end of dinner I was just happy that one of us would be getting the opportunity to intern for one of the largest Marketing and Advertising conglomerates in the world, but I sure as hell hoped it would be me.

The next morning, we met outside the hotel and walked together through Midtown a few blocks to the company headquarters on Madison Avenue. It was beautiful. The morning sun shining down on the slick business suits and ties and shoes whose inhabitants didn't have time to give a fuck about how wonderful it all was, but I took it all in. I loved every bit of it and I wanted to be a part of this city. This living organism comprised of all walks of humanity. It seemed to me the only place where I'd been that the amalgam of the people of the earth all lived and

Finally Somehow Home

moved and breathed together that actually kindof worked. It was amazing to me.

We walked into the foyer of the building, it was a tall building, ominous almost, and kitty corner to St Patrick's Cathedral, which was a wonder all its own. We got our visitor badges and were ushered through the security gates and into an elevator up to the 10th floor. Mahogany grandeur awaited us at the reception desk, and we soon found ourselves sequestered and each in a flutter of nerves in a large conference room with coffee, fruit, and sandwiches, replete with more hardwood all around and big squishy office chairs surrounding a big, and very serious looking, red stained dark wood table. Everyone tried messing around on their phones or laptops for a few minutes, but to the last man we gave up on it and just sat there looking at each other and waiting for our turn to appear before the review board.

The board was comprised mainly of four CEOs from four of the conglomerate's Agencies (Companies that the holding company owned), within which the "chosen one" would be working for three months each, for a year, then they would be offered a job at one or another of the Company's Agencies if their internship went well. In

Finally Somehow Home

addition to that, there were several other CEOs with interest in the proceedings who would be in the room, and in addition to all of them, the big man himself, Dale, the CEO of the conglomerate, would be observing the whole show. So, no reason to be nervous, there were only 8-10 Fortune 500 CEOs in the room, and we each had about 20 minutes with them.

I just did what I had learned to do as a young kid getting my teeth worked on by the dentist in Indonesia, where there were no pain numbing agents, just the drill and the pick: No matter what...relax. That shit works.

I was called in a couple hours after we got there as one of the last candidates. The room was big and, yes, bedecked with hardwood and a grand table that matched the rest of the upholstery. Four men and women, presumably the four CEOs, sat across the table from my seat, with a few others scattered around the room. I walked in, introduced myself, and said, "You're probably wondering why I asked you all to come here today." We all laughed, I sat down, and it began.

The interview continued on in a jovial fashion as if we were all just bullshitting with each other, because in point of fact, we really were. That's all an interview

Finally Somehow Home

really is. They're just trying to feel you out and see what makes you tick to find out if you'd fit into their organization. I don't remember all of the questions they asked me, but I just told them the things I'd learned along the way about business and people and shit in response to their questions. I let them get a good feel for who I was, that's all. Somewhere in the middle of the interview a question came up about how I challenge myself and I went on a diatribe about how I like to make myself think about hard problems, such as: "Come up with an alternative for the wheel". Someone in the shadows of the room asked: "Well, did you come up with any?" "Yes," I replied. "I came up with at least two. Let me use this paper plate as an example". Fortunately for me, there happened to be a small paper plate sitting on the table with a few leftover crumbs of a sandwich on it. I showed how a downward facing axle on a vehicle could use a disk or multiple discs to control forward movement and steerage, and then I said, "Let me see if I can make this thing into a cone really quick." I did so by folding it over along its radius and heard the same voice in the dark recesses of the room say, "Ha! He did it." I then showed how multiple disks of incrementally increasing sizes could make up cones, which at a 45*

-302-

Finally Somehow Home

angle or so would function perfectly as opposing tires, or if inverted to 135* could make up a single tire with two opposing axles. I had read somewhere that MIT was working on new concepts for the wheel, and I mentioned it and said that they were going about it all wrong... which they were, they weren't looking at reinventing the wheel, they were reinventing the tire and its braking systems and whatnot. Anyway, we bullshat for a while longer, and my time was soon up. It was actually fun. I think we all enjoyed the chat. As one of the CEOs, Denise, escorted me from the room, she said something like "I've never been in a more interesting interview in all my life." I thought for sure I had the internship nailed after she said that, so I went downstairs and had a cigarette to decompress and feel good about myself.

When I was done, I went back up to the 10th floor and was immediately snatched up again by Denise who told me that we each had 30 seconds to pitch to the board as to why we thought we were the best candidate for the position, and it was my turn. I went in not really knowing what to say because I didn't really know what they were looking for exactly, so I told them that I couldn't possibly know if I was the best candidate, because all of them were so qualified, and I didn't really

Finally Somehow Home

know what they were looking for, but if they selected me I would do all that I could to rise to and beyond whatever standard was set for me. I thanked them for their time and told them that I did hope that they picked me and I excused myself and walked out of the room.

We all waited there in that mahogany boardroom in fear and trepidation for Denise to bring back the findings. She didn't keep us waiting long. I just knew I had it in the bag, so when she said that so and so, a young SEAL was chosen as the intern, I was heartbroken. Fucking SEALs. But then she said something that brought me back to life: "Jason, Dale is very interested in you as a direct hire. We will be in touch with you within a month if we want to proceed. Thank you all for coming, and good luck in your future endeavors." It wasn't a sure thing, but at least I had a chance. I later realized that it was Dale's voice that had come from the dark recesses of the room during my interview.

I was all set to head back to Uganda, but an old friend of mine from my Recon days had gotten ahold of me a few weeks prior asking if I would be willing to work for his company in the UG (Uganda) overseeing the building of a

Finally Somehow Home

University Campus there. I told him that while I was in the US I'd come down and talk to them about it, but I also told them about the opportunity in NYC and told him in no uncertain terms that that was my preference. So, I hopped a plane down to Dallas and met with Tad for ten days or so, during which time I was introduced to the people funding the project. I had no real experience in Project Management of this kind, but I eventually acquiesced to working for them, at least for a short time, to get things off the ground there. Viola! I had a job in Uganda!

While I was in the airport on the way back, I wrote this:

As long as you are OK, nothing will change for you.
Wake up and dream.
You have settled for the possible.
But you cannot do the impossible.
You can only become it.

You don't transcend by doing things differently, you transcend by becoming something different.

I got back onto a big airplane and headed back to Africa. It sure was good to get that orange-red dirt under my feet again. I flung myself into my writing once again

Finally Somehow Home

while also setting up the groundwork for the building project that I was working on. I became more and more obsessed with truth and more enraged at the things that would merely put on the guise of truth. I wrote this and posted it on a social media page where I used to post the rest of my writings:

The Call-out

Bloody and beleaguered,
man stands unsteady,
atop the rubble of the earth,
and cries to the gods:
"We get along?
NO!
You get along!
Fuck you!"

If the Masters of all the religions in the world are real, if all paths lead to God, then why are we destroying each other over their inability to reconcile? Tolerance. What a sick delusion. Would you tolerate your sick child being prescribed the wrong medicine? The existence of many powerful lies does not prove the inexistence of truth. It does matter what you believe. The defiance of man against lies is merited. Hatred toward the deceived is

Finally Somehow Home

abhorrent. Tolerance of enslavement to lies is disgusting. The truth alone will reconcile us to each other. Liars be damned, gods or no.

The closest thing to the truth is the most insidious lie. Someone told me a story once about how Eskimos hunt wolves. They take a knife and bury the handle in the snow with the blade up then pack snow drenched with seal blood around the blade. The wolves come and lick the seal blood until the blade is exposed. When they cut their tongues on the blade, they continue licking it, never realizing it is now their own blood they are tasting, and they eventually bleed out through their mouths. That's what a lie does when you believe in it. It kills you when you think it's nourishing you. Truth is exclusive. It either is, or it is not. Wishful thinking does not change that. Not with mathematics, or with navigation, or with anything. But when it comes to our own existence and purpose and life, we are told that truth is somehow subjective. I remember talking to a girl in Boulder, Colorado about this. She told me that a bunch of her friends and her had gotten together, picked out all of their favorite parts of various different religions, then decided to believe in it. They made it up. Then they believed in it. Now tell me that is not wishful

Finally Somehow Home

thinking. The thing about truth is that you will not find it until you are ready to give up everything else in search of it. I think that is what Jesus was talking about when he said: "He who has found his life will lose it, and he who has lost his life for My sake will find it." Seek the truth and you will find it. It may be where you'd least expect it. Be ready though, because wherever it is, and whatever it is, it will be very unpopular to believe in because it's probably not comfortable to believe.

Someone sent me this question on Facebook around that time and this is what I wrote in reply. You'll recognize some of it from the first part of this book:

17 June 2016 Entebbe, Uganda

This is in response to Adam's questions in Visitor Posts...

Reader's Post: Hello Sir, I randomly came across u and your writing via Howzit Jinja. So, I guess you accomplished your goal by posting on there. I have read 3-4 of your timeline posts. I find your perspective and writing thoughtful and to some extent fascinating. Mostly, I am fascinated by the fact that you write and post these thoughts in a public way. I have 2 questions for you: 1) how do you make money in UG? It almost feels to me, you've

Finally Somehow Home

written some of these things out of necessity, forceful passion. 2) what is the underlying reasoning for posting these things? I find it hard to believe that you just want to stir the pot. Do you feel you are contributing to the world via your posts and writing? If so, in what way? Feel free to not respond at all; as well, feel free to respond via PM

Reply: Sir, Thanks for tracking me down through the Howzit Jinja page and taking the time to look over my stuff. Mostly, thank you for the questions. They are direct, some are difficult, and all of them seem to have a reason for being asked. Those are good questions and I will answer them all with the truth they merit.

Firstly, I did accomplish my goal! But my goal was not to peddle my writing. I have met you, and I hope it will lead to meeting you and other Jinja-ites in person.

Some background: I was born in the US, but when I was 2 my parents moved to Indonesia. I grew up there until I graduated high school. We got there in 1979. My dad used to fly around over the jungle, hours by air away from any kind of civilization. He and his fellow missionaries would look for smoke coming up from the jungle below. If and when they spotted smoke, they would mark it on a map, then spend weeks hiking through Sulawesi's mountains

Finally Somehow Home

and triple canopy rain forests to see if they could make contact with the people groups whose smoke they had spotted from the air. These people were as primitive as you can get. They had only occasionally met anyone from the coast to trade rattan and rubber for leaf springs to make machetes and spear heads, wire and bicycle inner tubes for their spear guns, salt, and other necessities of war and life. Their whole world since the beginning of the earth had been only them and the jungle with the few other equally primitive tribes who they were constantly at war with. They called themselves the people of Bahasa Madi: The people of the language of "NO". They were all about 5 feet tall or less, each tribe's trappings were unique, but all wore only a loin cloth, a small pouch for their betel nut, a razor sharp machete, its handle adorned with human hair from the heads they had taken, each in an ornately carved scabbard tied with wicker weaved rope around their waist. Leather would rot in the jungle. Two bamboo tubes about a foot long tied together and filled with blow-gun darts. The poison for the darts was there, ready, in the recess of the bamboo lid in the form of a dark tar-like substance. The blowguns were 8 feet long and their spears 12 or more. Some carried short daggers with L-shaped handles and blades treated with poison, the blades intentionally rusted

Finally Somehow Home

so that the poison was within the powdery rust. They lived in houses which were at least 20-30 feet off the ground to keep enemies within their own or other tribes from spearing them through the floor while they slept. Constant wars and vendettas. They did have medicine. From the Dūkūng. The witchdoctor who communed with the demons and ancestors that dominated their daily lives through taboos, curses, and the like. In one tribe, for instance, it was taboo to cut the grains of rice from the stalk unless done from directly behind it. A trespass would be found out and punished severely, sometimes by death, lest the tribe bear the ever-present wrath of the spirits they worshiped. The spirits of the trees and mountains and rocks. I saw a look in their eyes I will never forget.

When I returned to the US at the age of 18, I joined the US Marine Corps. I was in a Special Operations unit called Force Recon. It's what people would call Special Forces. Altogether, I worked in units like this for 15 years, all over the world. In wars you've probably forgotten, or maybe didn't even know about. I've never been to France or Switzerland or Monaco, but I've been all over this planet. They don't send you to places like that. They send you where there is pain. But I have been to some wonderful places too. I was a businessman in Washington DC for

Finally Somehow Home

several years and have traveled all over the world, from one Business Class lounge to the next. Four Star Hotels weren't good enough for me, neither was a Toyota, or a Casio, or an ink pen that cost less than $200. Yes, I bought into it, hook line and sinker. A friend of mine spent $15,000.00 USD for two nights at a hotel in Dubai, just because, at the time it was the most expensive hotel in the world. I haven't been a millionaire, but I've come pretty damned close. Then I lost it all. Everything. In one day. I'm glad I don't have that life anymore. I don't like who I was. Don't get me wrong. I'm not apologizing for anything. Making money is one of the hardest things to do in the whole world. Everyone is trying to do it. If you're good at it, and fair, my hat is off to you, and I hope you enjoy spending it. I might still get rich one day. I've invented a few things that might be novel. But not right now. This is too important. I need to write. That's why I came here. One-way ticket. Just to write. No job. No money. Just an invitation from my best friend to stay with him and his wife in Entebbe. And write. It was a giant leap of faith. The bravest thing I've ever done. Everyone, even long-time friends and mentors, told me it was a bad idea. And it's been the most amazing time of my entire life. Read "The Heavy Kind of Pain", and you'll get the play-by-play.

Finally Somehow Home

Since then I've found a job supervising the construction of a University Campus here in Uganda.

But I won't stop writing. I can't. To answer your question, I don't get paid for any of my work. As of now I have not even tried to. I'd love to be able to make a living with just my writing, and I'd like to get there, but I don't even know what that would look like. Poetry hasn't been cool since Edgar Allen Poe. I don't think that will change too much. You're right about one thing specifically, and I'm very glad that you caught it. These are ideas. They may or may not rhyme, but they are not just cute little words that sound pretty together. I sure hope not anyway. The purpose of Art ought to be to facilitate the creation of new ideas in the mind of the reader. To see things differently, or to think about something in a way that you've never thought of it before. So, if you want to get people to get honest with themselves, that's the best way to reach them, but honestly, I'm a writer. That's it. It's all I've got. So that's what I use. So what's it all about? I guess it would look like I'm just trying to get attention, or stir the pot, as you say. I'm glad that you asked that because my motives for writing this stuff surely come into question by a reader, and I don't want that to distract them from the important stuff.

Finally Somehow Home

You know that look I mentioned in the eyes of those tribal people on the island of Sulawesi. Do you know why I'll never forget it? Or why I felt compelled to foist my life story upon you? It's because I've seen people in every stage of cultural evolution. From the tribal person in a loin cloth, to the businessman in a $10,000 suit. And everything in between. And in every context from war to opulent luxury verging on the ridiculous. We all have one thing in common. Some have more diversions than others, so it's harder to see, but it's there. It's right out in front for the people of Bahasa Madi, or that little girl gazing out into nothing, standing by the road in the war ravaged bedlam that was once the town of Ar Ramadi, Iraq. There are no diversions for them. They face it every second. They have to. They are afraid. They are uncertain. Of everything. They don't understand. And they have lost hope in ever finding an answer. It's in their eyes. And the reason I'll never forget it, is that I see it every single day. That same look is in the eyes of all of us. Of every human being who, at the very core of who they are, when all the rest is stripped away, are certain beyond any doubt of only one thing: They don't know the truth.

It doesn't matter if the truth exists, or if it doesn't. If it's possible to find, or not. They don't know it. All that they

Finally Somehow Home

know is that the fear is still there. The uncertainty. And the hopeless bewilderment. In its purest form it is expressed in the face of a newborn child who feels the sharp sensation of pain. With every possible facility of expression its bewildered soul cries out only one enormous question: "WHY?"

And we have no answer to give it. Because we have none for ourselves. And this is the human condition. And it breaks my fucking heart. Because I know what the truth is.

I have no fear. I know my destiny. And I don't like the answer, but I know "Why". My life is far more than the breaths that I take. Live is a verb. And it has been given to me as such. I am a free man. So when I see that look in people's eyes. And I know that I know what can set them free. What enrages me more than anything on this earth, is the power of lies against truth. That even if I lay the truth out before them, the lies they believe will reject it. Or embrace but mutate it into another lie. For if truth is "adjusted" one iota, it is no longer truth. It can't be. If it is not exclusive of everything but itself, it is not. There is only one truth. And its greatest enemies are the lies that it does not exist, that it is incomprehensible, and its own distortion. The less distorted, the more insidious is the lie that it becomes, because it looks so much like the truth. It is counterfeit. No matter how good the quality, it is still counterfeit.

So, I'm not trying to "Stir the pot", if you mean that I just want to be controversial. I don't give a shit about creating controversy. In fact, it becomes a huge distraction from my aim. Assumptions are another huge distractor. Assumptions of my aim, or of my message. You see, in many cases, there is no message. I just want to make you think. I'm not going to foist my beliefs on anyone else. Why should they believe me? Why not some other self-proclaimed prophet? My aim is to help them identify the lies that they believe in. We all believe in lies and don't know it. Whether it's about who we are, or our self-worth, our abilities, potential, or even about the nature of money. We all lean on false beliefs. Only when we remove them do we see actual change in ourselves and our behavior. You'll never be skinny enough, if you believe you look fat. Only when you see the lie and remove it, can you see yourself as you really are. In truth. See what I mean? The truth is there. We just don't see it because there is a lie in the way. That's why I don't feel that I have to tell you what to believe...not that it would work anyway. If I help show people how to spot lies, the truth will emerge. And it may even surprise you what the truth is. You may have looked right at it before, and missed it. Because you weren't ready to receive it. There was a lie in its place.

And I want people to know how to recognize the lies that surround the truth. So, if they choose to, they can reject what they know in their hearts to be bullshit because it doesn't make any sense. Truth is reasonable. It is logical. Many lies will tell you not to use reason, especially when it comes to things like God. They will say that you must rely solely on faith. That's a sneaky one because it's almost true. You definitely must rely on faith to be able to accept a being capable of willing this universe into existence. That kind of being is incomprehensible to us just as infinity is. But just as infinity is incomprehensible, it is not untrue. Reason shows us that infinity is true even though we cannot comprehend it. In the same way, we must rely on faith IN THE TRUTH to arrive at a true but incomprehensible being. Belief systems that throw out reason subvert any possibility to validate their claims of truth. Very sly. But the lie is easily spotted. If they proclaim a supreme being and source of existence, surely its attributes are represented within that which the being has brought into existence. And they are. The universe functions on order, logic, and reason. So to say then that

Finally Somehow Home

you must abandon reason in order to understand the source of existence of a logical universe is stupid. It makes no sense. It is a lie. Reject it. If such a being exists, it will by nature be fantastic and inexplicable. If it is not, it is surely a concept from the mind of a man. And if it is not, why believe in it? I cannot even comprehend my own mind, so if I can comprehend such a being, it is less than me. I will just believe in myself and be done with it. Religion does this. It makes God small enough for us to understand, but not big enough to be God. So people choose to believe in their religion instead of their God, because their God is impotent. Even those closest to the truth do this. Many of them know the truth, but they don't believe that it is true. They don't know well enough to be sure. They are just as afraid as everyone else. So they have made the truth into a religion. Then believe and place their trust in their religion, not in their God.

So the reason I write what I do is that I want to give people the courage and understanding to defy the lies. To seek the truth. And don't dare settle for anything less. If you seek the truth with all your heart, you will find it. This is True. And the Truth will set you free.

Chapter 23

Another wonderful month came and went in Uganda. I fished the Nile River and Lake Victoria, and from the lake hauled in a massive Nile Perch. I explored Mbale' and Jinja and Kampala and made friends all over, but the work I was doing made me uneasy because I didn't feel qualified to do it. I called a friend of mine back in the States who had done large-scale Project Management of the same nature and asked him if he wanted the job. He said he did, so I worked out a deal with Tad and his company to do a switcheroo. New York was also on my mind. The city had its hooks in me, and I very much wanted to pursue the job there if it were at all possible. I decided it would be more advantageous to do so from back in the States, so with mixed feelings, I left Uganda and went back to Oregon to stay in my parents' basement

Finally Somehow Home

– yet again – until, or if, rather, the New York opportunity worked out.

I arrived back in the States in early July and immediately reached out to Denise to let her know that I was back in the US as an excuse to check up on the status of things. She said that she had a meeting with Dale in two weeks and would let me know. In the meantime, summer was on, and the fishing was great, so I spent plenty of time on the water and decided to take up fly-fishing. Fly-fishing is like conducting the orchestra of nature. It is elegant and beautiful and deadly. Learning it taught me this: Finesse is deadliest. There's nothing else quite like it. I love all kinds of fishing. It's the only activity I know where one can just sit and wait patiently in eager anticipation for something good to happen. And it usually does. But fly-fishing is something special and inexplicably so. I was enamored with it.

I was standing in the middle of the large back yard at my parents' house practicing casts with my fly rod when I noticed a fly landing on a peach in a tree about 30 feet from me. There's a challenge, I thought, and proceeded to attempt to flick the fly off the peach with the fly on my line. At first I was way off, but soon dialed it in, and

Finally Somehow Home

thanks to the fly's obvious distraction to the world around him, I was able, within afew minutes, to tune my casting to the point of perfectly flicking the fly off the peach. Holy shit! The level of accuracy required to, not smash the fly, or touch the peach, but perfectly flick the fly off the peach was actually doable by look and feel alone. I wonder how difficult it would be to teach a machine how to do that, I thought. It's definitely possible, and probably pretty simple. I looked into it abit. Whip physics is actually a thing. When you crack a whip, or if you cast improperly with a fly rod, you'll hear a crack or snap, which is the sound of the wave in the whip or line breaking the sound barrier. With a fly rod, you'll invariably lose your fly if the wave in the line reaches that speed. I'm sure I could weaponize this, I thought.

It made me think of the creature in the book of Revelation - *They have tails like scorpions, and stings; and in their tails is their power to hurt men for five months... and their torment was like the torment of a scorpion when it stings a man. And in those days men will seek death and will not find it; they will long to die, and death flees from them.* It was fucking brilliant, actually. With a long line or cable of some kind on a hydraulic

Finally Somehow Home

boom, with the right control algorithms, one could quite literally reach out and touch somebody hundreds of yards away. How you touched them depended entirely on the situation. If it was an enemy fighter surrounded by kids, for instance, you could very accurately and surgically remove him from the equation without injury to anyone in front, behind, or around him. If your target was a building, you could reduce it to rubble with afew whips from a steel cable. It also made me think of an idea that I had presented in a large meeting of the minds when I was working for the government. We were talking about "Less than Lethal" weapon systems. Again, thinking of the critters in the book of Revelation, I brought up the Stonefish. The Stonefish has a venom released through spikes in its fins that contains the chemical verrucotoxin. This shit will fuck you up. Symptoms of a Stonefish sting include:

- Difficulty breathing
- No heartbeat
- Irregular heartbeat
- Low blood pressure
- Collapse (shock)
- Bleeding.

Finally Somehow Home

- Severe pain at the site of the sting. Pain can spread quickly into the entire limb.
- Lighter color of the area around the sting.
- Change to the color of the area as oxygen decreases.
- Abdominal pain
- Diarrhea
- Nausea and vomiting
- Anxiety
- Delirium (agitation and confusion)
- Fainting
- Fever (from infection)
- Headache
- Muscle twitching
- Numbness and tingling, spreading out from the site of the sting
- Paralysis
- Seizures
- Tremors (shaking)

And depending on the severity of the sting, this shit lasts for 24-48 hours with lingering side effects for weeks after.

Now, I know this is fucked up, and I'd hope to never have to do it to someone, but what better deterrent is there than prolonged pain and agony. Think about it. If a synthetic version of this were created to persist the pain for weeks or even months on end, do you really think that poor bastard is ever going to pick up a weapon against you ever again? Fuck no. He's gonna want no part of it. Not to mention the deterrent to all the other motherfuckers standing around watching him writhe in unending pain. No one is going to sign up for that shit.

My suggestion was promptly met with guffaws and ire as inhumane, which is completely understandable until you consider the alternative. The alternative is not only the death of the individual you kill, but in many cases, that death is looked upon as honorable, and a door to paradise and bitches. If you remove that from the equation and insert afew weeks of agony, the incessant line of young fighters waiting for their shot at glory, and incidentally bleeding out an entire generation of youth as we saw during the wars in Iraq and Afghanistan and Syria, suddenly dissipates. A great many lives would be saved as a result of a non-lethal solution such as this, and this Whipgun idea would be the perfect delivery system for it.

Finally Somehow Home

I then began thinking about the possibility of building enormous Whipguns in space, or on the surface of the Moon. Not as weapons, but as transport systems. Huge levers could be built in space and even powered with nuclear explosions to launch shit down the axis of the whip. Think of putting a donut around a whip. If the donut can stay within the wave of the whip, which is traveling above the speed of sound down a lever as small as my fly rod, with a massive lever, you could launch that bitch through space at incredible speeds with pinpoint accuracy.

A couple of weeks later I finally heard from Denise in NYC. They didn't have a place for me, and she thanked me for everything, and that was that. I was devastated. So here I was again, stuck in the middle of nowhere with nothing and no prospects for my future. Back to square one. I agonized about it for a week, then started looking for jobs. Suddenly it occurred to me to just look for jobs in Dale's organization back in New York. Why not? I had already interviewed with them, and things had gone well. So, I applied for a few jobs there and let Denise know that I had found several positions that I thought I'd be a good fit for. She said she'd ask Dale about it. It might be another month.

Finally Somehow Home

The next few weeks dragged by like a dog's ass on carpet. I wrote when I could and fished as much as possible and took long walks to make the time go by. My buddy, Snake, from my days in Iraq was in the Seattle area, so I went to see him for a few days. It was always good to see a fellow gunfighter and talk about the old days. While I was there, we visited a friend of his who was making apple cider. I had never seen an apple press in action before and it got me thinking. I wrote this a few days later:

PURE

I didn't know that pain had so many flavors.
Or that everything I can feel can hurt so bad.
All at once. For so long. Like waiting till you're told you can breathe.
When the pain squeezes so hard that it all just crushes out of you.
Like the apple press.
Dripping the bile and blood of my soul.
Pulp and peel are gone. Refuse. Waste.
I am all that is left of me.
I am pure.

Finally Somehow Home

Chapter 24

I wrote some other things during that time as well. A lot goes on in someone's mind while they're waiting. Especially under that kind of pressure. I was still wrestling with my demons. The PTSD was back. I was edgy and nervous and anxious, but I hadn't given up. There's a lot to be said for persistence. Denise got back to me and said that Dale wanted to fly me to New York for a series of interviews. I had a shot.

A few weeks later I headed to New York once again. I had eight 50-minute interviews scheduled, in a row, with eight CEOs from different Agencies of the 265+ companies in Dale's organization. I had ten minutes between each interview, and my lunch break was an hour with Dale and the President of the company. I was more than a little nervous, but every one of the people I

Finally Somehow Home

met with was very easygoing and I found myself back in conversation mode as if we were just having coffee together. I'm not sure of the purpose of those interviews. I don't know if Dale wanted to grill me, or to see if I would fit in well in any of those organizations, but somehow from the CEO of Public Relations, to the CEO of a Tech company, and every type of company in between, I found some common ground and was able to have a meaningful conversation with each of them. It was certainly an exciting organization, and I wanted very much to be a part of it.

At the end of it all, Dale came in and we talked one on one. He told me that I would be hearing from him and thanked me for coming out. I asked him if I could stay in New York and start immediately and he laughed and said I'd better head back to Oregon and wait it out, so back I went. And again, the waiting game resumed.

After several weeks I was beginning to despair of everything again, thinking maybe he had changed his mind again. A month went by. I would check my phone literally every few minutes to see if I had received an email or a call. It was agony. I took long naps. I took long walks. I waited. And waited. And waited. Even fishing

Finally Somehow Home

wasn't fun anymore. And then one day it came. An offer letter for the position of Vice President of Operations. It was surreal. Nothing in the world around me had changed, except for this one thing. After all the agony of waiting, I knew what it was that I felt all at once. It was peace.

I ran to my room and pulled out a poem I had started back in Uganda. I wrote the last line, and it was done.

> *I've been in the desert before.*
> *Walking.*
> *Through the sand.*
> *Hours.*
> *No water.*
> *120 pounds of equipment and a rifle.*
> *The God damn sun.*
> *All you could think about was water.*
> *It would defy any king's ransom to you.*
> *The horizon is so far away.*
> *And I don't yet see our destination upon it.*
> *And then it's finally over.*
> *And you can see the water.*
> *And know that it's real.*
> *And know that you are about to taste it.*

Finally Somehow Home

Then it rolls out like sex across the tongue.
And you swallow its filling wetness like the taste of life itself.
And you're whole.
And quenched.
Stupefied.
It's over.

That's peace.

So, on October 7, 2016 I boarded a plane to my new home, New York City. My uncle and his partner, both incredibly talented artists - a musician and a Broadway actor, respectively - lived in a beautiful Brownstone walkup in Queens, and they very graciously allowed me to invade their space and stay with them while I looked for an apartment. I've seldom in my life seen the love of Jesus modeled as well as the love I received from these two men. I slept on their couch with my suitcases and shit scattered about their living room in as tidy a mess as I could manage. They shared my excitement and joy in this new great adventure. Their peaceful company and cheerful kindness was never once interrupted by even a hint at the certain inconvenience of my intrusive presence.

Finally Somehow Home

New York blew my mind yet again. It seemed a tribute to mankind's oldest and most utilitarian innovation: the elevated flat surface. Think on it for a second. It's an easy innovation, but a very important one. It's not something they created, at first, but rather something they recognized as imperative and sought out in any prospective place of shelter or survival, probably most commonly in the form of big flat-ish rocks. The flatter, the better. These elevated flat surfaces provided a measure of safety and cleanliness as an alternative to sleeping on the ground, they functioned as a workspace, storage space, facilitated cleanly and organized meal preparation and consumption, and very likely contributed directly and commensurately with their form and flatness, to the prosperity of the humans that made use of them. This prosperity may well have been attributed to a divine entity, invoking some form of worship for which the elevated flat surface was used as an altar, as clearly evidenced throughout history. And millennia later, standing in the middle of New York City, unequivocally the most vehement endeavor of the cultural evolution of humanity, I was surrounded by them layered one on top of the other reaching up to the sky like massive alters to the innovations of

Finally Somehow Home

humankind. I couldn't help but to recognize that in my single lifetime I had lived in and sojourned across thousands of years of time within the human lives to which mine had been so deeply and thoroughly intertwined along the strange pathways I'd taken on my journey through humanity.

In the maelstrom and pulse of New York I began to understand what humanity really is. When you zoom all the way out on it you start to see it. Humanity doesn't know what it is. Humans don't know what they are. And outside of the context of that understanding lies great depths of belief traps that a mind can fall into. Humanity is an Organism. It's like an animal. It is connected together just as other living things are, but not in the same way. What holds this organism together is not the tissue of flesh and skin and bone. The organism of humanity is sewn and held immutably together through the tissue of human relationship and cascades multiplicatively within the context of time. But it somehow doesn't grow older or wiser with time, but larger, more knowledgeable, and more refined.

It is a flat Organism. In other words, it does not have a hierarchical construct like an animal or human body

Finally Somehow Home

does - with head, shoulders, knees, and toes and all the rest. It is, rather, entirely comprised of hierarchically constructed nodes of only two distinct types, each type differently vantaged and both together perfect in the perpetuation of humanity, and thus equipped with components of respective identical functionality. Not only are the nodes of it physically unattached to each other, but they seldom, if ever, even touch another, except in consummation of the extremes of sentiment – to destroy another, or to show affection and procreate. This amorphous organism, though alive, is not sentient. It does not know that it exists. It is a beautiful wild thing with no equal that we know of. It is fitting that all other existent things marvel at it.

Each relationally interconnected node, though comprised of components of identical functionality, is exquisitely unique and different in behavior, perception, and action. Procreation over time perpetually refines uniqueness of new nodes by orders of magnitude through magnification and exacerbation of paternal traits, characteristics, cultures, habits, beliefs, and everything else that a new human passively or intrinsically inherits from past generations through its parents and caretakers. And each addition to the

Finally Somehow Home

corpus of nodes represents of themselves the most acute strengths of all that is vested in them as eternally unique, and truly the best and most delicately refined characteristics that have ever been or will ever be in a single human at what it does best, the way that only it in all of humanity and history can do it, unto the corpus of human wisdom and knowledge within their unavoidable interactions with other entities. And every single one of these eternally unique components has influence over every other component in the swirls and tides of the ocean of sentiment within which we all humans drift and sway.

I think that's what it means in Genesis when it says: "God created man in His own image, in the image of God He created him; male and female He created them." It appears as though this is speaking not only of man and woman, but of mankind. Two different components connected through the bonds of a relationship that is as powerful and essential as the components themselves. In its original form, a Trinity construct, thus "In His image..."

When you see it like that, you see what an amazing organism humanity truly is. And you see what amazing

Finally Somehow Home

and goddish creatures humans are. And you see what an amazing thing that you yourself are. That's not happy-hoorah motivationally bullshit. That's really how it really is. And once you understand that about humanity, and humans, and of yourself, you begin to understand the nature and enormity of what is each gift that is a human existence - of that unique sharpness that is formed from the tremendous differences of each of us. We are NOT all the same. Not a single goddam one of us is the same. It is, in fact, the vastness of difference between each human that gives each one such great power. The more the same we are, the less power we each and all have. The more astronomical the differences between each component of humanity, the greater the distance between each human's different eternally unique attributes, the more titanic the power of each and the more truly stupendous is the power of the corpus of humanity, whether in whole or in part, whether in a family, a boardroom, a community, a city, a country, a continent, the world, or in the whole of human existence, the further we are from each other in similarity of those sharpest points of each of us, the greater each of us is for ourselves and to each other. The prevailing notion that the importance of diversity is to enable us to all be the

Finally Somehow Home

same together because we're really all the same anyway, is both logically contradictory, and exactly, 180 degrees antithetical to how humanity actually functions. This absurdity condemns the state of what naturally is and attempts to gather our near infinite dissimilarities and cram them all into single, ready-made, one-size-fits-all, easy to understand and control, boxes leaving us exasperated and hateful at those who don't fit into them, and applauding the self-castration of those who willingly do. The hatred comes from ignorance of the essence of this amazing organism. We hate what we fear. We fear what we don't understand. We can't understand something we hate. Understanding what humanity is, and what we each are unlocks and dissipates this vicious trap. In fact, it seems that most of the loudest and most "unsolvable" contentions of society simply evaporate in the light of this reasoning and its derivative truth.

The organism of humanity is existent and temperamental of the collective mind of its components. We can watch it stumbling, and flourishing, and thriving and decaying. It is even subject to attack by disease and pestilence. Massive plagues upon it, such as war, that make it destroy swaths of itself and leave jagged scars with both sides entwined as if trapped together in the socio-cultural aftermath. (Thus, why so much curry in Britain due to the many past conflicts in India.) And other diseases of self-destruction which cauterize future appendages off its own self like a red hot scalpel through flesh. Those things that singe and sear the future of it off and make it not grow there again and lose, in effect, an otherwise everlasting appendage of the exacerbation of each component's future unique contribution to the corpus. For instance, China's "One Child Policy" is going to bite them in the ass hard, because there were so many abortions required to comply with it that the Chinese worker to retiree ratio is nosing into a tremendous plunge, wherein, by around 2050 there will be only 2 workers supporting every 1 person of their elderly generations who can no longer provide for themselves, as opposed to almost 7:1 in 2015. (Makes you wonder about the true purpose for which China developed the COVID-19 Virus, as it specifically targets the elderly.) But, does that mean that the 14-year-old refugee girl with a baby in her belly by rape must be forced to birth and raise the child? I don't think so, but the killing of the unborn writ large is clearly a disease to this organism.

Finally Somehow Home

Until I saw Humanity in this way, I also didn't really understand homosexuality, which, writ large, cauterizes humanity's growth and future because it passively amputates this magnificent cascade of human existence. It cripples and destroys the organism like a ravenous cancer, bringing long and richly cultivated genealogies, bloodlines, and strains of genetic brilliance to an abrupt and irrevocable end. You can like or dislike that statement all you want, but it will not make it untrue or hateful. That's just how that shit works. A master craftsman hates what kills its most magnificent creation. So, after years of agonizing over it, I finally understood and most importantly, understood my place in all of it. And it gave me great power to know it, but left me without excuse, because, while I have never been attracted to men, I myself am drawn grudgingly yet inexorably to it by the allure of the exclusive and extraordinary sensations unique only to male homosex. It is a ruthless and persistent burden with a discernible uncanny power against which resistance without a reasonable understanding of its insidiousness is all but futile, especially in light of the prevailing belief that the physical enjoyment of it equates to an alternate identity which must be adopted at the risk of accusal of

Finally Somehow Home

inauthenticity. A complete but clever crock of bullshit. As if the enjoyment of chocolate by some requires the acquiesce and redefinition of their identity. The prostate, when massaged, brings pleasure to the brain regardless of the ideological disposition of its owner. To say that if one finds it enjoyable, their identity is forfeit is ludicrous. Yet, as I said, I've felt the grip of its great power, and completely understand how so many have, without a reasonable argument against it, sacrificed everything, including their very identities for its sake. Most things that kill your life are self-evidently destructive, but some things are like the tree in the garden from which you "may not eat". It makes no apparent sense NOT to indulge, as it is clearly "good for food", as Eve observed of the fruit, and in this case, brings great pleasure, and to many is a consummation of deep love, but when you zoom out of the microcosm of a single human life and see the cataclysmic destruction it brings, it is more insidious than war, plague, and famine to the organism of humanity. All that being said, it does help to understand why it is bad for me and for humanity, but it doesn't make it any easier to grapple with from day to day. If you aren't drawn toward it, then you should thank your lucky stars. It's a dark and

Finally Somehow Home

powerful force, and almost insatiable. Many have been lost by going only one step further into its maw, and now live lives completely eclipsed by nothing but sensation.

Racism is another of these unsolvable contentions. It exists because, again, we don't know what we are. Both individually and collectively, we have an untrue concept of ourselves. You are daft if you think the only difference between races is the color of skin. The differences go much, much deeper than that. Each has been built up from the beginning of humanity within their own disparate and unique contexts. Each's way of thinking has developed differently as each culture has evolved within their race and region. The physical components are much the same, the corpus of knowledge may be much the same, though that is highly improbable, but how all of this is processed by each culture, and more specifically, by each human within its culture leans heavily on the foundations beneath it. And each foundation is entirely different. Each foundation is different for every single human. Fractal problems may come close to explaining how humanity works. In mathematics, a fractal is a recursively created never-ending pattern that is usually self-similar in nature. Each human is a fractal, of a fractal of a fractal of a

Finally Somehow Home

fractal... reaching back each generation to whatever the beginning was. Furthermore, each family, tribe, clan, culture, and race is fractal and far different from its adjacent counterparts. They cannot be made suddenly congruent because the splits have been happening on multiple dimensions over time, reaching back through the entire course of the existence of humanity. Yet, while the influence of family, tribe, clan, culture, and race are each refined within each splinter, the splinters themselves increase and continue to diversify. When these fractals intersect others with a different history of cultural evolutionary multi-dimensional development, they influence each the other to varying degrees, which further adds to the gap in disparity one to the next and each to the other.

Racism occurs with the expectation that we are all the same. When different races are exposed to the same information or stimulus, and each responds differently, the tendency arises to be incredulous as to why. Well, if you believe that we are all the same, then the varying responses to the same influences will rightly seem confusing, and the perception will be that one race is more or less apt than the other, depending upon the context of the observer. For each observer, even, will

Finally Somehow Home

likewise judge the response of others according to metrics most important to its own self, its cultural evolutionary foundations, and subsequent worldview.

When human and humanity are viewed in the light of this reasoning, the tenets of racism are undermined. A clear example of this lack of understanding about race and culture is represented clearly in one of the youngest cultures in humanity: the culture of Black Americans. The roots of this culture are derived from the predominant race and cultures of Africa's indigenous population. Physical components (humans), and the concepts thereof, and of this race and culture where transplanted and exposed to tremendous pressure within the foreign context of a very different race and culture. The grafting in of the African culture to the culture of the United States resulted in the birthing of a brand new and unique culture all its own. The outcome is truly remarkable. Within the few centuries of this new culture's existence, it has undeniably and powerfully impacted every other race and culture in the world. Music, style, fashion, all of the arts, in fact; the very definition of how humans perceive themselves and the world around them, aesthetically, and in many other ways is now universally held to the standard of the Black

Finally Somehow Home

American culture. The fight for civil liberties across the entire globe is derivative of this culture's own fight for such. This newly born culture, out of the same information, stimuli, and context, derived that which the predominant culture in the United States, without its influence, would have and could have never been able to accomplish. And thank God for it, otherwise, we'd still be sitting around in our lederhosen listening to accordion music. These are but a few examples of how this, possibly the world's youngest culture, has drastically transformed humanity in a very short time, and will continue to impact it into the future.

Race is too often viewed in two dimensions. It's not like a line, it's like an n-dimensional sea urchin. Each unique culture impacts humanity in uniquely different dimensions and in different ways within those dimensions. However, the value of each is interpreted through the lens of the fractal foundations upon which the observer's perspective rests, and therefore, according to each's own metrics (which are, through ignorance, dismissive of values foreign to its own way of thought.)

Finally Somehow Home

To say that we are all the same is to dismiss the greatest, most powerful, most beautiful attribute we altogether possess. The very things that make us fantastically different from each other are the things that, when one day truly recognized by each of all of us, will finally unleash the full, dynamic, and fierce momentum now dormant within this supremely elegant and complex organism called humanity.

But by far the most compelling discovery in viewing humanity in this way is the discovery of one's own self. When you realize that your eternal uniqueness very likely points to your purpose in this life, the understanding of yourself in the context of humanity as a whole can show you where to look and how to find something that sets you apart from every other human that has ever been or will be on this planet. Because again, the thing that you do best the way that only you can do it, done the best that you can do it, is your very own superpower. That's just how that shit works.

Chapter 25

I grew listless and bored and sought refuge in my writing. It's funny how angst just rings the god damn brilliance out of you. I had been battling with PTSD ever since I hung up my gun belt and quit deploying and had a cubic fuck-ton of PTSD from what I had experienced in my marriage, and for some reason, right then, it all came on with a vengeance.

PTSD is not just waking up with nightmares in the middle of the night. I had some of that early on but that went away. PTSD problems are not easy ones to even pinpoint, let alone resolve. The things that became my undoing were much more insidious and the only way through it was to learn my way out of it. There is just no other way. Around that time, I wrote this poem:

Finally Somehow Home

chi

If you, the latest, brightest apple of my eye,
would condescend to meet again,
though I have wrought your ire,
I would that you would bring a friend
of Bourbon, or of Rye... but please come...

You see that all that you don't know of me
could fill the basin of the sea
and still flood intrigue on the shore
like beer froth spilling o'er the bar.

You've never met a man like me,
nor any man, that I can see.
They're all afraid of living still,
but none have seen the torture mill.
Or they who have keep to themselves
and laugh at all the world calls pain.
Cause we've been there and back again...

And coming back...Is so god damn beautiful...
It's like watching a flower blossom
from the inside.

Finally Somehow Home

And live. And God Damn live.
So...
If you're fucking up my chi, I'm out.

I didn't realize when I wrote it that it highlighted some very serious problems I was having with my PTSD. You see when you are engaged in the business of life and death every day, when you come back, you find that what others consider important you do not. In some ways it's funny, as in the case of the poem. But it's not funny when you blow off your bills because they are "fucking up your chi". See what I mean? You tend to start to dismiss out of hand the things that you do not see as important, and you miss the importance of them because they aren't life and death. I struggled with my finances, and I had since I had come back from overseas. There was no real understanding of cause-and-effect in that regard. Nor was there really an understanding of cause-and-effect for much of anything else, for that matter.

My failed marriage still laid very heavily upon me as well. I felt a tremendous amount of guilt for not being there for my kids. I thought about it every hour of every day. I felt an overwhelming burden of anguish and pain, and furthermore, I felt like I was trapped in a hamster

Finally Somehow Home

wheel with no way out due to my financial situation. It was shameful. Here I was this big-shot businessman, and I didn't have enough money to make ends meet from one payday to the next. I saw no way of getting out. Other than maybe writing. Somehow, I thought maybe if I could make it big as a writer, I could get out of this mess that I was in. I knew it was a ridiculous long shot, but it was all that I had. All of what I've ever written, or most of it anyway, are things that I have learned. I never really wrote just to make words rhyme. I always wrote my way through the things that I was learning. And ironically a lot of the stuff that I wrote, I would go through after I wrote it. It was almost like I was foreshadowing my life in my writing.

I was, of course, still working, but after I got off work I wouldn't go home. I would walk around the city at nights with a 6-barrelled weed pipe in my pocket and duck into alleys or the backs of clubs and take a hit and share with newfound friends. But mostly I would walk into a noisy club or bar, find a place in the corner at an obscure table, sit down, open my notebook and just write. I didn't care about the world swirling around me. After awhile of this I started to notice something new. I noticed how much more people pay attention to you when you block the

Finally Somehow Home

world out and focus on anything else but being noticed by them. I also noticed that I could write better immersed in the chaos of the world around me. I began to feel feverish and frantic that my writing be discovered. I knew I had something good. Something amazing and ready for the world to see. But I felt like I was screaming at the top of my lungs in the vastness of space... and hearing nothing at all. The silence of my own voice was deafening. I think I know why Van Gogh cut his ear off.

I was writing *How to love a man*. I'd been working on it for a couple of weeks and it was exhilarating watching it come together out of nothing and carry such intensity in it. I was writing at a bar in Greenwich village, head down, completely absorbed in it and blocking out the rest of the world as the bar began to fill for the rush that night. I was sitting at a high-top table by myself when three Mexican construction workers just off their shift and still in their work clothes politely asked if I'd share the table with them. "Of course." I moved my papers over to make room and let them banter on around me as I dove back into it. After a few minutes I could feel their curious eyes on me as they became intrigued as to just what the hell I was doing. I glanced up and they asked me

Finally Somehow Home

about it. "Oh, nothing. Just doing some writing." I told them, and got back to work. Curiosity slaked, they returned to their bullshitting, but I could somehow tell their attention had been captured by a table of girls across the bar who were, unfortunately for my new buddies, way out of their league.

I looked up and handed them the poem. "Hey, take this over there to them and tell them that you wrote it." I said. They liked the idea and took off toward their targets with poem in hand. I went to the bar and got a drink. By the time I came back, those three dudes were the most popular people in the place. The girls were passing the poem around and reading it in turn. It was interesting to watch them become as immersed into the piece reading it as I had been in writing it. It seemed to completely absorb each one as they read it to themselves. Their face looked far away and their brows furled in concentration. Then when they reached the last line it was as if they were coming up from somewhere deep to breathe air again. And their faces showed it all.

After awhile, my construction buddies spilled the beans and word got out that I was the poem's author. Soon my

Finally Somehow Home

table was swarmed with women and others who'd read it. People were waiting in line to read it. It passed from one hand to the next throughout that whole bar that night. One very attractive girl with long straight dark brown hair approached me as soon as she discovered who'd written it. She told me she studied literature in Graduate School. "Are you famous?" she asked with a little laugh.

"No".

"Well, you're going to be." She said as she whirled away from me.

That's the first time I'd seen that kind of response to my work. It was mesmerizing and intoxicating. It was one of the happiest nights of my life. I realized with *How to love a man,* that I could say anything at all that I wanted to say if the intensity of the rhythm and rhyme was enough to captivate the reader to the point of literally not giving them room to breathe.

Later that night the young beautiful brunette Grad student started dancing right in front of me, grinding her perfect ass into my crotch. I looked at her slightly amused because her boyfriend was standing right next

Finally Somehow Home

to me with a "what in the actual fuck" look on his face. He wasn't even mad. He was confused. "What's your deal, man?" He said. "Nothing bro. I'm just hangin out. Doing alittle writing." "Oh", he said as if it all suddenly made sense. "You're the writer." And he turned and left his girlfriend to rub her ass against my junk.

Here's "How to love a man":

How to love a man she said expressionless – hidden like a treasure chest – that question is a gem – how to love a man she said again – mischievous and then it broke but she still tried to hide it. That smile she hides behind her eyes sometimes, though she knows I'll always find it. No matter where it is. It's mine. There it is. I told you so. It's beautiful. It blossoms out across the face and skin and lips and eyes and mine is there to meet it – only just the faintest brush the lightest touch is just enough to change a life to stop in time to surge the tide of life inside and find that I'm still in her eyes with nothing I can hide behind. Like summer wind the kiss begins it's sweet and slow and soft as sin the lips and neck and back and breast and then the lips again the clothes are on the grass her skin is soft her back is strong her breasts are in my face again she draws me in I feel her wet her liquid flesh her sweetest pinkest softest

Finally Somehow Home

sin inside the wet the sex the slap and splat of cock and cunt the slurp and suck the sweat the lust the shit the fuck the look of pain the nails the veins the scraping flames her dirty gaping eyes roll back my finger finds the crack it's in her ass her vision blurs her mind explodes she shakes she squirts her face unloads emotion pain then red again her eyes are back her body tight her ass surrounds my cock it hurts at first but then she feels it deep and big and hard and pushes back I feel the surge the blood the buzz the world is red and blurred she pushes back she wants it deeper in her ass she squeezes hard she's strong as fuck I can't hold on I'm gonna cum but she's not done with me just yet - her fingers slide like lightning striking on the inside- blinding fast and deep inside my ass and blow apart my fucking mind it all goes dark I'm hard as fuck I'm blowing up I thrust again and shake a scream and quake and cum my seed erupts there's no control of anything the overload is too intense my soul's escaped to join with hers it surges through her holes and fills the temple of her soul that's hers alone on earth to give as all the holes and soul and skin of me are hers to do with as she'll please she'll play away and stay awake and lick and suck and stick her fingers in my butt and other stuff and I will do the same to her but never ever hurt the girl who trusts in me enough to let me treat

Finally Somehow Home

her like a slut to fuck her face and butt the crazy stuff. Without the trust it's just the lust and guilt and shame and doubt and pain and all that other shit again. The girl inside of her I trust as much as I respect the boy in me who loves himself and owns his shit enough to love to lift her up above himself – it ain't just love all by itself – there's other stuff – if she actually likes the motherfucker's most of it – that's enough – it gives him fire 'cause when he looks into her eyes and sees the only thing a good man needs that she believes that he's the fucking shit – the man – the best – a beast – the God Damn Bomb – the motherfucking Virgin's womb – the goodest man she's ever seen – he won't back down from anything or any fight or any chance in all his life to prove her right and he will bend the very path of light from straight to round if that is what it takes before he ever lets himself let down the girl who treats him like her fucking man.

I had been studying Van Gogh and Picasso and started painting a little bit myself. My first real painting was actually quite good. It showed the face of a woman. Lightning reflecting off her eyes and lighting up her hair and face as if in a terrible storm, but she had no mouth. I called it *Voiceless in the Storm*. Anyway, I was drunk one night and accidentally left the painting in a

Finally Somehow Home

bar somewhere in the city. I tried to go back and find the place but I couldn't.

One day I went into the Museum of Modern Art (MOMA) in Manhattan with a copy of *How to love a man* in my pocket. I walked up to the wall upon which *Starry Night* by Vincent van Gogh was hanging and pulled out a thumbtack and the poem and tacked the poem to the wall next to the painting. There was a little crowd around the painting, and they all gasped as I did it. I turned to the shocked onlookers and said, "I'm putting this here because it belongs here. Read it and acquit me." The security guard who was standing there gasped too. His eyes got really big and he started scrambling toward me. I took a few steps back into a corner well away from any works of art, pulled my 6-gun pipe from my overcoat pocket and fired up some weed. Incredibly, that act somehow quelled the situation immediately. The security guard started smiling. He was trying desperately not to laugh. I told him not to worry I was not going to do any harm to any of the priceless works of art. Everyone relaxed. The Security Supervisor showed up. She was a middle-aged black woman and after she was told what had happened, she was also trying not to laugh. She then escorted me down

Finally Somehow Home

the hall where I was introduced to one of the museum's directors. She looked at him and looked at me and said, "Tell him what you did" in a way that reminded me of a mother scolding her naughty child. I said that I had put my poem on the wall next to *Starry Night*. She said, "Now tell him what else you did." and she started laughing. So, I told him that I had pulled out my pipe and smoked some weed there in the Museum of Modern Art. I told him that I meant no harm; I just wanted to share my poem. He advised the security guard to usher me out the side door before the cops showed up. By the time I got back to my apartment, someone had taken a picture of *How to love a man* pinned up next to *Starry Night* and posted it on Reddit.

I went back a couple days later and spotted one of the security guards who had been there. He recognized me immediately with a big smile. I introduced myself and told him I was sorry for the disturbance. He was a cool dude from Harlem and we hit it off pretty well. Then he called over the Security Supervisor and we chatted for a while. It was good to see her again. So, I thought I was cool with the MOMA. Nope. A few days later when I went back, she told me that she was sorry, but she was supposed to call one of the other Directors if I showed up

Finally Somehow Home

again. She apologetically escorted me down to the main lobby where a policeman was waiting. The cop was a pretty built dude and had an Eagle Globe and Anchor on his forearm.

"Who were you with?" I asked.

"3/5 ," he said.

"Goddamn, you boys stirred some shit up in Iraq," I said.

He nodded knowingly. "We sure as fuck did."

So, standing in the lobby amid my newfound circle of friends, the Director walked up and told me very seriously and in no uncertain terms that I was not welcome there until "further notice" while my new friends and I struggled to keep a straight face throughout the beratement and banishment. As far as I know I'm still *persona non grata* at the NYC Museum of Modern Art. Sorry MOMA. I hope someday you'll let me come back. I still think that Van Gogh would have gotten a great bloody kick out of the whole damn thing.

Unfortunately, yet in a fitting coup de grace, I lost my job around the same time, and for the same reason. I had been sharing my writing with Dale and others, and after

Finally Somehow Home

finishing *How to love a man*, I could not help but to send it out into the world. Unfortunately, again, all the people that I sent it to did not see the poem the same way that I saw it at the time. Some saw it as pornographic. Which is completely understandable, but the headspace I was in then was all about writing and the creation of art. Either way, Dale got a complaint or two about it and we had a meeting early the next day. I had already, weeks before, left a note on Dale's desk telling him that I didn't think I was an asset to the organization anymore and that I didn't feel right about collecting a paycheck if I wasn't contributing to its success. The outcome of the meeting was a mutual agreement that I be let go with a severance package of three months' pay.

Finally Somehow Home

Chapter 26

I got my severance check in the first week of April, 2017. It turned out to be about 25 Grand. I was anxious as fuck about what the fuck I was gonna do with my life, and yet, simultaneously relieved to be getting on to the next chapter, whatever the hell that was going to be. I decided I was going to take a crack at being an artist full time. I was also seriously considering taking a trip to Indonesia and finally going home after 22 years. I figured I had enough to last me for at least a few months. So, I paid 2 month's rent to Banksy and hopped on a bus down to DC to see my kids. It was always bittersweet seeing them. I handed the Ex a big wad of cash when I arrived as I wouldn't have any income for the foreseeable future. David showed me all his video games, and I had promised Dani that we would do a photo shoot, so we

Finally Somehow Home

collected her a bunch of outfits and went to different places around their apartment complex and set up props and she posed for the camera as if she knew exactly what she was doing. I coached her through a little bit of it as I had done some modeling a few years before, but she was a natural. On the last day I saw them I arrived at their place to find that David had somehow suffered a minor burn on his hand and was complaining that it was hurting him badly. The wound was dressed but looked as if taped and wrapped too tightly with gauze. When I attempted to redress the wound, I was met with adamant and intense refusal by his mother. She grew very angry. It took all that I had to keep my cool. So, with no other options, and before I did or said anything I would later regret, I gave my kids a hug and told them "I am always loving you." and left the apartment. I sat there in the rain on the stoop of one of the apartment buildings and realized that not then, nor ever, would I be "allowed" to truly care for my kids. I was not invited. A giant wave of realization swept me suddenly away into a place of deep despair and I wept bitterly there on the stoop in the drizzling rain as if the only wonderful part of my life had just died.

Finally Somehow Home

I texted a friend who lived in the area and asked him urgently to meet with me. By the time he got to McCormick and Schmick's in Reston Town Center, I had already ordered three fingers of Lagavulin 16, neat, and was about to consume it when he snatched it out of my hand and put it back on the bar. It was about 10:30 AM. I asked him, since he lived in the area, would he facilitate an emergency backchannel communications plan for me with my kids because I had a keen suspicion that at some point my communications with them would be entirely cut off. He wasn't having it. I can't say that I blame him. I was wild-eyed, wet from the rain, and had obviously been crying. I was a total mess. He asked me if I was OK before he headed back to work. I really didn't know what to say, so I said that I was. But I was not OK. Not fucking OK at all.

I don't really know what it was. I don't really know if I just snapped or what. Maybe. Maybe it was more gradual, but I was living it and to me I was doing fine. But I wasn't. I didn't want to feel the pain anymore. I wanted to feel good again, and for the first time in a long time, I had the money to facilitate something like happiness. I had no concept whatsoever of my future. The past only brought me pain that I could no longer bear. Only the present was there for me to live in. And I didn't give a fuck if I spent all of my future on it for the sake of feeling good for a change. It didn't even cross my mind to be concerned about that. But all of this understanding of what was going on completely evaded me at the moment. I was living one second at a time again. Just like Ramadi.

I needed more Adderall. So, I got in touch with my connect in DC who I used to go through when I ran out of my prescription. She told me to meet her at The Camelot Showroom. But first I needed a place to stay, and I had a bunch of extra shit with me that I had bought when I first got into town and I was hauling it around in a shopping bag, which wasn't going to cut it. I needed a decent bag. I went directly to REI in downtown DC. I had basically equipped and clothed myself almost entirely out of REI when I was working in Iraq, so I still had an account with them. I picked out a turquoise water-resistant Patagonia backpack. Before I'd left for Africa, I had also stocked up on a ton of shit from REI, so as I was checking out, the cashier informed me that I had a bunch of points on my account that could be redeemed toward purchases. Good to know.

Finally Somehow Home

I looked for a good Hotel in DC. I found one. It was entirely red, with eight red angel statues in the courtyard. The room was red and black leathered. It was perfect in spite of the very strange feeling I had as I walked in. I didn't want to be around anyone that I knew from before in DC. It was as if something was driving me to forget, to start over, to have a new life. The only thing about mine that I cared about any more was my kids, and I felt as if that had just been taken away. So, I was done. It was all too heavy. Too much to bear, so I let it all fall to the ground around me and walked away.

I left my bags in my room and got a taxi to The Camelot. I met up with my connection, got the Adderall, ingested a couple, chewing the 30mg extended-release capsules and grinding the small pellets between my teeth to get the full effect of the drug as soon as possible. I found a good table in front of the main stage on the second floor of the establishment and decided I would play the blindfold stripper challenge. So, I got about $600 worth of ones, fives, tens, 20s and 50s and put them in a big, crumpled pile on the table. The first couple strippers came by and were delighted to play the game, but the next one just grabbed a bunch of 20s and 50s off the table and walked away. "Fuck No." I said. "Come and put that

Finally Somehow Home

shit back!" She got all pissed. "I did not give that shit to you. You just stole it off my table. That is my fucking money, not yours." After a while of squabbling with the thieving bitch, she finally returned my cash. I was fucking livid. I picked up all my shit and bounced, still pissed off, but at least not dwelling on my disasterfuck of a life. I poked around in some other bars downtown DC doing whatever I wanted for the rest of the day and eventually stumbled back to my hotel.

It's not that I wanted to forget about everything, I had been mulling over some very new and different concepts in my mind from the past year in DC, Africa, and New York, and all the cerebral explorations that I had done with my writing. Some of them simple little truths I'd been jotting down, and some of them much more complex that layered one concept on top of the next one, but while they were floating around as separate elements in my mind, I knew that they somehow all fit together, I just needed to clear everything else aside and figure out how. I needed isolation to do that. But most important to me right then was to forget. To be distracted. To be apart from my god damn life.

Finally Somehow Home

When I'd first started writing, my intent was to be a novelist or some such shit. But I didn't really know exactly, I just knew that I wanted to write. It had been supremely frustrating to me that I hadn't yet been able to generate anything close to a fictional work, largely due to all the angst and bullshit that was taking up all my attention. But I had notebooks full of little quotes and ideas and poems and other works of prose I'd penciled down, not to mention the crazy shit that I'd learned and had been preoccupied with regarding existence, purpose, God, war, and everything else that was swirling around in my mind. A few weeks before my trip to DC I was mulling it all over, and within the disappointment of my complete failure thus far to produce or even start on a book of any kind, it suddenly occurred to me that, holy shit, I already had enough material to create a book out of all these little fragments of shit I'd been dwelling on for the past year. Furthermore, I had taken a shine to photography and photo editing. So, I thought, what the hell, might as well take all this shit and dump it into one book. The title for the book emerged suddenly in my mind one day as I thought about the wild-ass roller coaster that was my universe, and I settled on it as soon as it occurred to me. The name of the book would be: *The*

Finally Somehow Home

Perfect Fucking Life. I hadn't even really started compiling the different components of it yet, I only knew what the title would be and had a basic understanding of its composition. Basically, it was a photo and literary memoir of April 1st 2015 – around the time I made the decision to be a writer and fucked off to Africa, to April 1st 2016. It would be an amalgam of everything worth a shit that I had written and photographed from the very beginning of my writing career, up to the present.

I'd been writing under the pen name, ADAM for the past few weeks. I still don't know why I chose that name. When I got back to the hotel that night, I opened my laptop, got online, and officially changed my name from Jason Lee Morrison to ADAM. Then I changed my social media account name to ADAMAFTERDAMNATION. Henceforth, I told everyone, my name would be ADAM. I'm not sure if the transaction failed to go through or what happened, because I never heard anything back from the agency I used to officially change it. It might well be that my legal name is still ADAM, I don't know.

I found myself back at The Camelot the next day as soon as it opened. Mostly just sitting there at a table in a dark corner with my notebook scribbling shit down. I was

Finally Somehow Home

thinking about Jesus hanging out with tax collectors and sinners. In fact, in the Bible, it says that he used to eat and drink with tax collectors and prostitutes. I wondered about the tax collector thing for a while, and then it suddenly made sense. The Roman Empire controlled the Levant at the time which included Israel. In order to excise taxes from the locals, the Romans used a proxy. In other words, they didn't send their Legionaries out on tax collecting duty. It would've been a waste of manpower. So, they contracted it out. Think about this, you have the Roman Empire who demands a certain amount of taxes from each province under its control. Now bring in a middleman and require that middleman to collect those taxes under your authority. The power and authority of the Roman Empire. Who do you think would slide right into that spot if that were the case today? That's right. The Mob. The Mob of that day handled the collection of taxes and would never miss an opportunity to take advantage of the authority under whose auspice they operated to take a little extra for themselves. That's why tax collectors were so damn rich, and so hated by pretty much everyone. Surely, even the Romans despised the crooked fuckers. They outright stole out of the pockets of the people they had the power

Finally Somehow Home

and authority to collect taxes from. So, basically, Jesus used to hang out with gangbangers and strippers. And not just in a casual and bantering way either, it said he used to eat and drink with them. Another use for that word in Aramaic is the word "drunk". This does not mean that Jesus was going around banging hookers and doing drive-bys. If that were the case, the religious leaders of the day would have surely brought it up in his trial before they killed him, but he did establish deep relationships with many people that everyone else of that day despised. The most amazing thing to me isn't that Jesus wanted to hang out with them. Most of my shady friends wouldn't piss on a guy who went around talking about God all the time, let alone want to be friends with him. The most amazing part of that equation is that the shifty motherfuckers wanted to hang out with Jesus. They loved the guy. I think he spoke their language. Most people forget that Jesus grew up in Egypt. From around the time he was 3 years old to possibly 10 or 11. He was a third culture kid like me. He had a very objective view of cultures and knew how to relate to people in their own context. Then he moved to Nazareth in Israel. I've been to Nazareth, It's a shithole. And it was a shithole back then as noted by Nathaniel, one of Jesus'

Finally Somehow Home

disciples, when he quoted a saying of that day "Can any good thing come from Nazareth?". I guarantee Jesus spoke the language of the streets, both from his time in Egypt, from the rest of his life till he was 30 (as far as we know) in one of the most notoriously shitty parts of Israel back then.

Some of the strippers drifted by my isolated table, curious as to what I was doing, and perplexed as to why I wasn't gawking at them like all the others.

"What's your name?"

"Adam."

"Adam what?"

"Just Adam."

"Really!? You don't have a last name?"

"Nope. Just Adam."

"Whachya' doin', Adam?"

Within an hour or so, three or four of them had gathered and were sitting around my table listening as we talked about the nature of our existence, purpose, and what we

Finally Somehow Home

really want. Most people don't know how to want. The hardest part isn't getting what you want. The hardest part is the discovery of what that really is. When you find that, you will come face to face with yourself for the first time. Then you will begin the adventure of the discovery of yourself. You'll have to. Because the only way to get what you really want is by awakening that person and using every fucking part of who you really are, all at once, on full afterburner. Only there will you find your peace. And peace is the only place deep and rich enough for your joy to grow. Fuck happiness. Happiness is a fat rail of blow, nutting in stripper's ass, ripping it on a dirt bike, whatever. That's all awesome stuff, but it only occupies the present. Joy can't grow there because it's eternal. Your joy is linked to your eternal soul. To who the fuck you really are. And when you awaken that giant in you, and begin to manifest yourself, become yourself, you are drawing from something eternal, something more acute, sharper, and infinitely unique than every other human on earth, that nobody ever born or to be born, can ever begin to rival. The outcome of this dormant creature's awakening, discovery, and full manifestation is the only hope you have of "what you really want". And the only hint you

Finally Somehow Home

have to find yourself and begin your awakening is the answer to that question.

So, what do you really want? You must think about it courageously. Be bold enough to want what you are afraid to. What you could never now become. If it's not far as fuck beyond your reach, it's the wrong answer.

I went outside the club and down the stairs leading to the entrance out on the sidewalk next to the busy street, pulled out a Marlboro 72 Gold and lit it.

"Hey man, could I get one of those off you?" He represented himself well for a homeless guy. He was black and tall and had a contemplative face that looked like he'd seen a lot of pain.

"Absolutely." I pulled one out and handed it to him. "Thank you." he said as he lit it off the scratched and battered Bugatti Zippo I proffered.

"What's your name?"

"Adam." I said as I exhaled the smoke from my lungs. "Did you know that Jesus was a gangbanger?" I asked him. He looked at me quizzically. "Well, not really, but he rolled with those dudes a lot. Gangbangers and stripper

Finally Somehow Home

types. He was from a little shithole town called Nazareth. In the middle of nothing on a big hill that overlooks the Valley of Megiddo on one side and The Sea of Galilee on the other. I've been there. It's still a shit hole." We talked for a while. There was a pause in our conversation. We both gazed out at nothing together as if we'd known each other a long time.

"How do I get out of this, Adam?"

"Out of what?" I asked, knowing damn well what he was going to say. But he didn't say anything. He just looked at me, his bloodshot eyes misting.

"Goddamn. I wish I knew, buddy." I said, putting a hand on his shoulder.

Every one of us has this whole big life swirling around us. A full universe that really does revolve around us. We can't help it. That's how it works. No matter how much you empathize with others, and love others, and invest in others, and share their grief and burdens, the center of your universe will always be you. Because that's where you are. The enormity of my own life and all the things and people and ideas that were part of it were no bigger than his at all. But his was all pain. And hopelessness.

Finally Somehow Home

And desperation. No way out. That he or I knew of, anyway. And a way out was clearly the thing that he thought of the most in between every second, thought, and breath he took. In every synapse of his mind, he searched for it, frantic. We were standing right next to each other, but he was in hell. "Goddamn." I said sadly, "I don't fucking know man. I'm sorry. If I ever figure that out, I will come back here and tell you." I left him a couple extra cigarettes and walked back into the club perplexed. The dark cloud of this enigma hanging over me.

I had spent all of my money. I woke up the next morning and left the hotel without checking out at the front desk because I knew my bank account was at least a little bit overdrawn. It was a grey morning in the city and a light rain was gathering. I took my bags and wandered around downtown not knowing what was going to happen next and accepting it matter of factly and without much worry. Instead, an overwhelming urgency seemed to possess me. Deeper than need and more primal than instinct. To do something. Something pivotal. Like a mandatory destiny which was still obscured to me in a thick fog of mystery. As if the burden of my entire life rested on what I did right then. Because it did. And I

Finally Somehow Home

knew that I would have to discover what "it" was for myself. I had nothing else to leverage. No way to postpone this confrontation but to cry for help, and if I did that, I knew I'd miss this one opportunity in my life to discover what it was I must do to survive. I knew if I cried for help, I was finished and resigned to die slowly in my old life. The mastless, rudderless hulk still breaking apart in all the jagged reefs and storms that raged around it. I alone understood the gravity of it all, but that's all I understood of all of it at all. Not as if nothing else mattered, no. But as if there were nothing else at all. Because there wasn't. Like the premonition of birth for one still in the womb. My only clue was this pervasive desire to codify all the swirling ideas in my head. To sew them together and somehow to make sense of them. And with them to create something I could stand upon. I had my laptop with me, two phones, clothes, and random other shit. Enough to survive on, so I knew I'd be just fine wherever I was. The thought of going back to New York seemed like an evasion. It wasn't an option. I knew I'd live or die there on the streets of DC.

The conversation with the homeless man outside The Camelot kept running through my brain like a prophecy coming true, "How do I get out of this, Adam?" And now I

Finally Somehow Home

found myself there. Facing the dilemma that had so captivated my mind only the day before. I wasn't in hell yet. But I was standing on its doorstep.

I found a park bench under a tree that shielded me from most of the gloomy shitty drizzle. My grey SARAR trench coat and its opulent collar protected me from most of the wind. I took stock of everything I had with me and finally gathered the courage to check my bank account balance on my phone. It was -$3226.67. Hmmm. Looks like I'm in for an adventure. I knew that whatever happened I was going to need food, so started racking my brain trying to figure out how to sustain myself for a week or so at least, not knowing what lay beyond that. REI! I grabbed my shit and walked a mile or so the REI and asked if I could stash my bags behind the counter. They obliged and I went off in search of equipment that I thought I'd need. It occurred to me clearly that it was nothing different than a recon patrol. Travel light freeze at night was not a new thing for me. And all the rest of the principles of patrolling pertained to my current situation. Planning, Reconnaissance, Control, Common Sense, and Security. The most important of these being Common Sense. I selected a lightweight bright green camp towel that compressed neatly into a small grey and green zippered

Finally Somehow Home

pouch. I grabbed an inflatable seat cushion for some measure of comfort and to keep all my body heat from escaping into the asphalt or dirt, and raided the Cliff Bars, chocolate bars, and other energy bars, maxing out what remained of my REI points and providing me with about a week of rations. There were plenty of drinking fountains around for water. I stuffed it all into my bags and set out to face my destiny.

Finally Somehow Home

Chapter 27

The rain had abated, but the air was still that humid cold DC muck that sticks to your bones. So, what was I gonna do? Working on *The Perfect Fucking Life* was my first inclination, but the shit weather ruled that out unless I wanted to fry my laptop in the intermittent rain. I still didn't have a clue as to how to get out of this mess, but finally I had nothing at all but time to think. I figured I might as well document my plight, so I sat down on a street corner against a building that blocked me from the wind, pulled out my phone, and started recording. The following is the transcript of over thirty separate segments throughout my time on the cold shitty streets of DC. It has been edited and augmented for clarity.

Finally Somehow Home

April 26, 2017

My name is Adam.

Today is the 26th of April 2017. So, this is the deal. I've learned a lot in my years on this planet about people and about all kinds of different things. And lately I've been talking to a lot of people who've gone through some hard times and I've been doing what I can to take what I've learned from my life and give it to them. But I think the best way to see the truth of the things that I've been saying, for me and for the people I've been saying them to, is to live them out and see if they actually fucking work.

So, here's the thing... Somehow, out of some crazy course of events. Today is my first day as a homeless man. I did not see that one coming.

But this is what I have available: I have a laptop. I have a phone. My phone is going to die soon, all the minutes and data are going to expire on it at the end of the month, and today is the 26th. So, I have those assets available until that time, internet, etc., for data and a hot spot for the computer.

Finally Somehow Home

There are a few probabilities that I have to take into account: The likelihood of all this equipment holding up for very long and the likelihood of me being relieved of my possessions at any given time. I have quite a bit of stuff. I've got my computer bag, and this little backpack, and - since I wasn't actually planning on being homeless, I was just traveling - and this other backpack that's got a few sets of clothes in it.

My bank account is overdrawn by $2600. (Several charges hadn't yet hit at this time.) *So, there's no way that it's going to sort itself out. I have a check from the VA coming in at the end of the month. It's like $1,100 or something like that. So, all that's going to do is just get it closer to zero. Either way, so, it's a bit of a challenge, here. The funny thing is, none of the equipment that I have with me is what's going to get me out of this. And it's not through selling it that's going to enable me to overcome this. Selling it is only going to make me have fewer capabilities, and basically just prolong the agony. And it's the same thing if I ask for help, if I ask for money or anything like that, or if I ask for someone to bail me out, or call a friend or family, it doesn't matter, obviously something's going on here. Otherwise, I wouldn't be sitting here. So, let's see what I can*

Finally Somehow Home

do about it using just this, my mind, to get me out of this situation.

I am Adam.

April 27, 2017

So, first things first, today I got up after quite a pleasant sleep under a nice overpass. But the night before, I realized that I had like 130 bucks left on my REI account - that just popped into my head. And with that, I went to REI, and I got a pad to sit on and a towel. I put the towel over my head to keep my body heat in, and wrapped another shirt around my neck, and then I was fine. I had leather pants on and a pair of jeans over top of those. I was a little chilly, and it rained a bit but I was under a bridge so I stayed dry. So that was the first night. There's a lot of snatchus-grabus going on around here. I saw a dude get his bicycle stolen last night. I was just sitting there across the street and saw a dude tiptoe up and did the sneaky-sneak on another homeless guy. So, yeah, you gotta keep you keep your eyes on your stuff. Anyway, I got up and came out here and charged my laptop and my phone outside of a good ole CVS that had an outdoor socket. That was nice. Then I was putting my plan together and figuring out what I was

Finally Somehow Home

going to do, and realized, holy shit, this is actually a pretty cool challenge, you know, like, fuck you Bear Grylls.

But how do you get from zero to one? And not just to survive, but to thrive again? I've got no money, I've got no job, I've got nothing, so even if I made it back to New York it wouldn't matter (I had forgotten that I had paid the next month's rent already), *so how do you make it out of this thing? It's not just about getting out of homelessness. How do you make it out of this whole mess? This Wholemessness? That's the word.*

Yesterday as the sun was setting, I kept noticing people walk by and could see them wondering, "What's that dude doing?" That is a fair question. That is the exact question that they should be asking. Like," What's that guy's deal? He looks smart. He looks well off. What's the deal with him? Why is he now homeless?" And the answer to that question is the answer that's going to get me out of here.

I saw some birds in the grass hopping around, eating, and just doing what birds do. And after awhile it occurred to me, that maybe the reason this shit ain't working is because I'm not doing what I was made to do. I'm not doing what I was made for. I think it's time to start figuring that out. What the hell am I good at, best? And love to do? There

Finally Somehow Home

might be an answer there. What do I need to do? What am I? What do I have available? I have experience and knowledge, and I have a brain. I can start tying things together. Some of this I've been thinking on over the last week or two weeks about these abstract things, and I'm seeing some power in them. So now I guess I get to try them out and see if the shit works.

Let's start thinking big. Let's start thinking about how I'm thinking. How am I thinking? Am I thinking the right way about me? Am I thinking the right way about the universe, about existence and all that? Well, that seems a little crazy, but actually that probably has something to do with what the hell I am. So, I might want to start thinking about that.

A good starting point is that this thing that I'm sitting on is big ball of mud. Actually, that's all it is. And there's another big ball of mud up in the sky and that one's on fire. And those things move around each other, right? Well, here's the thing, if I wait for those two balls of mud to spin around each other over and over to get me out of this, is that going to help me out? Actually, no, it's not going to help me out at all. It's two balls of mud. That's time. That's what time is. Just sitting around waiting for time to figure it out doesn't make any sense. Alright, so now we've ruled that out.

Finally Somehow Home

What do I think I'm supposed to think? Well, if I sit here and I look at myself the way everyone is looking at me, and I'm not poking anyone in the eye here because everyone means it in the best possible way because that's how we're taught to deal with things like this, people are actually upset and worried about me because I'm not buried beneath a tremendous mountain of shame, frankly. And I don't blame them. I look at it and it does seem exceedingly shameful. But isn't it strange that my greatest tendency, and the expectation of others, is for me to bludgeon myself to death at this time because of all the evidence of my ineptitude to be able to maintain a normal lifestyle? We all think, "He should be so buried under shame that he is paralyzed. How can he live with himself?" And I've actually been in that position before. And that's exactly what happens when you listen to the shame. Because that is what kills you.

The fact that I'm not freaking out and crying for help is worrying to those who love me. I've experienced this kind of pain before and that's how I responded to it then. And it didn't work. Shame is actually what kills you. Shame is what stops you and freezes you in your tracks from being able to deal with these types of trials in life because you're so busy beating yourself up, (and everyone else is kind of in agreement), at the very moment when you need to be your strongest.

How are you going to be at the top of your game if all your energy is directed toward feeling like you're a piece of shit? A prize fighter does not berate the shit out of himself and have people come and call him names before he goes into the ring. If you need to be at the top of your game, you need to believe in everything that you know about yourself that fucking works, and figure out how to make it work better, and get every single thing about you that works best to fire all at once in order to launch your fucking ass through this atmosphere. That's what I'm talking about. "Fire all of your guns at once and explode into space. Born to be wild." That's what it is. Because the things that you are best at the way that only you can do it, done the best that you can, those are your afterburners, those are your boosters. You may float to the top at the same floaty speed as all the other bubbles, if you want to try it that way. But if you explore yourself and find the things that you do best, that you do better than anyone else on this planet, those are your afterburners. So, let's start looking for those. Let's start looking for the afterburners.

Finally Somehow Home

Look. Get over this idea that we're all the same. Where did that come from? It came about because of an attempt to assuage some pain of abuse, but it's totally fallible. We're not the same. And that's what makes us amazing. I mean, you think about a human being, the thing that makes humanity freaking awesome is that we're not the same.

We're totally not the same. We're absolutely 100% of the best parts of both sides. I have two kids, right? So, my son and my daughter, they are each all of me. And they are each all of their mother. But that creates a new type of human being that is extra sharp at certain things which that human being does the way that that human being does things best.

Why? Because the things that you do best, the way that only you can do them best, and the things that when you really are honest with yourself, say, I'm really good at that. I actually really am. Or, I know that that skill, if I just sharpened it a little bit, it would be better than anyone else that I know.

Guess what?

Those things are things that you, your human being, your beast that you live in, those are things that that thing does

Finally Somehow Home

better than any other beast like it on this planet. What's that mean? The things that you are best at, the way that only you can do them, you are the best at doing those things in the entire history of mankind. In the history of the universe you are a rock star in those things. Alright, cool. So, there's a glimmer of hope and that's the truth. Now this isn't Joel Osteen happy-happy shit. I can't Joel Osteen my way out of this shit with happy-happy thoughts. I'm not saying that things those guys say aren't true, but I've got to get down to brass tacks here, that "Don't worry, everything's gonna be fine." that is complete bullshit. "If you just wait long enough and you deserve it, the universe is gonna bail you out." That ain't gonna work. So, at least we've identified the fact that there are things that I do better than anyone else on this planet because every single one of us, including you, has those things.

Finally Somehow Home

Chapter 28

April 28, 2017

I just woke up. I slept here. It was actually really nice in the morning. The sun was up and it was a lot warmer. Anyway, I have a pretty awesome hygiene kit too, which is nice. I was able to like, put some face cream and lotion and stuff on. See if I can keep myself from going to shit too bad. Anyway, just by the way, in case you end up in this situation, this is a good spot because look, it's along a wall, right? So, if you sleep along the long axis of the wall, then it reduces your silhouette. You just don't want to really draw too much attention to yourself. It minimizes your silhouette and you've just limited your exposure and avenues of approach by 180 degrees, right? So, if anyone's trying to snake off with your stuff, you'll see them coming.

Finally Somehow Home

Anyway, so back to the whole shame thing. Shame is powerful. Look, even in politics. The biggest, most powerful weapon in politics is shame. People will step down from their jobs because of it. It's pretty powerful, isn't it? Watch where that stuff's pointing. You might be pointing it right at your own head, and it's strong. It's stronger than you.

I wrote a poem called "How to Love a Man" a little while ago, I'll post it on social media. Read it. It is going to shock some of you. Some of you are going to think it's beautiful. And some of you are going to think it's raunchy and ugly, you're going to have many different takes on it, depending on one thing. If you remove the shame from it, it's beautiful, it's pure. This is about two people doing what two people do very intimately and beautifully. If it offends you, here's the reason. It's because of your shame. You are somehow letting your shame become involved in what you're reading. It's written in such a way that it is the shame of the author alone. You cannot take that shame upon yourself. Do not touch what is not yours. That is the shame of the author. Leave that alone and read it. It is pure and it is actually tremendously beautiful. It's the shame in you, not the shame in it. It's the shame in you, not the shame in the world that makes it ugly.

Finally Somehow Home

Humans aren't good or bad. Humans do things. Sometimes they're grouchy and grumpy and sometimes they're beaten down by others and it causes them to act in a certain way, but when you develop habits that cause other people harm and take away their clear vision of what life is, you could call that shit "evil". Evil is a byproduct of sin. "Sin" is the shit you do that kills you yourself. It's the shit that others do that gives you an excuse to "sin", which kills you and harms them back. And the deeper you go down that wormhole the more you'll be drawn into it. And, by the way, this isn't an excuse or an "out" for fucking up, but bludgeoning yourself strangely only ever makes you go further. Everything you do that's bad for you "sin", just makes it alittle easier to do the next time because you no longer expect "righteousness" of yourself in that particular regard because you know about yourself that you've already fucked that up before. It gives you a lesser view of who you are that you come to accept, so the next thing that's a little deeper down the wormhole that you'd have never even considered doing before you did the last thing becomes more acceptable to you and it just keeps on going. Thats how an innocent remark becomes adultery which becomes an affair which becomes living a lie, which is a living hell, or that's how being an errand boy for the

Finally Somehow Home

mob becomes filling shipping containers with teenage kids. No one ever starts out to end up there. It happens one small step at a time because of who you've allowed yourself to believe that you are. Life is good, right? Actually, life isn't good. Good is life. Good is life. The more life you have, the more aware of your life, that's good, right? The less aware you are that you are alive, the more you're distracted from it... well, what's the opposite of life? Death. Sin is death because you can't be truly and fully alive. Life is the ultimate good. What if you're fully alive and you're distracted from it and don't realize it for 70 years? That's sad, right? Because you're too caught up in the things that have distracted you from the good, from the life. That's death. Death while you're still alive. So, if you develop habits that bring you death, and in the lives of others, limit their ability to see the beauty of what they are living, then that's evil, evil is the spreading of death. But people themselves aren't good or bad. They do things. They wake up and put their shoes on and the rest of it is just responding the way that they've taught themselves to respond. The way they've taught their beast.

We live in a beast. You aren't a beast, but you do live in one. You must teach your beast. But you cannot just tell it what to do. It will flippantly ignore you. It will get what it

Finally Somehow Home

wants. Regardless of all the thrashing and guilt that you impose upon it. It really doesn't give a fuck about those things. And it is much stronger than you. If it thinks it needs heroine... it will get it. You are helpless against it. And if you ever fully concede your will to its strength. It will slay your will dead. With ease. All of you will become all of it. All of the best that you will only ever be, will be beast.

You secretly hate yourself because you hate what your beast does, and you think it's you. You must love yourself. Enough to seize the power to overcome your beast. You must love your beast to teach it. You cannot understand a creature that you hate and you cannot teach a creature that you do not understand.

The beast you live in is of the wildest things upon this earth. And your will alone cannot tame it. You must love it and learn it and teach it. Your beast is supremely pragmatic and supremely powerful in its element. It hates the thought of your control over it as much as you hate the thought of its control over you. And if you never tame it, you will always fight it on its terms. It will always win. The greatest strength of your greatest will is only effective against it upon your will's own battleground. The

Finally Somehow Home

battleground of your will is Reason. You must train your beast to love what is best for it. Make it a student of the pain that gives it its most power. And it will soon understand.

Only through studied wisdom and the knowledge of its deepest desires do you have a chance. It is your very greatest enemy until you make it your very greatest friend. And no strength of mind can overcome its might... its only weakness to your will is its laziness. But that is not victory. Its strongest desires are the key. It will never want what you want unless you guide it into the understanding that what your will desires is what is best for it... for its own sake. The most strivent reaches to the human in you are the strongest against it... but never on its terms... only with supreme elegance and purpose and understanding and love toward it can you ever succeed. And then you can ride it. And it will be your greatest violence against your greatest enemies in this life.

No amount of Tony Robbins chest beating bullshit can do this. Only you can. And by your wisdom of will alone. Because it is a wild thing. The wildest of all that is animal. For if you but let it, it has a human at its behest. Your ultimate humanity will never be realized without its brute ferocity... so when you do some day bring

Finally Somehow Home

it around... in that place only, will you find that most wild and reckless and dangerous peace of which you've always dreamed.

Finally Somehow Home

Chapter 29

Now let's zoom out as far as we can. We each live in a beast, but we are somehow all connected. We have this thing called humanity, and each node of that entire organism that is completely connected through relationship is its own uniquely best thing. And it's been formed over the generations of its cultural evolution by every layer of that cultural evolution. So, you are the best modeled version of humanity that's ever reached that level of cultural evolution. You are better at whatever you do uniquely best, than anyone else on the planet. That's a fact. That's how it works. It's not like an organism like me, where I'm hierarchical, I have a brain, heart, lungs, etc., each with a different function, The crazy thing about this organism is that it all exists on one layer. Every single element of that organism to reason and everything else exists on one

Finally Somehow Home

layer. And it's all influenced by the emotions and the sentiment and the behavior of the other ones. It's a butterfly effect. And the same thing with the sentiment going on in different parts of the world. It affects us all. Sometimes you can't feel it. You don't know what the effect is. But you sense things nonetheless through relationships with other humans. And it's such a tight relationship that it actually makes humanity one thing. A single organism. So, what substantiates this idea about the elemental nature of relationship is very interesting. I guess you'd call it essence. That idea came from a conversation I was having with a friend of mine who is a nuclear physicist. We were talking about the smallest unit of existence. I wrote a paper on it called "The Annihilation of Nothing and the Advent of Existence" which demonstrates that you can't have just one fundamental unit of existence. If that were the case, everything would just be the exact same thing. But you cannot have just two different things either, because with two different things, comes a third – the relationship between the two. Very interesting that nothing exists out of "nothing" if not in Trinity. And this Trinity seems to entirely occupy all that is existent, because, once it replaces "nothing", it takes up all of "everything". And whatever the fuck it was that could

Finally Somehow Home

suddenly exist out of "nothing", it's safe to call that thing "God", but what is even trippier is that there is no such thing as nothing. The word "nothing" is self descriptively impossible, so that means that whatever this Triune thing is, it has always been. It is truly eternal in nature, so yeah, if anything deserves that name "God", it's that thing. But there's a problem here. So, where the hell did the universe come from then, if this Trinity takes up all of everything, there's no room left for the universe to exist. Well, what if this Trinity thing projects, or radiates whatever else is. It kinda makes sense, because we ourselves project meaning upon shit around us. A dog knows it drinks water out of a thing that holds water, but a dog doesn't ascribe a name – a meaning, to that thing. Only we do that shit. We call it a "bowl". Somewhere along the line a human said, "Goddamn it, I'm gonna call that thing that my dog drinks water out of something. I'm gonna call it a bowl." Well, that's kindof our job. Part of what humans were made to do. "Out of the ground the LORD God formed every beast of the field and every bird of the sky, and brought them to the man to see what he would call them; and whatever the man called a living creature, that was its name." Genesis 2:19. Man projects meaning on the universe around him. That's what science is. So, it's not too far of a stretch to think that

Finally Somehow Home

maybe we are an emission of this Trinity thing. Of God. "God, after He spoke long ago to the fathers in the prophets in many portions and in many ways, in these last days has spoken to us in His Son, whom He appointed heir of all things, through whom also He made the <u>world</u> [αἰών / aiōn : continued duration; a space of time, an age]. And He is the radiance of His glory[lit."brilliance"] and the exact representation[χαρακτήρ / charaktēr :a tool for engraving] of His nature [ὑπόστασις / hupostasis : substance] and upholds all things by the word[ῥῆμα / rhēma :a word, by impl. a matter: discourse, fact, message, statement] of His power[δύναμις / dunamis: power, might, strength, ability, meaning]. Hebrews 1:1-3. So, you could read that this way after looking at the Greek meanings of those words: "God, after He spoke long ago to the fathers in the prophets in many portions and in many ways, in these last days has spoken to us in His Son, whom He appointed heir of all things, through whom also He made the universe, time, and the age of mankind. And He is the radiance of His essence and the exact representation of His substance and upholds all things by the fact of His meaning." Now that's pretty fuckin' interesting. Also," He is the image of the invisible God, the firstborn of all creation. For by Him all things were created, both in the heavens and on earth,

-397-

Finally Somehow Home

visible and invisible, whether thrones or dominions or rulers or authorities—all things have been created through Him and for Him. He is before all things, and in Him all things hold together. Colossians 1:15-17. (Now, flash forward to 2022 and look at the work of John Clauser, Alain Aspect, and Anton Zeilinger who won the 2022 Nobel Prize in Physics "for experiments with entangled photons, establishing the violation of Bell inequalities and pioneering quantum information science." – Basically, proving that the universe is a "simulation", or maybe another way of putting it is that it is a "projection".) *Huh... no shit!*

Anyhoo... all of this not only shows the essential nature of relationship, but it also serves to inform how we think about whatever that infinite Triune thing is. It serves to inform how we think about God Himself. So, now maybe start thinking of God like something like that. Just throw out all the other shit. Because if there is such a thing as something that exists, that's how it does. That makes a lot more sense than anything else I've heard about God, rationally speaking. So, now we're thinking a little bit differently about God.

Finally Somehow Home

Einstein said, "Science without religion is lame and religion without science is blind. They are interdependent and have a common goal – the search for truth." So, with that then, let's try something new. Let's look at what we know about God or the Bible scientifically. Because up until now, both sides have been poking each other in the eye so much that they can't use each other's Legos. But I bet you there's Legos in both buckets that build the right thing.

It seems as though there's been such a squabble between "science" and "religion", especially between creationism and evolution that they're kind of in a deadlock. Until you start looking and realize that the deadlock has been an emotional one, really. Well, let's look at Genesis again from a scientific perspective as if I was Indiana Jones and I had just uncovered this thing that was written around anywhere from 1200 to 2000 BC and no one has ever looked at it before, and I open it up and start reading it, well, the first part, not surprisingly if God wrote the damned thing, is going to talk about the creation of everything. So now we're going to approach this ancient manuscript scientifically.

Finally Somehow Home

Chapter 30

In order to do this, imagine you're the one trying to explain it in such a way that Og and Zog can understand it. In fact, imagine that you are a scientist with the task of explaining the concepts of Space, Matter, Energy, and Time to primitive people of the earth from several thousand years ago. They have no written language, and no words for these concepts in their spoken language. It would be no easy task, but that is exactly what is going on here. What, from their environment, would you use to communicate these concepts to them? Go ahead. Answer the question in your own mind, before you go on. You're sitting there outside of their shitty little cave around their little fire with them cooking some mammoth meat. What would you use to explain Space, Matter, Energy, and Time?

Finally Somehow Home

These seem to be the most reasonable metaphors for their context and understanding:

Space: the sky, the night sky especially. We'll call it "the heavens"

Matter: dirt or earth, water. We'll call it "earth" or "water".

Energy: the warming light of the sun. We'll use "light".

Time: The track of the celestial bodies across the sky/motion.

These things, of course, exist in their own right, so when you are referring to the actual things themselves, such as the heavens, the earth, light, and time, and not the metaphors, you would have to define them as themselves when the actual things come into your narrative, and thereafter, depart from the metaphorical use of them. For example, if I tell you that I'll be using the word "heavens" to mean "space", I would then be compelled to tell you when I depart from the metaphor and again begin using "heavens" only to mean "heavens".

So, with that being said, let's look at Genesis 1, the first book of the Bible. We'll use the standard convention of Verses in the Bible (e.g. V1) as references.

Finally Somehow Home

V1. "In the beginning God created the heavens [space] and the earth [matter]."

This makes sense scientifically, because matter cannot exist without the space that it occupies, therefore space would come before matter.

V2." The earth [matter] was formless and void, and darkness was over the surface of the deep, and the Spirit of God was moving over the surface of the waters [matter]."

The Hebrew word for "the deep" is תְהוֹם "tehom", which also means "abyss". It can also mean "sea", but "sea" is not defined as such until verse 10, later in the story, when it says: "God called the dry land earth, and the gathering of the waters He called seas." So, we will continue with "earth" and "water" as metaphors for matter until we get there. So, as matter is, of course, not just a solid, but also liquid, gas, etc, "the deep", or "abyss" could indicate some kind of primordial soup. This makes a lot of sense when we see that the matter was "formless (Hebrew: תֹהוּ "tohu" – chaos, confusion, meaningless) and void (Hebrew: בֹהוּ "bohu" – emptiness)". Therefore, it appears as though "the earth", "the deep", and "the waters" in this verse are all referring to the same thing. They are all being used metaphorically in an attempt to describe this "universal primordial soup".

V3."Then God said, "Let there be light"; and there was light."

In verse 14 it says: "Then God said, "Let there be lights..."" This is when the celestial bodies that give us light are defined, therefore, until we get there, we will consider the light in verse 3 to be our metaphor for energy because in verse 3 above, as no source of light is defined, and according to the laws of the Universe that God is creating, light emanates from a source, it doesn't make any sense unless it is being used as a metaphor for something else. I've heard people say that the light came from God Himself, but as God is everywhere, there would be no way for Him to separate light from darkness, as that would directly contradict the scripturally validated claim to God's omnipresence. So, now we have Space, Matter, and Energy, and we are still within the bounds of the Physical Laws of the burgeoning Universe.

V4."God saw that the light was good; and God separated the light from the darkness."

Energy, by its very nature, possesses a positive or negative force. This could speak to this delineation, but it could also speak to the "formless and void" statement in verse 2: formless (Hebrew: תֹּהוּ "tohu" – chaos, confusion, meaningless) and void (Hebrew: בֹּהוּ "bohu" – emptiness)". This light could mean more or different than simply "energy". This could represent the introduction of the dichotomy of meaning and chaos. It could well represent the "laws" within which the universe will function.

V5. "God called the light day, and the darkness He called night. And there was evening and there was morning, one day."

The 24-hour day is not defined, or even definable, which clearly indicates another meaning for the word "day" here, until verse 14:"Then God said, "Let there be lights in the expanse of the heavens to separate the day from the night..."" There can be no measurement of time without motion. Evening and morning indicate the advent of Motion although there is as yet no way to measure it until verse 14. Evening and morning are also indicators of time that the people of that age would be familiar with, and so it is used here as a metaphor, for their sake. Furthermore, while word used here for day (Hebrew: יוֹם, yom) is *commonly used to refer to a 24 hr period of time, it is also used in other places to mean "age" or "epoch" such as in Genesis 2:4 "¹Thus the heavens and the earth were completed, and all their hosts. ² By the seventh day God completed His work which He had done, and He rested on the seventh day from all His work which He had done. ³ Then God blessed the seventh day and sanctified it, because in it He rested from all His work which God had created and made. ⁴ This is the account of the heavens and the earth when they were created, in the <u>day</u> that the LORD God made earth and heaven." - Genesis 2:1-4, the word "day" in verse 4 clearly encompasses all seven of the days just described and refers to them as an age or epoch. Also in Daniel 12:13 "But as for you, go your way to the end; then you will enter into rest and rise again for your allotted portion at the end of the <u>age</u>." The use of the words "And there was evening and there was morning, one day", is also unique to this part of the scriptures and as it is first used here, it could hint at an alternative meaning to its most common use as a 24 hr day, which the Hebrews define as from evening to evening, not evening to morning. Notice that from evening to morning is from dark to light, from chaos to order. It could also mean the end of an epoch and the beginning of a new one which is most likely why in Gen*

Finally Somehow Home

2:1-3 where it talks about the 7th and final day, when God rests, it does not say "and there was evening and there was morning a 7th day" as it does with days 1-6. It is likely that we are still in the "7th day". This passage in Hebrews 4:3-7 could well point to this:

3 "For we who have believed enter that rest, just as He has said,

"AS I swore in MY wrath,

They shall not enter MY rest,"

although His works were finished from the foundation of the world. 4 For He has said somewhere concerning the seventh day: "And God rested on the seventh day from all His works"; 5 and again in this passage, "They shall not enter MY rest." 6 Therefore, since it remains for some to enter it, and those who formerly had good news preached to them failed to enter because of disobedience, 7 He again fixes a certain day, "Today," saying through David after so long a time just as has been said before,

"Today if you hear His voice,

DO not harden your hearts.""

Finally Somehow Home

The "rest" mentioned throughout these verses, and all throughout the book of Hebrews, in fact, could well be the same rest as the 7th day rest. It certainly seems so here: 4 "For He has said somewhere concerning the seventh day: "And God rested on the seventh day from all His works"; 5 and again in this passage, "They shall not enter MY rest.""" Therefore, it would appear that "Today" in Hebrews 4:7 is the 7th day. We are still in the 7th day, or 7th epoch.

V6. "Then God said, "Let there be an expanse in the midst of the waters, and let it separate the waters from the waters.""

BANG! In the book Industrial Explosion Prevention and Protection, Frank T. Bodurtha defines an explosion as such: "an explosion is the result, not the cause, of a rapid expansion of gases. It may occur from physical or mechanical change." Basically, God blows the primordial soup apart with an explosion.

V7. "God made the expanse, and separated the waters which were below the expanse from the waters which were above the expanse; and it was so."

The words "below" and "above" are actually the same Hebrew word: מן "min" or מני "minni" or -מני "mine". This

Finally Somehow Home

basically means that the matter was separated apart, one from the other – at its most fundamental level, within the expanse of space, or expanse of the heavens as outer space is defined in the next verse and in verse 15: "for lights in the expanse of the heavens to give light on the earth..."

There is an argument in the Creationist camp that if there were an explosion, all planets would spin in the same direction. This would be true with a centralized explosive where all the energy emanates from a single point, such as with a hand grenade where all the explosive is in the middle and pushes the fragments out uniformly, but that is not what is described here. There seems to be emphasis here, by using the Hebrew word "min" twice to describe an decentralized expansion of the matter which shatters the blob of matter entirely apart separating the "waters from the waters" as if the energy erupted from in between all of it down to its most fundamental level. Imagine a Claymore mine which is C4 packed behind and somewhat between a shitload of small steel balls. When a Claymore goes off, those damn balls are flying around spinning all kinds of different directions, so that little argument doesn't hold up here.

V8. "God called the expanse heaven. And there was evening and there was morning, a second day."

Not until verse 8 is the word "heaven" ascribed to its actual meaning of the sky and outer space (there is no delineation for the earth's atmosphere – it was likely still forming), but hereafter it carries that meaning because it has been defined as such. It is no longer used as a metaphor for Space. The second and ensuing days denote the continuation of consistent motion according to the same Physical Laws that governed the first day.

V9. "Then God said, "Let the waters below the heavens be gathered into one place, and let the dry land appear"; and it was so."

After the explosion, the universe begins to form from the sub-atomic level. Gravity begins to gather matter into what are now the celestial bodies. Order is introduced to what was chaos: "formless and void" v2. Specifically, on earth, this is happening, but it is also happening generally throughout the Universe.

V10. "God called the dry land earth, and the gathering of the waters He called seas; and God saw that it was good."

Again, earth and water are here defined and depart forever from their metaphorical meanings. While this is going on throughout the universe on other planets and celestial bodies, this is the definitive transition from speaking of the Universe to now speaking of the planet Earth. Why? Because this record is for the people of earth.

V11."Then God said, "Let the earth sprout vegetation, plants yielding seed, and fruit trees on the earth bearing fruit after their kind with seed in them"; and it was so."

V12. "The earth brought forth vegetation, plants yielding seed after their kind, and trees bearing fruit with seed in them, after their kind; and God saw that it was good."

V13. "There was evening and there was morning, a third day."

V14. "Then God said, "Let there be lights in the expanse of the heavens to separate the day from the night, and let them be for signs and for seasons and for days and years;"

V15. "and let them be for lights in the expanse of the heavens to give light on the earth"; and it was so."

V16. "God made the two great lights, the greater light to govern the day, and the lesser light to govern the night; He made the stars also."

V17. "God placed them in the expanse of the heavens to give light on the earth,"

V18. "and to govern the day and the night, and to separate the light from the darkness; and God saw that it was good."

V19. "There was evening and there was morning, a fourth day."

This passage denotes and defines actual sources of actual light, thereby permanently departing from the metaphor of Energy hereafter. It also denotes the first measurement of Time according to the continuation of consistent motion as governed by the Physical Laws of the Universe.

And there you have it. There is a Big Bang in the Bible, boys and girls. It took us till the 1900's to come up with and label the Big Bang Theory, but there it is right there in the first chapter of a book arguably written 2,500-3,500 years ago. A book that scientists won't touch with a ten-foot pole because "it's religious", and whose followers "don't believe in science, they believe in God." What the fuck. The result

Finally Somehow Home

is that no one has ever approached the book scientifically, or very few at least, because their minds are already made up about it in that regard before they ever open it. It's a goddamn 3,500 year old ancient manuscript. Again, if you were Indiana Jones and you found it in a cave somewhere for the first time, would you just throw it out because "it's religious"?! Yeah. I didn't think so. You'd study it scientifically and dissect it and look into all its nooks and crannies. That's the right way to approach it. If you don't, you're gonna miss some pretty important shit.

Finally Somehow Home

Chapter 31

After discovering this, I started thinking, well, maybe there is a lot more to this book that's been kind of misunderstood because when you really think about it, the Catholic Church was formed when the Roman Emperor Constantine had a dream that he went into battle with the cross before him and he won the battle in the dream and afterward he made everyone adopt Christianity and formed the Roman Catholic Church. Well, guess what happened? Just like the tribes in Indonesia, the tendency is not to discard previous belief systems, but instead to just add the new to the old. This is exactly what Jesus was talking about regarding old wine and new wineskins: " And He was also telling them a parable: "No one tears a piece of cloth from a new garment and puts it on an old garment; otherwise he will both tear the new, and the piece from the new will not match the old. And no one puts new wine into old wineskins; otherwise the new wine will burst the skins and it will be spilled out, and the skins will be ruined. But new wine must be put into fresh wineskins. And no one, after drinking old wine wishes for new; for he says, 'The old is good enough.'" Luke 5:34-39. Well, all those other religions were just kind of added to Christianity and mashed into Catholicism. So, you don't have the purity of whatever it was before, hell, even the Pope's hat is derived from adopted Phoenician influences. Jesus warned his disciples about this, he says, "Beware of the leaven of the Pharisees..." The Pharisees were the religious leaders of the day. What's leaven? Leaven is yeast. It's only something you ADD to bread. It's never something you take out. What does it do when you add it? It makes everything bigger. Right? So, what about that burden you are carrying that you can't quite keep up with anyway? Well, then you add a bunch more rules to it, how the hell are you supposed to keep your head above the water then? Right? "Beware of the leaven of the Pharisees." Beware of what people try to add to the truth. Fuck the leaven.

So, drawing from that, maybe there are some other things in this book, which – the book hasn't changed, that's historically proven by the way, what's changed is the way

Finally Somehow Home

we're looking at the book - that we've been reading the wrong way, because if all these other religions are influencing what we believe about it, it's going to taint the way we see things, not to mention the fact that we tend to understand them out of the historical context. We already misunderstood the first few sentences of it, so we might want to look into it some more to see if there's anything else we're misunderstanding. And when I started thinking about it, I realized, holy cow, that whole freaking book is all about child sacrifice.

Well, it's not all about child sacrifice, but a lot of it is. The first mention of it is subtle: Genesis 15:16 "Then in the fourth generation they shall return here for the sin of the Amorite is not yet complete."

According to historians, Abram ben Terah, later Abraham, lived from approximately 2150 BCE to 1975 BCE. This is the Abraham of old who is revered as the patriarch of Judaism, Christianity, and Islam. During this time people groups of the Levant worshiped many different gods. A good number of them, such as Moloch, demanded the sacrifice of the children of their followers. In some cases, it was done as a one-off sacrifice in order to gain something in return, such as when Mesha the king of

Finally Somehow Home

Moab sacrificed his first-born son, which occurred around 860 BCE:

2 Kings 3:26-27 "When the king of Moab saw that the battle was too fierce for him, he took with him 700 men who drew swords, to break through to the king of Edom; but they could not. Then he took his oldest son who was to reign in his place, and offered him as a burnt offering on the wall. And there came great wrath against Israel, and they departed from him and returned to their own land."

And again, in Judges where Jephthah ignorantly obligates himself to the Hebrew God YAWEH so that he may win a battle, and ends up sacrificing his daughter.

But it is no stretch at all to presume that most cases of child sacrifice to these gods was conducted regularly as ritual for the sake of the community. Imagine living your childhood in fear that you would be chosen as the sacrifice. It was like the Hunger Games but there was no game. One was chosen to die for the sake of the many, and that was that. Now imagine being the parent of that child and being fully obligated to surrender them because the neighbors next door had to do it last month and now it's your kid that got picked. It's your turn. And who would be the most likely candidate to deliver the child to their death? I would say

Finally Somehow Home

probably the father. The child's very picture of security and strength carrying them to the altar or to the fiery arms of Moloch. Without doubt the most horrible experience any human being has had to endure.

Now imagine this belief system's impact on the cultures of these people groups after nearly 1000 years. With the ritual killing of children a centerpiece of their religion and culture, this is the making of a sick and twisted society. This is the "sin of the Amorite" in Genesis 15. It appears as though God gave the people of the region of Canaan over 700 years (from Abraham to Moses) to get their shit together. This is also the reason God was such an asshole to the Canaanites in telling the Israelites to destroy every man, woman, and child of them when they retook the land. It was so that there would be no possible way for this diseased culture, its religions, and tenants to persist. It was in order to erase a very dark stain on humanity. A rotting sickness.

Deuteronomy 12:29-31 "When the Lord your God cuts off before you the nations which you are going in to dispossess, and you dispossess them and dwell in their land, beware that you are not ensnared to follow them, after they are destroyed before you, and that you do not inquire after their gods, saying, 'How do these nations serve their gods, that I also may do likewise?' You shall not behave thus toward the Lord your God, for every abominable act which the Lord hates they have done for their gods; for they even burn their sons and daughters in the fire to their gods."

So, what's the deal with God asking Abraham to sacrifice his only son? It is, in fact the second mention of child sacrifice in the Bible, after the sin of the Amorites.

Genesis 22:1-2 "Now it came about after these things, that God tested Abraham, and said to him, "Abraham!" And he said, "Here I am." He said, "Take now your son, your only son, whom you love, Isaac, and go to the land of Moriah, and offer him there as a burnt offering on one of the mountains of which I will tell you.""

Genesis 22:10-13 "Abraham stretched out his hand and took the knife to slay his son. But the angel of the Lord called to him from heaven and said, "Abraham, Abraham!" And he said, "Here I am." He said, "Do not stretch out your hand against the lad, and do nothing to him; for now I know that you fear God, since you have not withheld your son, your only son, from Me." Then Abraham raised his eyes and looked, and behold, behind him a ram caught in the thicket by his horns; and Abraham went and took the ram and offered him up for a burnt offering in the place of his son."

There are many reasons for this trial of Abraham. A very important one is that God was showing Abraham who He is. God had made a covenant with Abraham, but Abraham had nothing but personal encounters with God to inform him of who this God is, of His character. He had no scriptures to go by, no priest or teacher to tell him. All that Abraham knew about God is what was spoken to him personally or demonstrated to him through events such as this. A very large part of this is to show Abraham that this God is different. He's not like the other gods. He does NOT demand of his people the lives of their children, ever.

"That ain't Me."

Jeremiah 7:31 "They have built the high places of Topheth, which is in the valley of the son of Hinnom, to burn their sons and their daughters in the fire, which I did not command, and it did not come into My mind."

So, what's the point? What is the significance of this sick theme all throughout the Bible? Well, if there really is a God - this nebulous incomprehensible thing of ominous power and sentiment - and this God wanted to relate to mankind in a very meaningful and profound way, how would a God, more specifically, how would this God do that?

But wait a minute, we have not yet discussed the most significant case of child sacrifice mentioned in the Bible. Not of an infant but certainly of a child of a father, a son. The great significance of child sacrifice is that it is the most depraved act of humanity. And with the greatest depravity comes the greatest pain. Pain. The one and only thing that every single human on earth can relate to. That's where God chose to meet us. To relate to us. Because He knew that's the only way we'd all get it. And He chose the harshest and most brutal pain that any human has ever had to endure so that He could relate to every human being who will ever live. He gave up His son as a sacrifice. He, without obligation, carried His own son to the altar and laid Him on it. And watched.

This God seems to be able to relate to us.

In and through the darkest part of humanity He's there.

On purpose.

Finally Somehow Home

Trying to tell us something:

"I'm real, I get it, I get you, and I've got you... no shit"

That makes sense. Again, maybe we need to rethink how we're thinking about God. Forget the old guy in the clouds with the beard and all that stuff. In fact, presumably, if He is that triune infinite kind of force I mentioned before, and relationship is one of its fundamental attributes, then, clearly the thing is deeply relational, right? So, if He's going to relate to something that He made, then He's obviously going to want to do it in such a way that can be understood.

Finally Somehow Home

Chapter 32

The point is, there are some things that, if thought about differently, change how I view me. Because remember, back to me trying to get out of this little predicament... So, I started pulling this thread a little more, and this is just where it left me. And I started thinking, okay, so you've got the Big Bang, and the formation of the planets, because, think about it, what are we standing on? It's a ball of mud. It's a big ball of mud in space, like I said before. And I can understand how it was formed if something went Kaboom! in the midst of this "universal primordial soup of matter", whatever you want to call it. So, the thing blows up and then you have just crap flying all over the place and it starts blobbing together and spinning around and forming elements which are blobbing together. That's why a vein of gold is somewhat linear, for instance, because

Finally Somehow Home

that's how it was flying through space when it hit the side of the blob of mud that's the Earth, right? It's a big blob that keeps spinning and it gets whacked a few times and it starts slowing down, right?

And as it slows down some of the things trapped inside of it, especially liquids and gasses are drawn out by the centrifugal force and/or forced to the surface by internal pressures, and the lighter elements of it are trying to get away from it, trying to flow out back to space, then after it's gotten pretty damn big, all of a sudden this other big mud ball just down the road just ignites into flames because it was such a big mud ball and the matter within it was so dense and under so much pressure, that, Boom! it ignited. That's our sun, and any liquids that had seeped up to the surface or anything that was on the surface of this planet was instantly vaporized. It just flash-fried probably everything, maybe that's why there's a big burnt spot in Africa where the Sahara Desert is. So, Wham! Now you have an instant atmosphere on this planet, or at least the beginnings of one. So, okay, that makes sense to see it that way.

We need to stop mystifying everything, it's a ball of mud in space. It's going to change. And, yeah, we definitely have an impact how much it changes. If we're spewing things into the atmosphere they are caught up in that loop, because of the flash fry effect, that's what happens every day, the sun shines on the earth, and cooks it. That's why you till the soil, you flip it over and the earth cooks it, and it activates nutrients in the soil, and that's how it works. It's just a big slow cook. When we introduce toxins and stuff into that, of course it's not healthy. Overall, though, the thing is going to change. It might be a little pebble on someone's beach one day on another planet. There are holes in the ozone. Oh no! When it came brand new out of the box, there wasn't a hole in it. Now there's a hole. Who put the hole in the damn thing? It changes. It does. Things are still seeping out of the ground because of that big swirling effect, and it's still cooking things that seep out from within it, so certain things are released into the atmosphere at different times. So, it's gonna change the environment. But yeah, we definitely still need to look after it too.

So, then, when the earth was ready, God made Adam out of dirt. (This is kind of His M.O. He makes sure everything is ready, then executes His plan. "I go to prepare a place for you..." Same kind of thing.) So, then this triune infinite kind of God decides: I'm going to make this creature, I'm going to make it completely independent of me. It's not a projection of me like everything else. It's made out of the projection of me. It's gonna be its own thing. What do I got laying around? Oh, well, I've got a bunch of this awesome stuff that I made called mud that I made this awesome universe out of, and oh, there's some on the ground right now, so I will make Adam out of mud, or more accurately "dust". "Then the LORD God formed man of dust from the ground, and breathed into his nostrils the breath of life; and man became a living being." But Adam was its own thing, an entirely different thing than all the rest of the universe. And then Eve was made of Adam. Eve was made out of Adam's rib and not dirt again. Why? because it's the beginning of an entirely new thing: humanity.

But hold on a second. Why would a God like that make an amazing creature like that, then just be like, "Ok, dude, go name all this stuff, subdue the earth and do whatever the fuck you want." He actually made man to be totally independent of Him with no obligation to Him whatsoever. Really? He walked and bullshat with Adam every day in the garden, but man had no obligation to God, whatsoever. The only stipulation he put on Man was of the Tree of the Knowledge of Good and Evil. He said, "Don't eat of that tree, if you do, you'll surely die." End of story.

Finally Somehow Home

So, this supreme, infinite entity, makes this amazing creature whose purpose is just to be totally and completely free. Of everything. Including Himself.

Okay, why?

So, now think of a brand-new human being. What does a brand-new human being want to do?

It wants to do whatever it wants.

It just doesn't know what it wants yet. Hmmm.

In fact, what is it that every single person who's ever been or will be really want most? We want to do whatever we want.

Well, is that weird?

Because after a while, it learns to do what it doesn't really want to do.

And it does that.

You know... enough to get by and make a living. Sometimes it's what you gotta do. You've got to do what you don't want to do. You can't always do what you wanna do.

Finally Somehow Home

But here's the problem with that.

I think we were made to do whatever we wanna do.

I do.

Why else would you be best at that?

Why would you be the best at exactly the same thing? Like the best in the world at it? Why would you be the best on planet Earth at the same goddamn thing that you really want to do most once you find out what that really is and sharpen it?

Yeah, like, ah, OK, well, this is sounding alot like a one-way trip to poverty for the rest of my life, for sure. But think about it. I'm the only one who does what I do best the best in the world, the way I do it the way I do it best.

Hmmm.

Maybe that's what I'm supposed to be doing.

Maybe. You know, maybe. Because apparently there's a reason I don't have any freaking money and I'm homeless and I don't have a job and if I went and got another job doing the same stupid shit... I say that, but the jobs that I have had, the things I've been doing, actually haven't been stupid. They've been amazing. I'm fortunate, I've had some really cool jobs. I've learned a lot. Why am I not still doing that then? Well, it seems as though, even though it was fun, it was awesome, I made a lot of money, and I was really good at them, it seems like those were not the things that I was made or intended to do. However, I can't help but notice that even in the jobs that I had, the parts I did best, what I really excelled in, were the things I liked doing the most. The things that used the parts of me that I was best at doing. That's where I invariably did my best work. Those experiences probably made whatever I'm intended to be much stronger, but that wasn't it.

Funny how that adds up. Okay, so back to our story.

So, you had these two humans now. Whose job basically was to do whatever they want to do. And according to the Bible, you've got the tree of life. Right? Not the tree of Good – the tree of Life. And then you've got the tree of the Knowledge of Good and Evil. Not the tree of death. The tree of the knowledge of good and evil. And again, he said, "Don't eat from that tree, if you do, you'll surely die." What's with the names of these trees? They don't make any sense. Is there something in there we've been missing?

Finally Somehow Home

Here's the something there. The tree of the knowledge of good and evil - the fruit of tree of the knowledge of good and evil was the lie of the knowledge of good and evil. The tree of the knowledge of good and evil is actually the Tree of Death. Because it is the lie. The knowledge of good and evil is the lie because it obfuscates the truth. It obfuscates "Life and Death" with "Good and Evil". The knowledge of that lie is the fruit of that tree. The knowledge of that lie is the fruit of that tree. When you believe a lie, you eat the fruit. When you eat the fruit, you believe a lie.

And that's where the shame comes from. The shame was the thing that sold the deal. How did the serpent get them to eat the fruit? Because they were buddies with God who had told them about eating out of His tree, and "It's His garden and, you know, we're His friends and we're kind of His guests, and you know, I know it looks tempting, but no man, we're not going to take anything away from our relationship with this guy who's been real square with us, so, no thanks."

And then this is the lie. "You don't really have to... you don't have to do it that way. Yeah, He told you not to do this, but it's cool. Just go ahead and eat it, because you don't have to offend Him. You can actually pay for this yourself. Just a

Finally Somehow Home

little bit of shame. Just a little bit of shame. And He'll see, oh, they feel bad that they did it. So, if they feel bad, they feel ashamed, they feel poorly of themselves, that will assuage any offense. That's how you can do it. It's kind of a way of borrowing. That's what it is. It's really no problem. You've got credit through me."

So, this is what blew my mind about this: The feeling I have in my stomach when I sign a car loan or a home loan or owe a big debt. Just that feeling I get in my gut.

It's the same feeling I have when I think about how bad I am.

It's the same feeling, Exactly.

But when I'm signing, it's like, "This fucking sucks, but, but I gotta do it to live."

So, I just do it.

We do it. Well, it's funny because that's kind of how we do the other thing too. It's how we do it. We do, we pay for our sin with our shame. And that's what sold the deal for them. So, they believed the lie that they could pay for it with their shame. And that's where all this other crap came from. Hell, that's where shame and evil on this earth came from,

Finally Somehow Home

before they believed it, it wasn't real. Evil is real now, but shame is still a scam.

Here's how I found out. I'm driving to work one day after cheating on my wife. And I'm feeling so - beating the crap out of myself - just wishing I was a better person, and I suck, and man I just can't live with myself, and all this stuff. And then I heard a song on the radio, it was Mumford and Sons, and it said "...It's not the long walk home that will change this heart, but the welcome I receive with the restart..."

And I was like, You're right! It's not the moping around... moping around don't do you no good. It's not the moping around that gets you back on your feet. It's the welcome you receive from the one who you've offended. And then I remembered this little kid's song I used to sing: "Rejoice in the Lord always, and again I say rejoice." And I thought, you know what, right now I'm just gonna be happy. Like, this is weird, I shouldn't be doing this. I felt so awful. I shouldn't be happy at all, because I just did this horrible thing. But according to the Bible that I've been raised and taught on, it says "Rejoice always, again I say rejoice." So, I'm like, oh, okay, we're going to try this out and see what happens, because, you know what, that's what it says, so

Finally Somehow Home

that's what I'm going to do, and I'm going to try and break this thing or see if it works.

And dude, you know what was weird?

That gave me such control over the emotion that was throwing me around in life right then, because I was unhappy in the marriage and still doing these horrible things and all that. But it separated me from the emotion of it entirely. It wasn't really until that moment that I got actually started being able to deal with that bondage in my life. It was a long road. But that's what it was that actually saved me from my darkest demons. It's not feeling guilty about it.

Think about it.

Just don't feel guilty about it.

Just choose not to.

No, I'm done with it. I'm not doing it anymore.

Do it.

Look at how messed up this is, the entire masculine population of the evangelical church today has been

Finally Somehow Home

totally rendered inept over their guilt from the fact that the beast that they live in has a set of balls and they masturbate. That has debilitated the men in the church for generations. That's all they ever talk about. They're fixated on it. Try me. Go to any evangelical men's bible study and you'll see. The self-loathing is palatable.

"I masturbate... I struggle with watching porn.... Ughhhhh."

Okay, I'll tell you what. Just quit feeling guilty about it. You're not supposed to. Stop feeling guilty about it. And you'll beat off like crazy for a little while probably if you're kinda nutso about it, but you know, after a week or so, you'll actually get bored of it.

Dead serious.

Try it.

That's the only thing that actually helps you overcome things the beast wants.

Finally Somehow Home

Chapter 33

I wrote a pretty cool poem called "Dragonrider" a long time ago.

I'm riding this life.
I'm riding this thing like a dragon.
See, the dragon is just doing its own thing.
And me?
I'm just hanging on for the ride.
It IS like riding a dragon.
Each life has a life all its own.
We meet the ageless beast somewhere early on.
And we ride it for our life. As others have before us.
Some of yours are dragons, like mine.
And some of yours seem doves to me.
But no.
We each ride a dragon.

Finally Somehow Home

And then, a little while later, I learned some more about it.
I re-wrote it and called it "Dragon":
I'm riding this life.
I'm riding this thing like a dragon.
See, the dragon is just doing what dragons do.
And me?
Well...
I'm just hanging on for the ride.

It is like riding a dragon.
As if each life has a life all its own.

We meet the beast somewhere...early on.
Before time begins.
And we ride it for our life.

Some of yours are dragons like mine.
And some of yours seem doves to me.

But no.

We each ride a dragon.

Or fight it.

Finally Somehow Home

Or both.

Early on I know this much:
I must break it.
I must.
Or die.
Or kill us both in trying.
Better dead now from living somehow,
Than dead in a life of dying.

It shrieks and roils and bucks
and flies like fucking HATE on fire.

To break me.
It must.
Or die.
Or kill us both in trying.
Better dead now from living somehow,
Than dead in a life of dying.

It is Ten-Thousand Hells of Violent Fuck
- this BEASTFIGHT lode.

Finally Somehow Home

Idle stands the Devil by.
Transfixed.
Somehow beaten.

But then one day in sadist taunt,
I of a sudden let it go.
To watch it try to kill me I suppose.
I do not now sure know.

He flies like the roil of the hurriflame wind - hard, hot, mad, and quick - like the flick of the tip of a wick with a whip - Sharp. Violent. Perfect.

It's then, I find myself in awe of him.
My spurs and crop and beating-chains,
and all the shatter-smashed remains
of the environs where we've fought -
when he would try to scrape me off,
all hurt him. Bad.
Tough Motherfucker, I'll say that.
That's what makes him reckless and brave,
The beast knows he can take a beating.
His greatest power is in his bleeding.

Finally Somehow Home

Scorn bears his iron screams:
FUCK FEAR.
"It's but the fantasy of Pain," I sing.
FUCK PAIN. He shrieks again.
"For when it's gone I will remain" - I sing along.

I push him on. Lift him up.
And he flies even faster.
And turns even harder still.
Like wild grace. Terrifying. Mesmerizing.
So, I urge him on. With all that I am.
Then the fear: If all of me is spent to lift him up, then who is there for me?
And the answer surges beneath me, in power.
And I learned that when we strive in unison.
To lift the other up, it becomes a dance.
A beautiful, wild dance.
Like sex.
Striving together as one for the sake of the other.
Becoming one.
And then I knew what love is.
And then I loved myself.
Because, then I understood it: I am the dragon.

Finally Somehow Home

It is like riding a dragon. And beating the crap out of the freaking dragon ain't gonna do shit. It just makes it more pissed off. And he's just as strong as you. You've got to do it another way.

You know, you might be a little like, "So, don't feel ashamed about stuff anymore, huh?" Sounds like some loose cannons run around, right? How are we gonna control ourselves then? Well, think about it. The concept of sin is actually the thing that we resist against that makes us human. Because the more you sin, the more of an animal you are. And the more you don't, the more human you are. Sin is actually what we push against that makes us human. Well, what do we push against it with? We feel bad about stuff that we do, so we don't do that stuff we don't want to feel bad about, and that makes us human. Our shame is actually the thing that makes us not do bad shit. We use it to beat the shit out of ourselves to not do stuff that makes us feel bad, and we make ourselves feel so bad that we're sure that we will never do anything that will make us feel bad again. So, we feel bad all the time for no reason and it still doesn't work. But that's what we do with it. And we beat the shit out of each other with it too because we motivate people by just plunging them into guilt and

Finally Somehow Home

shame and that is the makings of a wonderful type of relationship if you've ever been part of one of those.

So, what do we use then to keep our shit together? Remember I talked about that poem I wrote called "How to Love a Man"? Here's the interesting thing about it, it's like shame versus beauty or something, right? But this is how you know which one is a lie. Because when you read that poem shamefully, it's not that the beauty comes out of it. It's that when you read it without shame, the beauty is already there. It has been there the whole time. The shame is what's covering up the beauty. So which one do you think is the lie?

That's the thing. With sex, if you have a crappy sex life, you need to deal with some shame stuff. That's what sex is all about, okay? It's not bad, it's not evil. And that's the point of it. That's how it's supposed to work. That's the physical act of love - the striving with all that you are to just make that other person feel like the most amazing person on the planet and they're doing that for you. Well, holy shit, maybe we should start thinking about that when it comes to relationships. If you believe, and this is actually in that poem too, but if you believe about a man that he is the biggest piece of shit that ever washed up, that's exactly

Finally Somehow Home

what he's going to be, especially for a man. Girls, if you believe about a man that he is going to take care of me and love me and keep me safe more than anyone else on the planet - yeah, this is my man - I wouldn't hang out with him if he wasn't good enough to be my man - that dude will do everything within his power to prove you right about him. That he is a good dude. He is a good man.

How do you think you get Marines to charge up freaking Mount Suribachi? "Man, you'll probably never make it. Probably never do it, don't have what it takes..."? No, you give them strength. You encourage them, you lift them up.

Guess what?

I guarantee you, if I stood up and said, you know, none of you knows how to love a man, I would get laughed at. "Oh, you don't have to know how." How's that working out for you? Because everyone I tell this to, tells me, "Well, that's not how it is with my boyfriend. My boyfriend, you gotta beat the shit out of him."

How is your relationship?

Is that dude doing everything in his power to make you feel like you're the queen of this planet? No, hell no he's not.

Finally Somehow Home

Why? Because you beat the hell out of him all the time, that's why. What I'm saying is, it's easy. It's easy to have a good man.

Picture in your head... and this is me, the homeless frigging dumbass giving you love advice, it's hilarious. Anyway, picture in your head the most awesome person you can ever imagine in the universe. And picture them in a room and them looking around, and what kind of person would they want to be with? Now you be that person and you'll be fine. They'll walk right up to you. But you be that person. Here's the thing, it sucks because you've gotta be that person when they show up. You can't start being that person when you see them, like, ok now I gotta get my shit together. It's too late. You gotta already be that person when you bump into them. That's how you find someone that's worth giving a shit about. Only one relationship in your life will ever be a success. So, keep that in mind. Some things are worth saving up for. So, make sure it's a great success.

Okay, anyway, total rabbit trail. I'm going to circle back.

Chapter 34

I was telling you about seeing the world without shame. It's so cool, man. It's so cool. We were talking about when you read that poem without shame, the beauty has been there the whole time. The shame is what's covering up the beauty. So which one do you think is the lie? When you remove your shame from how you see this world, it's suddenly beautiful, when you remove your shame from how you see your life, it's suddenly beautiful, when you remove your shame from how you see yourself, you're suddenly beautiful. Try it. You'll see.

It's weird. But that's the only way that you can actually walk through it and use it like it's your very own. And you can. You can use this whole thing, this whole universe however you want to use it. However you want to use it. The hardest part is figuring out how you want to use it.

Finally Somehow Home

Remember, what you really want are the things that are best for you and give you life. It's not about good and bad, right and wrong, it's about life and death. What is it that gives you life, or what is it that brings you death? Remember, that's what sin is. It's not a rule like in a game: if you break it, you get punished. It's a law like in science: if you do it, it'll fuck up your life. If you continue to believe the lie, you'll be burdened with more shit that distracts you from life, so it's not a free pass. The "punishment" isn't from God zapping you when you fuck up, it's baked in. It's not a free pass to be a fool. It's a removal of the blinders, it's the ability to see things as they really are in the light of the truth. It's a free pass to an abundant life.

It's not that you don't see the shame, or are not tempted to grab onto it. It wants to restrict you. Like me walking around right now on the sidewalk talking into a camera with people all looking at me weird, I should be so ashamed. And guess what, if that happened, I would never make this and this would never happen and it would preclude me from doing what I have to do to get out of this situation. So, you see how much it limits you? It holds you back. It doesn't even exist.

Finally Somehow Home

So, here's the thing about shame. The whole animal thing in the Bible, when Adam and Eve said, okay, we'll do this shame thing, and then God shows up and He's like, guys, if you eat from that tree, you can't live in the garden. If you eat from a tree of lies, if you choose to believe in lies, you won't eat from the tree of life. You won't eat from the truth. So, the whole freaking thing about shame and all that is that when Adam and Eve thought they could pay for their sin with their shame, that was the lie. Remember what I said when I signed the loan, that's how we do it now? But that ain't the right way. It doesn't work. You can't shame yourself into being happy. That's how we do it now and no one is happy. But remember, when you remove the shame, the beauty has been there the whole time? Why do you think you're attracted to beauty in the first place? It just draws the eye, doesn't it?

It's powerful.

It lifts you up from the top. If there's no shame in the way. And here's how.

When you love you,

Finally...

Finally Somehow Home

The dragon thing I was talking about, fighting the dragon, beating the hell out of it, beating it to make it fly faster, or just to make it go in the right direction. And it's all over the place, but then you let it run and let's see how crazy awesome it is. That's you. See what you were made to do. Yes, it's wild and scary and shit. But let it run. Let it go.

Encourage it when it screws up. How many of you when your best friend comes up to you, and says, "I just screwed up big time." How many of you say, "You're damn right you did you, you idiot!"? If you do, that's not your friend. Quit doing that to yourself. Start literally patting yourself on the back and encouraging yourself, instead. Start listening to see if you're believing the lie that beating your beast up will fix you. You can't flog it to make it do amazing things. Lift it up and be its best friend and feed it and take care of it. You gotta train it. And then you realize it's like sex. Two people striving together for the sake of the other. And then you realize that, holy shit, I'm the dragon. And I will only be able to perform at my maximum potential if I love me. If you notice I'm not beating the crap out of myself for being in this situation. But that's how we live life is beating the shit out of ourselves whenever we screw up. Knowing that if I have to be at the top of my game, I need to believe that I'm not a piece of shit, right? Because if you

Finally Somehow Home

believe that someone is an amazing human being, they'll try like hell to prove you right. You are the same with you. But if you think you're crap, then you can't set yourself up for anything to live up to. Where do you begin? You're screwed. You have to be your own very best friend. If you're on opposing teams, ain't nothing gonna happen. Because here's the thing. If you want to get to a point where you can actually be happy, because you no longer live with shame, well, you can't do that if you ain't friends with you because you and you are going to be miserable together. You can't be happy if you don't like you anyway. So, you've got to figure you out. Fuck the shame. Let it run. Learn how amazing you are.

So, when Adam and Eve did all that stuff, remember, God brought the animals out and he sacrificed the animals. Why? What the hell was that all about? Seems horrible to kill two unblemished innocent animals because a couple people fucked up. It is. It's supposed to be. It was a life for a life. That was the beginning of death on earth. The death of the animals acted as a covering for their shame, (God literally covered their nakedness with the skins), as an atonement. Until a worthy sacrifice was available. Remember, when you believe the lie, you eat the fruit. When you eat the fruit, you believe the lie. The lie is the subterfuge of "good and evil" which obscures the reality of the exchange. The lie is: Sin = Shame. The truth is: Sin = Death. The collateral for your line of credit is your fucking life. The lie is the belief that your shame is sufficient to offset your offense. It's not. It's another subterfuge. Your shame don't do shit but rob you of your life on this earth. It's not even a real thing. But we all believe in it. Because we believe the lie. So that nebulous triune God made a temporary way for Adam and Eve to not have to carry their shame. From day one. Because he knew we couldn't deal with it. We just couldn't handle it. So that's why the whole animal sacrifice thing took place. And then he saw we were having such a hard time with the shame because we were piling more and more rules on top of ourselves to shame ourselves into behaving the way we wanted to behave, because that's how we do it now. We bought the lie hook, line, and sinker, and we buy it every day.

That's why the whole coming down, dying on the cross thing happened. The only sacrifice worthy to pay off and settle up the line of credit, was God Himself. His own Son, back to the whole child sacrifice thing. He's communicating with us. He goes, trust me, I got it. And He did it. "For the wages of sin is death, but the free gift of God is eternal life in Christ Jesus our Lord." Romans 6:23. "The

Finally Somehow Home

wages" – what you have earned – You have earned death. You deserve it. You made the deal and now you're trapped in it. "But the free gift" – that which you didn't do shit to earn, and you cannot afford but it's given to you anyway – that's life! This is mercy and grace. Mercy is what you deserve, but you're spared from, and grace is what you don't deserve, but you're given anyway, and real, true grace, the grace from this infinite triune being, is never bounded. It is limitless. If there are limits to it, then it's not real grace. It is the most precious thing in the universe and can be found nowhere else in existence than in the person of Jesus Christ. Look for it. I dare you. You will not find it anywhere else. I've spoken of unloading your shame. The unfortunate truth is that of yourself, you cannot. You are bound to the contract you signed when you ate the fruit – Your life for your offense. It's a zero-sum game. Someone has to pay, and that someone is you. And no religion or person or god that exists or is in your imagination will pay it for you. Because they can't. Their pockets aren't deep enough. Except for Jesus of Nazareth. Because He's the only one who will give you the grace that only He can and is willing to give. If you really want to be free, He will take your sin debt on Himself and the shame that comes with it, then instead of demanding payment for it, He'll tear up the note of debt. That's the grace of Jesus which he earned the right to give to anyone He wants to as much as He wants, and He wants to give you all that you need. He proved that when He earned the right, when he was wrongfully accused and murdered by the highest authorities of government and religion of Humanity. When the only one who's ever lived a worthy human life was killed by all the rest of us, because we didn't like what that enormous contrast revealed – that we are each and all despicable motherfuckers compared to all that a human should be. And when earth rejected Him, Heaven did too because of all the human shit he chose to carry with him – your death and shame. The only place left for Him to go was Hell. So, defenseless he went into the maw of His enemy, and there deposited the shame that you carry on your ledger at the feet of him who demands the payment from you. And while He was there, he told the poor bastards in its captivity that He had paid their debt too, because they would have never otherwise known they were free. And the moment all the debt of all of humanity was paid in full, Heaven proclaimed Him worthy. And suddenly there was in Hell, all that infinite power of that nebulous force that is existence itself, manifested in Him at once, bursting Hell asunder which could not contain Him, and setting free all

Finally Somehow Home

its captives that believed what He'd told them, leaving Hell in shattered ruin, He returned to His body on earth to plant His Church before He went home to take up His rightful place on the throne of all that is at the right hand of whatever that mysterious source of existence is that tells us to call it God the Father, and just as He was there in the beginning preparing the earth for humanity, so He is preparing another place for anyone who chooses to believe that the weight of their massive debt that is killing their life has been paid for in full, and by His grace you are free now to do whatever the fuck you want if you can discover what that is, free of shame, with no obligation, and armed to the teeth with the essence of the relationship that comprises that infinite triune existence, which He tells us to call the Holy Spirit of God, who He has sent to teach you how to get your shit together and be fulfilled and find peace and joy, and finally hear the music in this new and abundant life that you never knew you were missing. This is the Good News of Jesus Christ, God damn it! And that's the truth.

So, what do I have to do to get this free gift? Well, when Adam and Eve were standing there at the tree of Death, how did they buy into it? They believed the lie. Well, to eat from the tree of life, the cross of Christ, you must eat of its fruit. You must believe the truth. That's how you receive it.

Finally Somehow Home

By believing it. What is the truth? "Jesus said to him, "I am the way, and the truth, and the life; no one comes to the Father but through Me." John 14:6.

And what does He want us to do now?

Go back to finding that thing that I gave you, that life, and you enjoy that thing as much as you possibly can. You become the freest that you can ever become. Because that's when you're really you. And if you're not free, you can't do the things that only you can do the best, the way that only you can do them.

Because I believe the truth, all the things we just talked about. I see the world in a different way now. I see the world in a way that frees me, it removes the shame and lets the beauty draw me up. It frees me from the death, what we call sin. It's like reaching out and unplugging yourself from a source that's feeding on lies instead of truth. Exactly what caused all this mess in the first place. It is. Let's start seeing things how they really are. It's not God beating on you every time you sin. Every time you sin, he misses you.

So, I think I'd better kind of wrap this up pretty soon.

Finally Somehow Home

I think I've got it. I think I can, in good faith and conscience make a phone call and ask someone to get me a train ticket home. I think I can go now. Because I have found that thing that I love to do the most, the best, and most beautifully the way that only I can do it when I do it at my best.

Here's the thing about God. He's not a zapper. He doesn't need to miracle up a lightning bolt when you ask him for a sign. That's just an insult to Him. Make a lightning bolt!? He's like, "Cumon, all this stuff is made out of me, I can do way better than that." He never hands you a friggin' inner tube and a friggin' jet pack. Because that doesn't do you any good. If I would have gotten an inner tube or a jetpack out of this situation, I'd have never learned anything and it would've been a total waste. He is the great figure-outerer. He helps you figure shit out. When you ask him for his help, he's like, Yeah, let's do it, man. Start thinking. Do you know how I know?

Because you guys and me, we just watched a miracle. You watched me figure this out. Not just how to get out of this, this homelessness, but how to get out of this Wholemessness.

Finally Somehow Home

And now I know what I do best. And this is my first movie, book, work of art, whatever you want to call it. I hope you enjoyed it. I think I can go home now.

Chapter 35

It was just getting dark when I called Gary. He showed up soon after in his little white Prius and gave me a couple hundred bucks. Enough to get me to New York and a little extra. I was elated. I felt as though I had just slain a fucking dragon. The world made a lot more sense to me now. I'd found what I had been looking for. I didn't even realize it until it was over, but me filming myself making sense of all this life shit for myself and attempting to convey my line of reasoning to others was me doing exactly what I do best the way that only I can do it best because that's what I love doing the most, because that's what I was made to do. Hell, that's what this whole book really is. Until that point in my life, as I said before, I really didn't know what kind of shit I wanted to write, and in the pursuit of my mysterious destiny, immersed in the bravest and most difficult thing I'd ever done in my life up to that point, I unwittingly and instinctively

Finally Somehow Home

began doing exactly what it was that I was so frantically searching for to do. It was the bravest thing I'd done thus far because I knew damn well that everyone I knew would think I had legitimately gone insane, pity me, feel ashamed for me, and otherwise recoil at the cringiness of it all, especially because as I made each short video, I was posting them on social media. But under any other circumstances I would never have learned what I did. The tremendous shamefulness of the experience forced me to discover some very important things about shame that I would have otherwise missed. I was in the middle of it, submerged in it so completely that I quite literally had to reason my way from death to life. It was one of the most intense and epic battles I've ever fought. But it was all abit too much for the many friends and family who watched it unfold in real-time like a bad dream. So, as I was arriving at the apex of one of my life's most monumental victories, every other person on the planet who knew me was arriving at the conclusion that I had certainly gone stark raving mad, and all of them were deeply concerned for me. I can't say that I blame them, the videos show a man in disarray, distraught, and seemingly rambling on and on about existence and the universe and other such non-sense. I was dirty and

Finally Somehow Home

disheveled with a giant cold sore on my lip from the strain of it. Their emotional response to my appearance and disposition impeded any attention at all for the actual meaning of the words coming out of my mouth, but I didn't care. Inside, I was flying.

Gary dropped me off at Union Station downtown DC and I wandered around the massive courtyard relishing the cigarettes I'd just purchased with the money he'd given me. I had a few hours until my bus was ready to depart. I went into the dingey bathroom and washed up a little, put on a fresh shirt from my backpack, and combed my hair. I had some CREED Aventus cologne with me, so I doused myself with it. It felt amazing to be somewhat clean again. I went back outside for another smoke. A couple homeless black guys bummed cigarettes off me. One was crippled in a wheelchair and the other pushed his friend around dutifully. Goddamn, I thought. It's hard enough being homeless, let alone crippled and homeless. And I knew it wasn't easy for his friend who looked after him either. Homelessness is a full-time job, so the fact that he was willing to take care of his friend really grabbed at my heart as well. I sat down on the clammy concrete and we bullshat for awhile, and smoked. "You guys want something to eat?" I asked. I

Finally Somehow Home

walked with them into the food court. "Get whatever you want, guys. Get something to drink, too."

"No, Adam. This is plenty." They said, refusing any more than they needed. I grabbed afew extra cigarettes out of the pack and handed them each a couple. "I gotta run guys, my bus is leaving in afew minutes." I said as I grasped each one by the hand. "You guys stay safe, ok?"

"Stay Black, Adam." The crippled one said as I turned to go. I touched my fist to my heart and nodded, acknowledging the magnitude of what he'd just said to me.

"Take care guys."

The bus arrived at the New York Port Authority just after the sun came up. I had a new life ahead of me and had escaped the doom of my old fate. I felt free again, fearless and eager for whatever lay ahead. Banksy was her usual calm and unfluttered self when I showed up to the apartment. I assured her that I was OK and told her about my adventures. She'd been watching everything unfold on social media as well, so she was worried at first, but supportive and happy that I'd made it through my ordeal safe and sound once I gave her the straight skinny on it.

Finally Somehow Home

Everyone else, though, was not similarly disposed. Pretty much everybody was convinced that there was something seriously wrong with me and in various ways tried to convince me of the same. I became incensed and exasperated trying to explain, that yes indeed, some shit was very wrong, but me living on the streets for three days was the confrontation and resolution of it all. I'm fucking fine, God Damn it! I'm actually fucking GREAT now! They didn't get it. Some thought the "tough love" approach the best route: "What the hell is wrong with you!? What are you doing!? Your friends and family are worried sick about you!" I know there is a place for tough love, but most of it that I've ever seen in action is just laziness on the part of the accuser to really understand the situation. Mostly, I was accosted with cyclic salvos of nauseating pity. People were beside themselves with how much shame they knew I just had to be wallowing in. It pissed me off and made me sick to my stomach. I started to realize that few, if any, actually listened to what I was saying in the videos, so they missed the whole point of it. Not surprising in hindsight, but at the time I was livid. I had just accomplished what few other people in the world would ever have the sack to take on, and instead of celebrating the great victory of it, I was

Finally Somehow Home

lambasted with their fear and conviction that I needed mental care. Looking back on it, I understand. For one thing, the account and line of reasoning recorded in the videos I posted were not nearly as clearly stated as they are in this book. The previous chapters are, admittedly, a more fleshed out line of reasoning than what I could do then, just on video and from memory. Some redundancies and less relevant points have been omitted, and some of the salient points have been added to and reinforced in order to communicate to you, the reader, the ultimate findings of my curbside cerebral exploration. My parents, God bless them, were quietly beside themselves with concern. They asked that I go to a VA hospital in New Jersey and get evaluated, which I did. But they were still not satisfied because after speaking with the doctors and explaining what had transpired, the VA saw no reason to admit me for inpatient treatment.

Bansky reminded me that I had, in fact, paid another month's rent in advance before leaving, so I was able to stay in the apartment and see where life led me next for another month. My parents got in touch with Gary who bought me a plane ticket back to Ontario, Oregon. It was a good and well needed rest and I soaked in the peace

Finally Somehow Home

and calm of it for afew days until my parents asked if I would please visit the Boise VA hospital for a further mental evaluation. I was expecting to be interviewed and possibly stay in an inpatient evaluation program for a day or two, but they decided, instead, to lock me up for five days in the psych ward with a handful of recovering meth junkies and other cats and dogs. I was pretty fucking pissed off by the time I got out, but I knew my parents had recommended I go out of love for me, so I held no hard feelings. I did, however, take exception to the VA doctors' diagnosis of bipolar disorder, as I have never otherwise exhibited bipolar symptoms. I started to slowly believe that maybe they were all right. Maybe I was mad, but I knew that I had discovered some great and meaningful truths in the course of my adventure that had truly saved my life. I really don't know. Maybe there was a little bit of both going on. Stands to reason that the human mind in its normal state is not capable of exploring where the mind of a madman can. So, I was OK with either case, although the bipolar diagnosis seemed like a cop-out on the part of the VA docs. They prescribed me massive quantities of lithium and sent me on my way.

I arrived back in New York wondering what the hell I was gonna do next, but still reveling in my latest victory

Finally Somehow Home

and in the power I had found in it. So much more of life made sense to me now and I was strong and alive again – far more so than the pathetic and confused state I was in before I'd left to DC. I started working on *The Perfect Fucking Life* and compiling bits of writing from the many notebooks I'd filled with ideas over the past year.

A few days after I got back, I said, "Fuck this", and abruptly stopped taking my prescribed lithium medication. I don't know if that has anything to do with what happened next or not. I still don't quite fully understand it. I don't know if it was God or the Devil or both, but I find it hard to believe that, if there is a God and a Devil, they were not somehow deeply instrumental in the following events. I thought that if God is real, and the Devil is real, they had certainly noticed me by now, mental stability notwithstanding. Whether I really was mad or not, they would both undoubtedly be inclined to weigh in, in some form or fashion. Sometime before I had traveled to DC, I remember walking through New York City, a conversation raging in my head. I'd had enough. I felt thrown about and torn between the two rivals as if I was a ragdoll in the middle and remember saying clearly in my mind "Why don't both of you just fuck off and leave me the hell alone." Hell, maybe that had something to do

Finally Somehow Home

with it. I don't think it had the desired effect. If they hadn't noticed me until then they certainly did after that.

I had started a casual and bantering relationship with a pretty girl I'd met at a Ramen shop one evening. We mostly just texted back and forth until the subject of God came up. I told her, as succinctly as I could manage, what I believe. "I wish it wasn't true", I said. "But I cannot deny that it is." That was the end of our short relationship, but the sentiment held true. I've heard a lot of people say shit like, "I sure hope there is a God." Not me. I wish there wasn't one. I wish I could just do whatever the fuck I wanna do in life. And I think this is the highest and most fervent desire of humankind. But the strange thing is that, only because there is a God, can I do whatever the fuck I want to do in life. If there wasn't one, I'd be getting stepped on by everybody else doing whatever the fuck they want to do in life, and so would they, and it would just be a giant snarl of bullshit fuckery and mayhem. But the evidence before me seems to indicate that there is one. Thank God, he's a good one. If He wasn't we'd all be fucking dead by now. But at this point I was just sick of the whole fucking thing. And I think that was the point with the tree in the garden. To keep us from something

Finally Somehow Home

far beyond our comprehension and ability to deal with. Like making a three-year-old file taxes. That whole realm, and those dimensions are so far beyond our capacity to understand, it's pretty clear that we really aren't made for that world. Yet we somehow got all fucking tangled up in it. And I was fucking sick of it, thus the whole "both of you fuck off and leave me alone." But I guess it's got to work some way and that's just the way it works.

When I was a kid, probably about 12 years old, I distinctly remember to this day, being gripped by a sudden terror, almost a premonition, that I was the Antichrist. It was a severe and enduring mindfuck for me. Because, when you look at what the Antichrist does in the prophecies of Revelation, he actually does a lot of really good shit. The world comes together in peace. Everyone likes him. And then he takes a turn for the worse and goes toe to toe with God. Fuck that. I never ever want to find myself in a position where I'm opposite that guy. For more than just the reason that I would inevitably get my ass kicked. Mostly, though, because I really like Jesus. And He likes me. In fact, that's the thing about Jesus that is seldom, if ever, mentioned, and it's something I have clung to no matter how big of a shit I

Finally Somehow Home

think or realize that I am. Yes, we've all heard the song, and we've all heard people say: "Jesus loves you." He does. But the thing that blows my mind is that Jesus likes you. He thinks you're cool. He really wants to hang out with you. He is enamored with you. I think with the idea of God, at the end of the day, that's what really wins me over. Not to mention all the shit that He's done for me in my life. And I see his fingerprints everywhere throughout it. I know what they look like because it's the parts of life that are kind of blurry. The parts that I can't quantify in any way. The rest of the things of life are fairly easily explained. But all the shit that He's involved in is shrouded in impermeable mystery. That's why I think that He was involved in all this, although, to this day, seven years later, I still don't know what it was all about. Maybe I was crazy. Probably, I was. But honestly, I don't think I was as crazy as I was just wrong. But even if I was just completely insane, like I said before, if there really is a God and a Devil, there's no fucking way either one would be able to resist getting involved in this shit.

A few years before this, when I had been working in DC, I, of my own volition, and on my own time, blueprinted a powerful technology system capable of supercharging Artificial Intelligence, bringing Internet of Things to

Finally Somehow Home

reality, and far surpassing present Advanced Analytic capabilities in use by the DOD and Intelligence Communities, among other things. When I was the lead Subject Matter Expert for Advanced Analytics at CTTSO, it was my job to know and understand the state of the art in all such systems, and drawing from the meeting years ago at USSOCOM with the Green Beret Colonel named Stu and his challenge to create a system that would facilitate intelligence analysis and enrichment across multiple languages for Allied and Partner Nation collaboration, I had done just that, but had never gotten the funding to actually build it. Part of that blueprint was something called a digital identification. The idea behind this was that if a computer knows who you are and knows certain attributes about you, it can then more rapidly and accurately push information to you that is relevant to your operational context and to you yourself. For instance, if an Infantry Platoon Commander has orders to secure a road intersection, and sensors pick up a column of enemy tanks moving toward his position, if those sensors are plugged into a broader system of some kind, instead of the computer overwhelming every person on the battlefield as to tanks approaching that intersection, it could instead, send exactly and only the

Finally Somehow Home

pertinent information to the specific digital identification that is in that location presently and is in a position of authority as well as send that information to those digital identifications in his direct chain of command to inform them also as to what is transpiring. That lessens the Platoon Commander's burden of communications to his higher headquarters in the middle of a battle allowing him to focus on the battle itself, and also streamlines and simplifies communication flows throughout a complex environment, such as a battlefield. Digital identification, in this blueprint, would first have been incorporated into a form of identification already in use, such as a Common Access Card, which is the standard form of ID carried by US government and military personnel. A small microchip in the card would hold the information of its owner and, when linked to devices such as a GPS and communications equipment, would be able to act as a Blue Force tracking device as well as inform the system of the operational context of its owner. Coincidentally, this digital ID could be inserted subcutaneously, thereby ensuring that, in the heat of battle, it is always collocated directly with its owner. I trademarked this idea as $DIGID^{TM}$ with the US Patent and

Finally Somehow Home

Trademark Office. Well, while I was in New York I decided to modify the trademark for branding purposes and changed it from all capital letters to the simple lowercase, and replaced the two "I's" with colons so it looked like this: $d{:}g{:}d^{TM}$. The problem that occurred to me instantly after I wrote it down and saw it on paper, was that this subcutaneous identification or Mark bears a striking resemblance to "666". And I own the trademark to it. Not only that, but years ago I had already unwittingly blueprinted the system which I've described, which, when nested in a globally accessible virtual economic ecosystem, such as my "WAGGLE™" concept, would, at scale, provide education, training, employment, and commerce across the globe agnostic to national borders, perfectly facilitating all of the capabilities described in the prophecy of the book of Revelation that includes "The Mark of the Beast". *And he causes all, the small and the great, and the rich and the poor, and the free men and the slaves, to be given a mark on their right hand or on their forehead, and he provides that no one will be able to buy or to sell, except the one who has the mark, either the name of the beast or the number of his name. Here is wisdom. Let him who has understanding calculate the number of the beast, for the number is that of*

Finally Somehow Home

a man; and his number is six hundred and sixty-six. Revelation 13:16-18

Furthermore, I had just weeks ago been ranting about the idea, which I still believe to be true, that we all live in a Beast, and on top of that, had described myself as a Dragon in at least two poems I'd written. (The Dragon is another part of the prophecies of Revelation, and it's not a good dragon like Toothless, it's an asshole dragon that does some pretty cringey shit.) *And the whole earth was amazed and followed after the beast; they worshiped the dragon because he gave his authority to the beast; and they worshiped the beast, saying, "Who is like the beast, and who is able to wage war with him?"* Revelation 13:3-4. Not a single aspect of this was premeditated, except for maybe the idea I had mentioned before about pain inducing weapons based on Stonefish venom, which were indeed derived directly from the book of Revelation, but my idea behind that was to preserve life, not to destroy it. Add to that the idea of the Whipgun, and you have another prophecy of the book of Revelation fulfilled. *They have tails like scorpions, and stings; and in their tails is their power to hurt men for five months.* Revelation 9:10.

Finally Somehow Home

I could feel it building. This strange and inexorable momentum toward something that I knew would utterly destroy me. Maybe part of me wanted to pull God's punk card. To see if - if someone really claimed to be God, what would happen? Would God show up? What the fuck has to happen for God to actually show the fuck up? I wanted to see it. I wanted to see Him. I felt as though it was on my plate. Like a destiny waiting for me. I didn't think I was worthy of being God. That's not what it was. It's not that I thought that I was so god damn good. It's that I knew I was so god damn wretched. I still don't understand it. But this is what happened.

Around that time there was a huge jackpot on POWERBALL for over a billion dollars. That would easily cover the cost to build the enterprise I had envisioned. I bought a ticket with whatever I could scrape up and posted on social media that if I won the lottery I would change my name to "Jesus Fucking Christ". I woke up early the morning after the drawing and walked the half mile to my closest 711 in West New York, NJ. When the Pakistani dude behind the counter told me I was not a winner I was shocked. I asked him to check the ticket again. No luck. No divine intervention there.

Finally Somehow Home

Regardless, that night I made the subconscious decision to finally own my shit. I'm not sure what got me there, but I knew what I had to do. The next morning, I woke up early and went to Times Square as the sun was coming up. A couple of guys approached me and asked me to take their picture. I took several pictures of them and could see them talking between themselves about something. "Are you someone that we should know about?" One of them asked. "Kind of." I said.

"What's your name?"

"I just changed it this morning and I'm not really comfortable with telling you that right now." I replied. They thanked me and said that they understood and wished me the best of luck. I walked around downtown for a while. Passing by a subway station there were always groups of young black kids out rapping and hustling their beats on CDs they'd hand out. One of them asked me for a cigarette. I happily obliged and lit it for him. "What's your name, man?" he said. "Jesus." I said. He looked at me, reading my face to understand if I was joking or not. "Right on, man." he said when he saw that I was serious. Claiming the name of Jesus gave me resolve. I walked on. I saw an Asian family walking toward me.

Finally Somehow Home

The one in the front seemed to be the youngest, in his late teens or early 20s. It looked like his older brother was next to him, guiding him, making sure he didn't bump into anything because he was blind. I made a beeline for the blind guy and put my hand on his shoulder. There was a look of confusion and fear on the face of his brother for a moment and bewilderment on the face of the blind man. "If you believe, you can be healed." I said. "Be healed." "You're scaring him." His older brother said. I can still see the look of hope and terror on the face of the blind man. I nodded to his brother and walked on. I took a short break and emailed Gary. "The blind see." I said.

Those days were filled with power. It was the most free I have ever been because it's the most courageous I have ever been. I was absolutely lucid and reasonable, and I knew damn well what I was doing was thought be insane by all who saw or heard me, but I claimed to be the Son of God, and in so doing, believed that I was. There's no experience like that. When you absolutely believe, beyond any shadow of a doubt that you are the Son of the Almighty God. It was like another dimension of reality.

Finally Somehow Home

I took selfies and posted them on social media saying "the new face of God". I claimed to be Jesus come back to earth, and the Antichrist in one. I never heard any voices. But it was as if thoughts were being placed in my head. Not just thoughts but almost visions. One of them was Judas. He explained to me that Jesus had despised him on the cross. Which was the reason that God had rejected Jesus' sacrifice. Which was why Jesus said, "My God, my God, why have you forsaken me?". On that basis, I reasoned, Jesus must return to earth once again, and I was it.

I've thought a lot about Jesus when he was here on earth. When did he realize that he was God? When did he own his shit? He may have known it growing up because his parents probably told him what they'd been told by the angel before his birth, but when did he actually take the step and claim that identity for himself? There had to have been a definitive moment of some kind for him. Maybe it was at the wedding in Cana where he turned water into wine which was his first miracle. But I doubt it. But it had to have happened at some time in his life. That actually took place. A man of this earth from the womb of a woman claimed to be God, and he was right. And I could not deny the tremendous feeling. Like a

Finally Somehow Home

destiny I was hurtling toward that I was indeed Jesus Christ the Son of God. But I knew that the church would reject me as such and label me the Antichrist.

I saw Frank Sinatra. He was a nobody in the other world. Like the first guy who introduces himself to you when you first arrive at a new company or unit, the guy who tries to be your friend right off, because he's a loser and has no other friends. That was him. Longing for attention. I blew him off.

There was the drummer in the subway. The kid with no arms. He'd attached drumsticks to the nubs of his arms and was beating on cans with them to earn a little money. "If I told you I could heal you, would you let me?" I asked him. He paused and peered into my soul. "I don't think so." he said. "Why not?" I asked. "I just don't think I could handle the disappointment," he said, "if it didn't work."

Then there was the homeless black lady. It was about four thirty in the morning and the sun was just starting to come up. I was walking along the street and sat down to share a cigarette with her. "Who are you?" she asked me after a bit of small talk. "I'm Jesus Christ." I told her. "I just came back." She looked intensely at me. Frozen.

Finally Somehow Home

Then she got up very slowly and backed away one step at a time, then turned and fled.

It went on for about three days. Most of that time I wandered around the city. Adderall kept me awake all but 3 to 4 hours each night, and probably a little mania. I posted it all on social media. Then on the morning of the fourth day I woke up. I got out of bed and sat there suddenly aware that I had been claiming to be Jesus Christ, the Son of God. And I knew that I was not. I knew because God had publicly endorsed Jesus as His Son with the dove at the Jordan. He had not similarly endorsed me. I opened my desk drawer and grabbed the forsaken bottle of lithium, took two, and tried to go back to sleep to make it all go away. As I lay there in my bed, strange but real pains gripped me in a cold sweat. Something I had written months before came crashing into my mind and I knew I was living it out right then, sweating and thrashing from agonies of every kind within me that I could not define.

THE DRAGONRIDER'S SONG

Finally Somehow Home

FUCK FEAR. IT'S BUT THE FANTASY OF PAIN. FUCK PAIN. WHEN IT'S GONE I WILL REMAIN, SO LONG AS BLOODY NOSTRILS FLAIR, AND BURNING LUNGS CAN FILL WITH AIR, THE BLINDING SHREIK OF SOUL AND MIND ARE ONLY NOW. AND NOW WILL SOON BE LEFT BEHIND. FOR ONLY IN THAT LENGTH AND BREADTH OF TIME AND DEPTH OF PAIN IS THERE A FORGE SO HOT TO MELT THE DROSS AND PURE THE SOUL AND SMELT AND SMITH THE MIND AND WILL TO HOLD AN EDGE THAT'S SHARP AND HARD – ENOUGH TO CUT THE SHARDS OF DARK AND SHEER THE BARBS FROM SHATTERED DARTS STUCK DEEP AND HARD IN DEEPEST PARTS OF BLOODY BLUDGEONED SOUL AND HEART AND CUT THE INKY DUNGEON DARK AWAY WITH FLAME – IGNITES THE PAIN – A POWDER KEG – AND SPARKS THE CONFLAGRATION THROUGH THE VEINS AND BOILS THE BLOOD AND BURNS AWAY MY FACE ERASING MY IDENTITY – THAT OTHERS SEE – THAT WASN'T REALLY EVER ME AND EVERY SINGLE THING'S AFLAME AND BURNED AWAY EXCEPT A NAME AND EVERYTHING THAT ISN'T ME HAS DIED IT'S GONE I'M PURIFIED I'M STERILE-CLEAN, I WASN'T GETTING WEAKER ALL ALONG – I THOUGHT I WAS – BUT ALL THE WEIGHT OF FEAR AND HATE AND PAIN

Finally Somehow Home

AND FAKE ARE GONE AWAY I'M STRONG AND LEAN AND FIERCE AGAIN I'M MORE THAN FREE, I'M LESS THAN I HAVE EVER BEEN, I'M NOTHING ELSE AT ALL - BUT ME.

And I didn't hear a voice, but I felt something leave. And as it left me out the open window of my bedroom the words rose in my mind as if placed there:

"Fine, go back to your impotent God who never does anything."

I sent Gary another e-mail. This is what it said:

"Please erase that email I sent to you. Someone else could use it. It's powerful. Adam was someone else. He left yesterday. I "woke up" laying on the couch saying "Jason, wake up. You're ok." out loud to myself. Looking forward to new things."

It was all finally over.

Finally Somehow Home

Chapter 36

The poem was right on the money. I had destroyed myself. I had become a pariah. I was nothing. *Nothing else at all but me.* I had died for my sins. I did. I had committed the ultimate blasphemy against God, and as a result my past life was over. Do you see how that works now about sin? I had killed it. Killed it dead. All credibility was gone. All reputation. Everything stripped away. Everything that wasn't only just me was fucking gone. Except for who I am. And in spite of the hot water I knew I might be in with God, it felt so good to be free of the dead life I'd been dragging behind me. It did. It was as if I was breathing fresh air while everyone around me was choking on coal dust. I had overcome crippling shame only weeks before, and I was free. Of everything that wasn't me. The courage I had erroneously used to proclaim that I was Jesus Christ had

-478-

Finally Somehow Home

not left me. And it was just as strong. Shame conquers courage, but for me, reason had conquered shame. I saw my courage for what it really was then... just like in the Dragon poem, "...his greatest power is in his bleeding...", courage is a wild and dangerous thing, and its magnitude is exactly proportionate to how much pain you are able to bear, and I knew shame was a scam, so I could bear a lot of it. Courage is power. Your courage is your power. I had mustered all of my power on full afterburner and flown straight into the side of a fucking mountain. I had just failed like a fuck in front of everyone again. Shame is a scam. It ain't real, if you have grace. But I didn't know if God would forgive me for this one. Historically, one doesn't get away with Impersonating a Deity. That's gotta be at least a misdemeanor. I thought that I was doing what I was supposed to do. I felt tricked. Fooled by God Himself. Betrayed almost. I thought I was manning up, having faith like Abraham, withholding nothing, going all in, stepping into my destiny, in spite of the fact that I knew it would destroy me. Everyone I knew had watched it all go down. And for those who didn't witness it firsthand, my ex was kind enough to email every person on my Contacts list of the computer I had left with her and tell them all about it. My kids knew about it

Finally Somehow Home

too. Rent was due. I had no money. I had no job. I had no place to go. I had no vindication. And I never would, from this.

While I had been roaming the streets telling everyone I was Jesus, my Marine Corps and other Special Ops buddies were monitoring the situation. They had gotten in touch with Banksy to make sure she was OK and were standing by to help however they could. Some of them had actually been planning a snatch-and-grab, but I'm glad that didn't go down. Not sure that would have worked out well for any of us and thankfully I snapped out of it before something like that was necessary. I was the boldest and most confused I've ever been. All I wanted to do was to be a part of whatever that nebulous triune Source is up to in this universe, and as a result of my boldness and willingness to do so, I was completely destroyed. The only thing that survived was only all that I've ever been, and I had only just figured out what that was on the streets of DC. I was the strongest I'd ever been in my life, and at the same time, had no credibility with anyone on this earth that knew me. My only choice was to be silent. To shut up and color like the rest of them and act like I had not found peace. And I think that's what made people so frantic. My life had just exploded in a

Finally Somehow Home

public, self-inflicted, completely deserved thermonuclear disasterfuck and I was ok with it. In fact, I seemed strangely happy.

If you ever do find happiness, I have a sad revelation for you. You will be standing there alone and lonely in it waiting for someone else to show up. And you will look at them all and hear all of their excuses for not being happy, and you will long for them to abandon them, but they won't. They will invariably demand that you exit your happiness and dive again down into the grime and take offense at something to relate to them. And if you don't do it, they will not understand and say you can't relate, and if you blow off their excuses as they should, you will make them angry, because their excuses against their own happiness are the most important things in their lives. It's true. Our most sacred treasure is our most vicious pain. Clinging to it gives us the right to do shit. It justifies our anger and our hate. My pain was gone. At least for the moment. As if the fire that burned everything away had gone deep enough to get the nerves. Like the charcoal of a third degree burn there was no sensation left. Only the dawning realization that the healing would be the most painful part of it.

Finally Somehow Home

So, I was supremely alone in my happiness. Because no one would approach me as if I were happy, because no one that knew me believed that I could be, because I had just sacrificed all the shit they were striving for which didn't make them happy and they all thought more of that if they could get it would make them so, and I knew it wouldn't and I didn't give a fuck about it, so I felt obligated to act unhappy around others so I could relate to them. But I didn't do it. And I don't think I'll ever do it again. So, I was alone.

But whether I was happy or not, I was still in deep shit. Once I put the word out on social media that I didn't think I was Jesus anymore, my phone started blowing up. And it wasn't church friends calling. It was my War Brothers.

Monkey was a SEAL. He looked and acted like a roided out version of Joey from *FRIENDS*, which was another of his callsigns over the years. I had worked with him in Iraq. He was on the Baghdad team, while I was in Ramadi, but for some reason, whenever we were together, we always got into a shitload of trouble. It was March of 2005, and I was rotating out for a one-month break with abunch of guys from other sites. We got into Amman,

Finally Somehow Home

Jordan from Baghdad late that afternoon, put all of our gear and bags in our hotel rooms, and proceeded to go out and get completely fucking annihilated. But on the way to the bars we all stopped at pharmacies and stocked up on steroids, Ambien, Valium, Cialis Viagra, and anything else we could get our hands on. My hotel roommate had an early flight out to South Africa that morning and I had set my alarm to wake up for the flight that most of us were on back to the US. Unfortunately, the alarm clock thing didn't work out for me. I woke up to a flying elbow to the face. Monkey had noticed that I was not present in the lobby when everyone else was getting ready to go to the airport and had come up to my room to check on me. First, he filled the ice bucket with ice water and threw it in my face. No response. There were two queen beds in the room about 5 feet apart, so Monkey took a running start, launched into the air off the first bed and brought his entire 240 pounds down on my face with his massive elbow. "What's going on!?" I asked in a bewildered stupor.

"Dude, everyone's getting ready to leave. We're all in the lobby. Hurry the fuck up." I jumped out of bed, grabbed all my shit, and headed to the lobby with Monkey. As we got on the plane Monkey asked me if I had any Ambien.

Finally Somehow Home

"Of course, bro. And here's another one for your next flight." I was still hungover as fuck and tired, so I took a Valium and an Ambien and passed out in my seat. About five hours into the flight, I woke up. Some girls were giggling and laughing behind me. I looked back over my shoulder to find Monkey sitting in the middle seat of the middle row between 5 or 6 hot Lebanese girls with his huge arms stretched out around them. I didn't think anything of it and got up to go to the bathroom. On the way to the bathroom, I noticed people looking at me strangely, sniggering, or turning away and trying not to laugh. God Damn it. What the fuck. I got into the bathroom and looked into the mirror. Dicks of various sizes and shapes were drawn all over my forehead and face with a permanent black Sharpie marker. I looked like a coal miner who'd just found the Dick motherload. God Damn it, Monkey! After a half hour or so I managed to get all the dicks scrubbed off my face and came out of the bathroom to find Monkey sitting in my seat and grinning up at me and swaying slightly from side to side. "You motherfucker. Payback's a bitch." I said, laughing. "Now, go back to your fucking seat and get some rest, bro. Take that other Ambien."

"I need more, I already took those."

Finally Somehow Home

"Jesus Fucking Christ, Seth. Here's two more. Now go to sleep."

I went back to my seat to try and finish out the rest of the flight in peace and closed my eyes. The cabin was dark and chilly and dry, and the incessant rumbling of the jet engines had put most of the passengers to sleep, all wedged in different states of disarray in their seats. I awoke to the sound of a small, subdued commotion behind me from which I distinctly heard Monkey's voice. "It fell off."

I could see his shadow coming toward me now. Shuffling down the aisle carrying something enormous, the form of which I couldn't quite make out. "Monkey, what's going on?"

"It fell off." He mumbled again.

About the time the flight attendant came around the corner from the galley, is about the same time that Monkey emerged from the shadows with an entire overhead luggage bin in his hand. The flight attendant's face looked like it was being stretched causing his eyes to pop out alittle. "What-What-What happened?"

Finally Somehow Home

"It fell off."

The little flight attendant was about to lose his shit.

"He's very tired", I said as I grabbed Seth and hurried him back to his seat, over which dangled the remains of the components that had once secured the overhead luggage bin to the rest of the airplane. "Now, go to sleep, Monkey, God damn it."

I didn't see him again for a couple of months, and when I did see him, he had no recollection whatsoever of the events on the plane, but he told me what had happened next. Dawg, another SEAL who I worked closely with later based out of Bagram, and who'd been in the Teams with Monkey, had gotten him to his connecting flight once we landed in the US, and his girlfriend picked him up from the airport, drove him home, and poured his big ass into bed where he passed the fuck out for a while. When he woke up the Ambien had worn off, but happy-go-lucky Seth was in deep shit. He could not for the life of him explain how his pockets were filled with the phone numbers of so many Lebanese chicks.

I ran into Monkey a couple of years later on a classified program. We were going through the initial screening

Finally Somehow Home

and selection course. Monkey was another of the students and picked us up at the airport. I didn't know he'd be there, so it was an awesome surprise to see him again. We threw our bags into the rental car and headed to the hotel. "Bro, I'm off the sauce man. I'm all natural from here on out."

I was truly shocked. Monkey ate at least one bowl of Dbol flakes with Tren-sprinkles for breakfast every morning. "No shit! I'm proud of you, brother. How long you been off juice?"

"Four days."

"Wow, that's pretty good, Monkey. Keep it going, bro." I figured I could buy his liver another day of rest if I said something encouraging like that, but no telling what kind of experimental horse steroid was still coursing through his system from four days earlier. I'm not sure how many extra days he made it, but I doubt it was more than two. Monkey was a goddamn machine. We were in the wrong lane. Monkey's dumb ass was in the lane to go straight at the light and the hotel was to the left. "Don't try this at home," he said with a wry grin on his face, as he hit the gas and spun the wheel and smashed directly into the car in his blind spot.

Finally Somehow Home

"No one man, in full kit, can pick up a fully equipped shooter and run them off the battlefield," the instructor said.

"I can." said Monkey.

"Bullshit."

"I'll show you."

"Let's see it." Said the instructor as he pointed at a 6'4", 260-pound student. "Go put your body armor on and get your M4. Lay down on your back over there and stay limp. You're wounded."

"OK, Monkey, go pick him up." Monkey, in full body armor, with his rifle slung, got a running start at the student lying on the ground. He grabbed him by the front of the body armor, and rolling, somehow emerged at a dead sprint with the massive dude on his back, arms and legs flailing. Monkey sprinted 100 meters with him before the instructors told him to stop. Monkey was a god damn beast. I fought him on several occasions. It was all fun and games, but we punched each other in the face a lot when we'd get drunk.

Finally Somehow Home

Monkey got in touch with me immediately and offered to help however he could. I was out of money, so he sent me some. He said he had a buddy in Pennsylvania that I could stay with, and he might even have a job for me. It was my only real option, so I jumped at it.

Remember when I told you about Moshpit? Moshpit had been Philthy's Team Leader and Mentor for several years in the Marine Corps. When Moshpit was hit by the IED that ignited the fuel cans in the back of his gun-truck in 2009, Philthy took it very hard. He got good and shitfaced for a few days, then he got busy figuring out a way to help his brother. He and Potsy were running a very successful private security company out of Florida, and even into Haiti and the Dominican Republic, but Phil made the time and started running marathons, hosting golf tournaments, and talking to anyone who'd listen to make it happen for Moshpit. Like a man possessed, Phithy created the Brothers In Arms Foundation and began to build it. Within weeks he was distributing donations to Moshpit's family as well as the other families of those hit in the same ambush. Within two years BIAF, along with a couple of other fundraising partners, had raised the money and begun construction on a beautiful and accessible home in San Antonio, Texas

Finally Somehow Home

for his wounded Team Leader. But Phil kept going with it, expanding the Foundation's reach. The Brothers in Arms Foundation is a resource for veterans and families of veterans in crisis and serves the US Marine Recon and Raider communities as well as others in need. They cover expenses that the VA and others can't, such as burdens upon family members within and outside of the immediate family, family friends, girlfriends, or little things, like, what are we going to do with the pets while we go to the funeral, all the way up to hotel rooms and transportation, which brings up Raider Air. Raider Air is any kind of air support up to and including a 747's time and crew donated in support of Brothers In Arms Foundation support activities. The Foundation is one of the few, if not the only Non-profit Organization with a Memorandum of Agreement for transportation of active duty troops and their families by air with DOD.

Philthy got ahold of me right off the bat. He sent me some cash and helped me get a Uhaul to go to Pennsylvania. I packed the entire apartment up in one night. Partially because I had to be in North Bend, Pennsylvania by 10:30 the next morning, and partially because I knew Banksy was low key pissed at me and it bummed me out. I felt like shit for putting her through all that I had. She was

Finally Somehow Home

supportive as hell of me from day one, in my work, in my art, in everything, and I had become a cringey pain in her ass. Before I left, I sold her my $16K sofa and chair combo for 2 Grand. It was the best I could do to say thanks and still somehow plague her eternally with the memory of me. I was sitting on the ramp of the Uhaul with everything inside, packed up, ready to go, toothpaste in all the holes I'd left in the walls of the apartment, all done. I saw Banksy's light come on as her bedroom window turned gold in the early morning light. I should run upstairs once more and give her a big hug and say goodbye, I thought. I took another glance at the window, flicked the cigarette onto the street, got into the Uhaul, started the engine, and drove away. Shame fucks you like that.

You don't get smarter by taking tests. All that a test will teach you is all that you don't know about something. It's the knowledge of what you don't know that is the gold from the test. It is all the answers you get wrong that show you the way ahead. They show you your blind spots. How you were looking at it wrong before. Be a student of your errors.

Finally Somehow Home

But that only works if you stop and turn and look back and study them. And that is not an easy thing to do. But I had to do it.

I had been duped. By God, by the Devil, or by myself, I didn't know. It seemed like a combo of all three. Maybe I was in one of those situations that Job in the Bible was in, but for Job it was all, "Check out my servant, Job. He's righteous and awesome and whatever you do to him, he won't curse me, ha!", but for me it must have been something like, "Check out Jason over here, he's a complete fucking shit-show, and stupid, but He loves me. How much you wanna bet if he thought I wanted him to claim to be Jesus, he'd do it? The motherfucker will literally do whatever I say, ha!" And He was right. And I did. But there are a few things I should have caught on to before I went that far. The truth really does set you free. It was because I hadn't been endorsed by God that I snapped out of it all. That was truth destroying lies. Furthermore, I realized that I could never be the Antichrist since I will always bow the knee to Jesus. He is my Captain, my King, the Lord of my life, and the Son of God. "Though he slay me, I will hope in him..." Job 13:15. And the book of 1 John emphatically states that the Antichrist will deny that Jesus is the Son of God: "Who is the liar but the one who denies that Jesus is the Christ? This is the antichrist, the one who denies the Father and the Son." 1 John 2:22. So, there's no way I could actually be the Antichrist. I heard a pithy quote that describes my condition quite well at the time: "Don't believe everything you think." That is exactly what I was doing, and with alittle mania sprinkled in there, you can start to believe all kinds of shit if you don't backstop it with truth.

The question must be asked: If I didn't believe in all this "religious mumbo-jumbo" would I not have gone through this? Was I just a victim of my own bullshit belief system? Yes and no. Yes, I would have gone through some existential crisis anyway, but I would have been stuck there had I not had access to the truth to set me free from it. Anyone who goes mad will go mad in the direction of their greatest vector of thought and imagination, and this kind of shit is the kind of shit I think about most and most deeply. So no, I would not have gone through it in the same way, and I would have never uncovered all the truths I did that have set me free had I not believed in all this "God hooey". Some things are worth the pain of them.

Finally Somehow Home

North Bend was enchanting. My hosts, Mike and Denise, lived in a house on Main Street built on a lot that Mike's dad had won in a poker game against a family rival. Right Hand Young Woman's Creek flowed into and through town from the North and another small Creek joined it that cut through the center of town from West to East out of Skunk Hollow just before Right Hand Young Woman's Creek emptied itself into the West Branch of the Susquehanna River that ran from West to East below the town. The air was fat and wet and the drooping black and grey clouds hung low over the dripping green mountains like dirty, burnt, fucked up cotton. The rain was thick and splatty like in the tropics and dumped on the soggy mountains around the little town in turns, sending drops and rivulets into the draws and hollows where they met to make trickles and streams that swirled into the creeks where the trout were rising after the June hatches adding to the rain rings on the clear water.

There's something about fishing. Even Jesus seemed to like it. Hell, after Jesus was crucified, his disciples said, "fuck it, we're going fishing." and went fucking fishing.

Finally Somehow Home

There's just something about it. Especially with a rod and fly. There's nothing else in the world like the sudden soft shudder and tug of the line down the pole into your fingertips when the trout rises to your fly and takes it, and if you don't do something right, right then, you'll lose him, but you must be as gentle as the fish is or you'll snap your 3 lb tippet, then the measured soft flick of the wrist even though you really want to pull with all your might, and a tenth of a second later, once the bend of the pole has put the pressure on the line and stretched it, the hook bites in and you know because you feel the fish's confusion turn to rage and then the dance is on. And you're touching each other through the rod and line. You can read him, and he can read you. And in those moments, if you're good enough, you know what he is thinking, and the only thing you hope for in all your life right then is to land him in your net, and that's the only thing in his that he's trying to fight, and you are one with him, and he with you in the most elegant contention for life itself that you will ever experience. And there's fly line everywhere in the rushing water and your rod is as straight in the air and as high as you can hold it while bending your knee and with the other hand scooping the beautiful, slick, gleaming, shimmery, exhausted

Finally Somehow Home

creature into your net and the world is right, and you've just won something monumental but you don't know why, you just know it was beautiful, and you let him go back into the cold current between your knees and see the big swish with his spotted tail right before you never see him again in your life and he's gone and no one knows but you and him forever the depths of all that you felt when you felt all of him fighting all of you for all of his life, when all you had to win with was pure elegance and finesse, and you did.

Mike was a sportsman and outfitted me with a fly rod and flies and I spent a lot of time on the creeks and rivers with him and his brother, JR. JR could tell you anything you wanted to know about anything outdoors. Especially when it came to fly-fishing. He and Mike helped me hone my art tremendously and I'm a better man for knowing them. Ray was a bona fide Pennsylvania mountain man and lived next door to Mike and Denise's. We would all get together most nights and have a fire out on the back deck and smoke cigars and drink and throw knives and axes and listen to music and bullshit about nothing. It was good for my soul to be there. It was like being a kid again.

Chapter 37

That was seven years ago. And just what was it all about? I still don't know all of it. But I have a sneaking suspicion that when I got on my knees on that shitty carpet with the French swirls in it at that hotel in Denver and asked God to do whatever it takes, no matter what, I think that mighta had something to do with it. Did I get success or fame or fortune from any of it? No, that's not what I was asking for, but it does bring up the question: So, what gives me the right to give anyone any advice at all? Hell, according to what everyone else is striving for to make them happy, I didn't get any of that. I have all the shit that everyone doesn't know that they want but does, and none of the shit that everyone is going for but never gets enough of. I have love, joy, peace, patience, kindness, goodness, faithfulness, gentleness, and self-control in my life and for me alone. And don't forget the "F" word.

Finally Somehow Home

The thing that no one wants to claim that they want, but what actually gives them the most beautiful things in life. Yes, a Family. But it didn't start off like that.

I went back to Oregon, to my parents' basement. I finally went through all of my notebooks and fully compiled the first draft of *The Perfect Fucking Life*. I worked construction for $15/hr cash under the table. And every second of every day at work I wondered how the fuck I'd gotten there. I wondered if that was it for me. I had no way out. I owed $2500 per month in child support and over $150K to the IRS with interest rising at $1000 per month. I couldn't even get to square one. I made about $500 every week in cash and would Western Union half of it every two weeks to the ex, but the court didn't know or care, and I couldn't afford a lawyer, so the arrears kept accruing. And for all my other debt, I couldn't afford to declare bankruptcy.

I moved to Snohomish, Washington. My buddy's sister let me rent a spare room from her there, and I figured with all the tech companies in the Seattle area, I'd be able to land a decent job and get back on my feet. The first job I got was as an electrician's apprentice wiring low volt shit for $14.50/hr. The job mostly consisted of climbing

Finally Somehow Home

up a ladder, drilling a big hole in a 2x6 above your head with all the sawdust and bullshit falling into your eyes and down the back of your hoodie, climbing down the ladder, moving the ladder 2 ft, climbing up the ladder, drilling another hole in another 2x6, climbing down the ladder, moving the ladder two feet, climbing up the ladder... that's pretty much what it was for 8 hours every day. I was a 40-year-old electrician's apprentice working the same job as high school kids. The very first day on the job, I got down on my knees in the porta-shitter, and staring down into the blue water full of other people's shit and piss, asked God with tears in my eyes just what the fuck His plan was in all this. Within 4-5 weeks, the State caught onto the fact that my wages weren't being garnished for child support, and quickly amended the problem. Instead of $14.50/hr I was now making $6.53/hr before taxes. I tried to make it work as long as I could, but as all the job sites that I was on were far away from Snohomish and took a lot of gas to get to and back, after two weeks I told my boss that I couldn't afford the gas money to get to work and had to quit. As I was driving home, not knowing what to do next, I passed a car dealership in Kirkland that sold Maseratis, Alfa Romeos, and FIATs. I went home, took a shower, grabbed

Finally Somehow Home

my fanciest duds, printed off a resume, and went back to the car dealership.

I've heard that the equivalent of being a stripper, for a guy, is joining the military. I thought that was true until I got into selling cars. The GM's name was Steve. He was a cool motherfucker and we hit it off right away. From day one, I fell in love with the Italian craftsmanship. From the stitching in the seats and dash to the sound of those Italian engines ringing through their exhaust, it was all beautiful. Even FIAT, with the Abarth and the Spider, had a fun and sporty side. The Alfas were beautiful and mean as fuck, especially the Quadrifoglios. The Quadrifoglio is a four leafed clover represented in a white triangle on all Alfa race cars to this day. In the early 1920's, one of Alfa's drivers, Ugo Sivocci, kept coming in second place to a certain Enzo Ferrari. One day in 1923, before a race in Targa Florio, Ugo painted a white square on his new car with a green four leafed clover in it and began winning races. A few weeks later, while test driving a new car before his crew was able to paint the lucky four leafed clover on it, he crashed and fucking died. So, never missing a chance at melodrama, and to immortalize Ugo, the Italians lopped off one of the corners of the square to commemorate his death, and

Finally Somehow Home

every Alfa Romeo race car since has borne the green four leafed clover inside of a white triangle as the Quadrifoglio. The Giulia and Stelvio Quadrifoglios of today carry a Ferrari 2.9 Litre Twin Turbo V6 with 505Hp and 443 ft-lb of torque, and in RACE mode, they sound like the Devil's whorehouse with otherworldly grunts and screams and groans emitting from the quad pipes.

The Maseratis were exquisite. Like a big-titted stripper that's out of your league. Every inch of them was a masterpiece of craftsmanship. Because Maserati shares a building with Ferrari, there's a lot of cross pollination from both sides that goes into creating these blistering fast and loud works of art. And one of the many things I love about Maserati is that you can blow the doors off a Corvette with your whole family in the car.

I sucked at selling cars. Well, at least the slow ones. I sold more Maseratis and Alfa Romeo Quadrifoglios than any other sales rep, but the run of the mill cars and SUVs and the little gutless FIATs I really didn't give a fuck about, so I wasn't good at selling them, though I desperately needed the money. It was commission-based pay, of course, so while it was only as consistent as my car sales,

Finally Somehow Home

which was abysmal, for some reason the State left me alone and didn't garnish my scant earnings.

Every month on payday, I would go to my favorite Indian restaurant in Mill Creek and get a giant steaming plate of Lamb Biryani to go and a couple cigars from the tobacco shop nearby. That was my ultimate and only luxury in life. I lived in a small room with a queen mattress on the floor and one small dresser. All I had brought with me were my clothes and my laptop. I didn't think about writing. I didn't think about Africa, or New York, or DC, or Pennsylvania. I didn't want to think about any of it. All of that seemed far away to me. As distant as if it had never happened. Or like it had happened to someone else in another life. Maybe it had. I was someone else, and though I was in the same mind and body, it was not the same life.

There were a few bright spots. But not many. One of them was Dr. Teresa Cheng and the organization she founded called Everyone for Veterans. My teeth had been giving me problems and were in complete disarray, and I had no dental insurance. Somehow, I got ahold of Dr. Cheng and discovered that E4V is a network of dentists provides free dental work for Veterans across the

Finally Somehow Home

United States. I was able to get into Minahan Dental in Kenmore, Washington, and get a complete overhaul of my teeth at no cost. I don't think Dr. Cheng and her staff at E4V, or the folks at Minahan Dental, understand how much that means to someone in the position I was in at that time, but I am forever grateful for it. If you're a veteran and you need dental work done, look into Everyone for Veterans. They're eager to help.

Every spare moment I looked for work at Microsoft, or Amazon, or Boeing, or one of the many other massive tech companies in the area. "Not enough work experience." "Not technical enough." "Overqualified." "Underqualified." One of my clients at the Maserati dealership was the HR Director at Microsoft. Even with her help setting up an interview for me, nothing. The only reason I wasn't just wallowing in despair is because that had gotten boring a long time ago. Hell, the reason I'd quit writing is because I was sick of writing about the misery I was in. I took long lonesome walks down the bike trail that ran through town. Five miles or more, some days. I tried fucking around with my photography, but mostly out of boredom. Every once in a great while I'd have an extra eight bucks or so, which was enough for a drink and a tip for the bartender at one of the many

Finally Somehow Home

watering holes in the quaint little town. If I stretched the drink out long enough, I could spend a half hour at the bar as if I had a normal life like everyone else. But it didn't matter. Even if I did happen to make friends with anyone at the bar, I had nothing to offer them. I could only afford to breathe and sleep, and I often went hungry. I used to keep a jar of peanut butter in my desk at work and eat spoonfuls of the stuff because I couldn't afford lunch. I talked to my kids occasionally, which was awesome and horrible, because invariably, David would ask me why I wasn't sending Mommy any money. That kind of humiliation is the worst I've ever felt. The gloom of the Seattle sky was nothing compared to what I felt inside. I was worthless. To myself and to everyone else. No wonder a certain someone had told me that it would be better for everyone if I just killed myself. I couldn't understand how, after all that I had been through, and learned, and experienced, and seen, and done, how was I still so fucking worthless. Nobody wanted me. For anything. Nobody. I couldn't even give myself away if I'd tried to. Too much baggage. And all I saw in my future was that I might make it, just barely hanging on, if I was lucky, until I died there in it. There was no light at the end of the tunnel. There was no tunnel. Just a caved-in tomb.

Finally Somehow Home

"You're a great guy, and we all really like you here, but you just aren't putting up the numbers. I'm sorry, but we're going to have to let you go." About a year after I'd gotten to Snohomish, I lost my job at the car dealership. It was actually sort of a relief. I hated selling cars. Especially in the grey areas where one was expected to be unscrupulous to get the deal. I left with a perplexed sigh of relief.

I got a job at the Double Barreled Wine Bar in downtown Snohomish. It was in the Spring of 2019 and the grey winter skies were beginning to clear and let through stray beams of sunshine. The vibe at the Double Barrel was mellow and light and I spent most days pouring wine for the older ladies of Snohomish and avoiding the overt flirtations from many who became regulars. It was easy work and gave me room to breathe and think. I decided to start writing again, so I went to the bookstore and bought a red MOLESKINE notebook like the ones I used to write in that was small enough to fit in my pocket and started carrying it around with me. But for the life of me, I could think of nothing to write about. So, I wrote about whatever. I wrote about not being able to write. Some of it was great. Some of it was garbage, but I was writing again. A few days later I was working in the wine bar and

Finally Somehow Home

overheard the two ladies I was serving talking about writing. And I don't remember what it was, but the color red came up in conversation. "That's funny," I interrupted, "I'm a writer and I write in a red notebook. Here it is, right here." It felt great telling people I was a writer again. We chatted for afew short minutes. "May I write something in your notebook?" asked one of the ladies.

"Of course."

This is what she wrote:

WRITE HAPPY
WRITE SAD
DON'T ERASE!

Fail! Grow! Love!

Be OK with change.
Get rid of nothing.

Keep your passion.

Accept your past to be in the future!
The past is small compared to the all!

Finally Somehow Home

- Jenny

"Now go home and write." She said.

And I did.

That's the day I started writing this book.

Don't ever be afraid to encourage someone. You have no idea. Your kind words might be all that it takes for them to change the world. Thank you, Jenny.

My daily walks began to take on purpose. As I walked along for hours reliving my life in my mind I would take voice notes on my phone. That past Christmas I had gone back to Oregon to spend time with my folks, and brought another dresser, my desk, and a chair back with me. Once I'd get back to my room, I would sit at my desk and work the notes on my computer until they became a part of the story that was taking shape before me. It is humbling to write about yourself. You tend to forget all the things in life that you've fucked up but reliving it all to write it down makes you go deep through all of it again. The great triumphs and the great defeats and failures alike, all come back to you in full strength if you're doing it right. And you know you aren't writing it true enough

Finally Somehow Home

if you gloss over anything because the story fucking sucks. It sucks because it's not relatable. You can only relate to others insomuch as you are willing to be as fucked up as them; vulnerable to them, and to be truly vulnerable to them, you must be honest with yourself about yourself. If you aren't, they'll see right through you, but it doesn't matter, because they won't read your story anyway, because your story is shit because it's not real.

Chapter 38

Snohomish was a beautiful little town on the north bank of the Snohomish River. It was full of antique shops and bars, and that's about it, and there was a shit load of both. From what I heard, the reason for the large number of bars in Snohomish goes back to the prohibition days. Because of the little town's strategic disposition on the Snohomish River, bootleggers found it a perfect drop point for their hooch. The reason for all the antique shops... no idea. I didn't have much interest in antique shops, although I did peruse them all out of intrigue, for the sake of exploration, and honestly, mostly just scanning for hot tourist chicks, but, as you well know by now, I've always had a fascination and deep love for bars. I loved all of them in town with great fervor even though I rarely if ever could afford to walk into one. But

Finally Somehow Home

whenever I could afford to walk into one, I walked into one. My favorites, in no particular order because I loved them all for different things about them each, were The Old Inn Tavern, The Snazzy Badger, which was later renamed Who's on First, The REPP, and The Oxford Saloon. The Old Town Inn is the best and most quintessential dive bar I've ever been in. The Snazzy Badger was a sports bar with pool tables and dart boards and just a cool, slick vibe about it, the REPP was rumored to have prohibition tunnels running to it under the street from the river because there was a Speakeasy in the building back in the day, but that's just what I heard, not sure if it's true, and The Oxford Saloon had been around since 1910 and was haunted by a high class hooker named Kathleen that used to occupy the upstairs rooms and offices, as well as at least four other ghosts.

I got to know the son of the owners of The Oxford Saloon during his intermittent visits to the Double Barrel Wine bar. Noticing the interest of the older ladies that frequented the Double Barrel because of yours truly, he asked if I would be interested in working at The Oxford Saloon. Frankly my popularity among the older ladies in town became something of a hilarious nuisance. There was a well-respected local Motorcycle Club in the area

Finally Somehow Home

comprised completely of former Marines. The bike club was called The Marines MC. Over my time in Snohomish, I had run into several members of the club and gotten to know the President. When they found out I was a Force Recon Marine, they wanted me as a Prospect. The President's name at the time was PC. He was a good man, and something of a horn dog from what I gathered. On one occasion PC and I were standing outside of the Snazzy Badger having a conversation. He was trying to get me to join the club. I was tempted. I needed the camaraderie and would have loved to swing my leg over a motorcycle again, so I was seriously considering it. During our short conversation on the sidewalk, we were interrupted twice by drunk older women hitting on me who knew me from the Double Barrel. PC was annoyed at the interruption, but impressed, nonetheless. He redoubled his efforts, offering me a spare bike of his to ride until I got my own if I'd prospect for The Marines. At the end of the day, as much as I wanted to, I told PC that I kind of had a problem with authority, and didn't think it would work out for me to be a part of the club, in spite of his generosity and our shared bond as Marines. I sometimes wish I would have taken him up on the offer, but it's probably a damn good thing that I didn't. Who

Finally Somehow Home

knows what kind of wild, awesome, stupid, shit I'd have gotten into in such a wonderfully enabling environment. Anyway, the point is that I'd always wanted to be a bartender and now I had my chance at The Oxford Saloon. And that's how I met Lila.

I had been working at The Oxford off and on for a couple weeks by then. The Oxford was vintage Old West as fuck. The building looked like something you'd see in an old grainy brown and white picture with loggers, gunfighters, and cowboys milling around the street and a hitching post in front of it because that's exactly what it still was. The main floor held a large dining area with 20 ft ceilings, a large oak bar along the righthand wall with a huge mirror behind it, and the stage and dance floor in the back. There was an upstairs, as I mentioned before, of offices and empty rooms, mostly abandoned, and in the basement where I usually worked, were pool tables, darts, a dance floor, and another bar with a more modern motif.

The only thing I'd had to do with women for the past two years was to gaze lustily at them from a distance whenever I got the chance. I didn't expect any to give a shit about me and I was right. None of them did. Hell, I

Finally Somehow Home

couldn't even buy a girl a drink if one did pay attention to me, let alone be any kind of a decent provider or boyfriend for anyone. I was having a hard enough time doing anything for myself. Several months before, on one of my walks, I realized that I was in a dangerous position. I knew that because I hadn't been with a woman in any kind of relationship or any other way for so long, that knowing me, I'd fall in love faster than a Lance Corporal in a Strip Club with the first chick that even looked at me. But there wasn't much chance of that anyway, I laughed, because I had less game than a blind duck hunter to begin with. I was hopelessly fucked. So, I prayed about it: "God damn it, Lord. I just wanna ask two favors of you. First of all, I'm gonna fall in love with the first girl I date, so could you please make sure she is a good one? And second, I have no game whatsoever, so if you wouldn't mind, could you please have her initiate things?"

I was still learning the tricks of the trade in bartending. The owner's son, upon hiring me, made it clear that I was never to accept phone numbers from patrons nor give out mine to any. I had a sneaking suspicion it was because he wanted all that action for himself, as he was one of the bartenders as well.

Finally Somehow Home

It was a weekend night, but the rush had died down and it was getting on near closing time. I didn't see her walk in, but in the dim light soon noticed two girls sitting at the other end of the bar who were being served by the owner's son. A few minutes later, as I scanned around to make sure everyone was happy and content with their drinks, one of the girls waved her hand at me. As I approached her, she looked up at me with enormous bright eyes, her thick hair was dark and long and flowed down in billows almost to her waist. She was and still is one of the most beautiful women I've ever seen in my entire life. "Are you married?" she asked. I laughed, impressed that she obviously didn't give a fuck if I had a girlfriend or not.

"No."

"How old are you?"

"How old do you think I am?"

"38" she said immediately. She had clearly already been discussing it with her friend.

"Nope. 41. How old are you?" I asked her. "I'll be 26 in afew months." She said. "What's your name?"

Finally Somehow Home

"Jason. What's yours?"

"Lila" she said with a fetching smile.

"It's very nice to meet you, Lila." I said.

"It's nice to meet you too, Jason."

I got back to work at my end of the bar feeling good about myself that such a gorgeous woman had taken notice of me. About 10 minutes later she waved me down again, this time making the sign as if she wanted the check by making air scribbles with her hand. I walked over. "I'm sorry, I can't cash you guys out, let me get your bartender." I said as I waved the owner's son over. "No, I want your phone number." She said, just as he arrived. Without hesitation I grabbed a beer coaster, wrote my number on it, and handed it to her, all under his malicious gaze. Fuck this nerd, I thought to myself, knowing full well he was pissed at me. And that's the last day I worked at The Oxford, and the first day I met Lila, May 4th 2019.

I got a text later that night: "Hi, this is Lila from the bar."

"Hey you. What are you doing? Home already?" I replied.

Finally Somehow Home

"Yes, good night." "I love you too." "OH SHIT, that was for my mother." "God damn it."- were the four texts that followed. I liked her already.

The Pacific Northwest is haunted with clouds and rain continually at war with the sunshine above that sometimes breaks through as if on raids of the tall, thick, lush pines that comprise the massive rain forest in the region and all down the PNW coastline. On the South side of the Snohomish River was Harvey field. Harvey field was originally a homestead, established in the mid-1800s. In 1944 the property was converted to an airfield and is now home to a shit load of airplanes, helicopters, and hot air balloons, as well as Skydive Snohomish and is still owned by the descendants of the original homesteader, all of whom are aviators. Though I had no hope of being able to afford to go skydiving, I couldn't help but poke around and explore the place. In so doing, I somehow discovered that Skydive Snohomish was hiring parachute packers for the SKY SNO tandem program in the summer, and holy shit, I knew how to pack parachutes from my time in the Marines, so I gave them a call.

Finally Somehow Home

Tyson was a cool dude. He was one of the sons of the family that owned the airfield and was the owner of Skydive Snohomish. I didn't realize it at the time, but SKY SNO was a world class drop zone. Literally. Since it started in 2000, they had developed a very impressive name for themselves including accolades from the *Travel Channel* which voted them one of the world's 9 best places to go skydiving. The list also included drop zones in Dubai, New Zealand, Switzerland, Australia, Nepal, and Thailand. *Backpacker Travel* said they were among the number one world's best skydiving locations, and *Awe365* named them among the top ten DZ's in the US. Tyson had his shit together. And I had no idea what I was getting myself into.

I showed up, bright eyed and bushy tailed on the first day, ready to learn how to pack tandem rigs. They were quite similar to the chutes we jumped in the Marine Corps because we hauled so much weight with us in equipment, guns, and ammunition that we needed very large canopies to handle the load. The same was true with tandem rigs, of course, because there were two people hanging beneath the god damn thing. The main difference was that in the Marine Corps, and in the Military Freefall community in general, we flat-packed

Finally Somehow Home

our chutes, whereas the civilian world generally pro-packs theirs. I had pro-packed before but needed some refresher, and to get the job, I needed to be able to do it in less than 20 minutes consistently, and the faster, the better. No big deal, I thought. This should be easy and a great way to spend the summer. And the greatest thing about it was that the more chutes you packed the more money you made because you were paid by the parachute.

I was wrong. I had definitely forgotten how strenuous it is to pack a parachute. Especially when you are hustling to get it done as fast as you can, which is always the case. And especially when you do it for 8-10 hours straight. Tyson had me practicing for a few days to prove that I could get it done right and fast enough to meet the requirements. The reason we had to pack so fast is because we had to beat the loads going up in the airplane. In other words, we always had to have enough chutes for the Tandem jumpers ready before the airplane made it back to the ground to load the next stick of jumpers. You wouldn't think that would be much of a problem because generally it takes a while for an airplane to climb to 12,500 feet, put out jumpers, then land. But skydive pilots are fucking maniacs, and the primary SKY SNO

Finally Somehow Home

airplane was a Cessna Caravan with an upgraded 850hp Blackhawk engine in it that could climb like a cat on meth with its tail on fire. Once the jumpers exited the aircraft the pilot would point the nose of the airplane almost straight down to the runway and usually beat the jumpers to the ground. The tandem instructors would hit the ground, release their tandem student/passenger, run back to the shed, grab another chute, suit up, and standby to get back on the airplane for another jump. It was turn-n-burn all day long. And if you were too slow to beat the loads you didn't get a break because as soon as you finished one, an instructor was dumping another one on you to pack. And packing a parachute is like doing fucking burpees or 8-count bodybuilders all fucking day long. It was one of the most enjoyable yet most physically strenuous jobs I've ever had in my entire life. Here is a poem I wrote about it after a long day of packing for SKY SNO.

The Pack

Pack and pack and pack and pack the pain is in my lower back but we keep packing never waiting, only ever hesitating when the damned chutes drop in and only if and only when we're done with all that's on the floor and

Finally Somehow Home

after that we pack some more, the only way to make it stop is sweating harder bigger drops upon the wretched parachutes, fucked and flipped through, lines a-shit, kill line probably fucking ripped and rubber bands all broke to fuck, "we need two more before the bird goes up", the god damn team loads never end until the day is done my friend, it's six-six-six, the devil's number, eighteen tandems, four damned packers, two of us are turning two on every load except the new guys, turning one and shitting bricks and sucking on a bag of dicks, because they ain't had any break all day, they're too damned slow to beat the loads and then the people want to talk and ask them questions while they pack: When do you replace the rubber bands? How come the airplane always lands before the chutes, and on and on and all the screams and Whoops of joy like salt rubbed in the fucking wound.

Only really sick fucks enjoyed it, and the packing shed was rife with really sick fucks. Some of the best people I've ever worked with in the civvie world. Most of these guys were 18 to 24 years old. By that time, I was almost 42. It was like being in hell with all your favorite people and your lower back aflame the whole time.

Finally Somehow Home

But it was perfect for Lila and I. After we'd met at The Oxford we didn't actually get to see each other again for two weeks. Lila had an 18-month-old son named Ryker who had just started walking. She came from a rough past and was making it work however she could, living with her grandparents in Lynnwood. Riker's dad wasn't part of the picture anymore for reasons I won't go into.

I was sick with a cold or some shit and Lila couldn't get away from the little one for a while, but after two weeks we were finally able to go on our first date. In the meantime, we texted each other endlessly and got all the preliminary awkward bullshit out of the way and straight on to the infatuation. It was the perfect love story. One of those where there is no sudden wakeup call from that first warmth of meeting someone you could fall in love with. No sudden wearing off of the affection we soon had for each other. It just kept going and building. We had both been through our own versions of hell and I think we just didn't have room for pain or unkindness or drama like that in our lives anymore, so neither of us let shit like that in, or dwelt on perceived wrongs or misunderstandings. We gave each other the benefit of the doubt about everything. In spite of all the shit she'd been through since she was a little kid, she had

Finally Somehow Home

miraculously escaped the bitterness that so often comes along with it, and was instead endowed with a heart that somehow glowed with kindness and the kind of tenderness that never wants anyone to feel the agony that she herself had endured in this life. We fell in love immediately. She would come over with little Ryker and the three of us would lay there on the queen mattress and play Bon Iver softly late into the night. She brought to my life a sanguine peace I had never felt before with anyone. She loved me, and believed in me, and thought I was cool, and handsome, and strong, and it gave me power that I hadn't had in many years. Lila taught me to love myself. I figured, if she could love me as much as she did and for all the reasons that she did, maybe I wasn't such a worthless shit after all. I had value again, and if it was only to her, I didn't care. Her love was all I needed. She didn't just change my life; she gave me a new one that I'd never had before. She made me into something more than myself, or more than I'd ever been before anyway. And I knew that, without question or hesitation, I would unleash all of who I was in the kind of violence that leaves indistinguishable shattered bits of people in its wake if ever anyone laid a finger on her and or tried to

Finally Somehow Home

hurt her. I was more than in love with her. I was fully and eternally devoted to her.

We were both broke as fuck. I began to relish the rainy days because, much to the chagrin of Tyson and the SKY SNO crew, and to my utter delight, we couldn't jump with cloud cover over the Drop Zone, so I always had rainy days off. We'd get together and pool our meager cash - "We've got $85 for the weekend!! We're rich, biotch!!!" - then go on simple and lovely adventures to the beach or the river and lay there on a blanket in the sand and drink IPAs and relish this peace and love that neither of us had heretofore known. Two weeks after our first date we were on the front step of the house where I lived, smoking Marlboro Reds. I knew it was stupid and silly and dumb, but I also knew beyond any doubt that I had found beauty and joy in life again, and when I was with her I felt home, and I never wanted to be without that feeling ever again in my life, so I got down on my knee and took her tiny hand in mine and asked her to marry me. She looked shocked and laughed. "Are you serious?"

"Fuck yeah, I'm serious."

"Then, Yes!" She said as she jumped into my arms.

Finally Somehow Home

I had no idea how or when I was going to be able to pull off a wedding let alone being married and providing for a family, but it didn't matter. I wanted her to be in my life forever. There's this idea out there that when you're looking for someone to spend your life with you must find this person who has all their shit together and believes and agrees with every single thing that you believe or agree with, and never makes mistakes. Not only is that boring as fuck, but it's total garbage. There are many things that Lila and I don't necessarily see the same way in this world and neither of us had our shit together when we met. But there's no one else in this world I'd rather be around every minute of every day than Lila. We have fun together. We enjoy each other. We think each other are beautiful. We forgive each other when we do stupid shit. We are truly best friends, and I don't mean that in the bullshit way that many couples say it then can't wait to get the hell away from each other. I mean that she is the best friend to me in the way that gives me power and cuts me slack and wants only the best for me. And I am the same for her. I have no idea where I'd be today if she'd never found me. She saved me. And I saved her. Alone, neither of us was enough to make it, but together we saved each other.

Finally Somehow Home

We were married in the Double Barrel Wine Bar on September 15, 2019, and moved all three of us into the spare bedroom I was living in. She was working as a dental assistant again by then and I was making a shaky and miserable go at selling life insurance. In the intervening months I had been busy writing and had finished the first portion of this book. But I was still too close to all the trauma and mental anguish I had been through, and I still didn't understand what the fuck it had been all about. I was simply unable to write about my divorce, my kids, DC, New York, or anything else that had happened only a few years before, but I had a good start.

Finally Somehow Home

Chapter 39

In 2020, when the COVID-19 pandemic struck the world, we suddenly found ourselves without a place to live. We were given notice, literally overnight, to pack up our shit and get the fuck out. I'm sure our little family was an inconvenience to the lady we rented from, but the COVID scare on top of that broke the camel's back. So, with no place else to go, I returned to Oregon and my parents' basement with our little family in tow. We stayed there briefly until we found our own little two-bedroom apartment right in the middle of the quaint little meth town that is Ontario, Oregon, right on the state line, about an hour from Boise, Idaho. Lila immediately landed a job as a dental assistant, and I got to work on whatever my hand could find to do.

Finally Somehow Home

A few months after we settled in, I learned that Monkey died due to post surgical complications following a routine cervical surgery. It was a horrible tragedy and dealt me a vicious blow. I felt like the wind had been knocked out of me for weeks. We hadn't spoken in a couple years. He was pissed off at me about something and I had no idea what it was, and he wasn't returning my texts or calls. I'd figured we'd just work it out in time, but I didn't know that time was the one thing we didn't have enough of for that. I felt like I'd let him down for not getting my shit together faster. For not letting him see a return on the investment he'd made in me. It still hurts deep to this day. I hope I'm making him proud, wherever he is right now.

I secluded myself in my office for several weeks before the funeral. Maybe that's what started it. Probably. I dug up the manuscript and images that I'd compiled to create *The Perfect Fucking Life*. It hadn't seen the light of day in over three years. I determined to publish it, but I had no idea how, so I started calling friends to see if I knew anyone who knew anyone who could help. Adria and I were introduced several months before through my good friend Chris who I'd met while brokering deals for Personal Protective Equipment during the COVID

Finally Somehow Home

pandemic. Adria's trade was finance, and she managed the financial portfolios of some of the world's wealthiest families. But her art was that of the catalyst. She, of her own volition began to leverage her massive network of the world's elite for philanthropic purposes by making critical introductions to families, organizations, national governments, and other world leaders. In so doing, she founded The Vine Global Impact Foundation, authored the book *The Vine*™ and created ZERO-AI™, a social impact platform that uses an AI concierge system to build bridges of trust for global communities. She always had time for everyone and took a sincere and genuine interest in each of her countless friends and acquaintances and the problems they each faced, and if anyone ever needed anything imaginable, she invariably knew someone who could help. No great surprise, Adria came through and introduced me to some options for publishing. Hope, at last.

When the editor of the publishing company read the title, she was intrigued and asked for the manuscript. "We don't publish picture books." Was the curt response. God Damn it! Back to square one. After feeling pissed off and sorry for myself for a few days, it suddenly occurred to me that I could just strip the pictures out of

Finally Somehow Home

it, add more content, and Viola! I'd have the makings of an actual book. So, I did. It took me afew days, but by the end of it I had just over 200 pages of content. I sent it back to the Editor. "We can work with this, but it needs editing." I scraped up the $500 fee to pay the editor and sent it off. Within afew days I opened my newly edited manuscript of *The Perfect Fucking Life* and was immediately sick to my stomach. She had gone through the thing as if she were a 9th grade English teacher. As soon as I saw the words to the first sentence of the first article, I was livid. Those were not my words. Some of them were, but others had been added in. No telling what other changes had been made to my body of work. It was completely ruined. I couldn't help but to think I might just have to sell out to these fuckers if ever I was going to get a book published, but I couldn't bring myself to even consider it. No fucking way. God Damn it! Back to square one.

I was at Sturman's Smokeshop, a cigar joint in Boise, one day enjoying a fine stick and bullshitting with the other patrons. An older gentleman, seemingly in his mid-60's was sitting next to me, likewise enjoying a fine cigar. He introduced himself as Ed, and I soon discovered that he was the Editor of the Boise Beat, a local online periodical

Finally Somehow Home

that covered nightlife, cuisine, music, and more in the Boise area. Ed had come to Boise via Los Angeles where he'd been heavily involved in the entertainment industry in many different ways. While in LA he had written for the LA Beat and had started his own spinoff once he moved to Boise. I told him about my sputtery writing career and he agreed to look at and critique some of my work. I was ecstatic.

As soon as I got back home, I pulled up a few articles I'd written and fired them off to Ed. "Let's meet and discuss." came Ed's reply and we set up a time and place in Boise to meet. I was aflutter with nerves as I pulled onto the freeway for the hour-long drive to Boise, but was soon distracted by a sudden rattling, a cloud of smoke and parts of my car bouncing along the oil-slicked road in my rear-view mirror. I called Ed to let him know I'd be late, had the tow truck drop the busted car off at the junkyard, got a ride back home, and was back on the road in my other piece of shit car in an hour.

The birth of a true artist is marked by moments of delightful affirmation in which the artist actually realizes he's being born and that he's actually good. That night at the bar in NYC when everyone read my poem

Finally Somehow Home

was one of them. This was another. Ed spoke to me matter-of-factly as if I were his protégé. He is the first professional writer who took my work seriously and saw real potential in me, and I owe him a great debt of gratitude for it. It was an amazing feeling. One of wonderful recognition comingled with an awareness that I had a very long way to go, and really ought to ignore the fuzzy feelings for the moment, shut the fuck up and listen. Although the Boise Beat had its own distinct niche' and voice, Ed offered to let me publish some short articles in it if they were good enough. A few weeks later I was a published author.

But I was still stuck n' fuckt with *The Perfect Fucking Life*. Another of the people Adria had introduced me to was Tyler who headed up a publishing service called Authors Unite, but the price tag was something I couldn't dream of affording in my present circumstances.

"Adria, what do I do?"

"Why don't you go to some non-profits and see if one will fund your book?"

"I'll give it a whack. Thank you."

Finally Somehow Home

I had met Pep several times before. The first time in San Diego, CA in 2000 when we were both awarded the Force Recon Team Leader of the Year Award, him representing 4th Force and I from 5th Force/3rd Recon Bn. The second time we met was in Washington DC in 2002 when I was with 2d Force. We had been training in Quantico, VA and made the drive up to DC for the Force Recon Association's Marine Corps Birthday Ball, wherein Pep was receiving yet another Force Recon Team Leader of the Year Award. We couldn't help but notice that some of the Vietnam era Recon Marines attending the Ball had brought along members of their extended families, including at least two beautiful young ladies, and we further couldn't help but notice that Pep and crew had swooped in on them before we even arrived and were parading them around like trophies, so we resolved to amend the situation.

As with any Marine Corps Ball, the rule of thumb is: "Drink until failure, or your cut off." Not wanting to tarnish the legacy and tradition of our beloved Corps, we complied with this explicit directive as best we knew how... and we knew how pretty well. While we're on the subject of the Marine Corps Birthday Ball, I'd like to take a moment to formally submit the following toast as a

Finally Somehow Home

permanent and official fixture in the Marine Corps Birthday Ball Ceremony:

To our tattered, bruised and battered, bloody knuckled band of bastards. Vagabonds, rapscallions, Lords of war's disaster. Make your toast, then man your post, there's killin' to be done. Climb down the ropes, and man the boats, and kill until it's won. And if you should fall, don't fret at all, your brothers will come find you, and take you back for medivac, or otherwise assign you. You'll man your post with all the host of those who life has known, and sip your scotch on overwatch of those who drink alone. So cammie up, and tape your frags, and jam your magazines, and know you'll never drink alone, United States Marine.

-Jason Lee Morrison, Sgt/USMC

I had to put that in there in case the Commandant of the Marine Corps ever reads this shit... but now back to the story...

As the night went on, me and a couple buddies from my Platoon started maneuvering on the High Value Targets (HVTs). Pep, as any Force Recon Team Leader would, picked up on it immediately and began executing his DRAW-D plan (Defend, Reinforce, Attack, Withdraw,

Finally Somehow Home

Delay). I noticed a weakness in the enemy's defensive posture and infiltrated their lines. Within a few minutes, the pretty girls were sporting the Dress Blue blouses and covers of myself and one of my teammates over their Ball gowns. They looked absolutely adorable in them too. We had the enemy on the run. I could see their red star clusters going up as soon as they fully ascertained the gravity of the tactical shift and saw Pep's hasty planning cycle kick into high gear as he and his buddy attempted to repel the assault. It was now a Close Quarters Battle scenario with neither side budging. The HVTs acted oblivious to the battle raging around them, but it was obvious that they were seriously contemplating a defection, and as with any such Operation, it was my prerogative to facilitate as seamless a transition as possible from enemy to friendly lines, but this was no easy task. I needed a SPIKE. A SPIKE is an Operation that infuses energy into the tactical environment to cause an asymmetrically exploitable response by the enemy. I saw my opportunity and pulled the trigger. We were in a large ballroom with several smaller rooms and passageways adjacent to it separated by glass double doors. I nonchalantly began to move toward one of the adjoining rooms with the ladies and my buddy in tow,

Finally Somehow Home

Pep and his team hot on our heels moving as fast as they could casually amble behind us. I pretended not to notice them, and as soon as we passed through the glass doors, I reached back and flipped the lock. I could see Pep clinching his jaw as he heard the latch flip and watched him try the door handle. I knew my decision was a risky one. The HVTs knew exactly what was afoot and looked at me as if to say, "Ok, you've got us here, if you want to keep us here, whatever you do next had better be good." Fuck. I hadn't had the time to build a compelling enough narrative for their defection in the other room, and now that they were faced with the decision I was foisting on them, I realized I'd pulled the trigger too early. Furthermore, we were now in a room with no booze in it, or anything else, for that matter. It was a valiant effort, but a fruitless one. I unlocked the door and we all walked back into the main ballroom where Pep and crew were loitering. Fuck it. We were in the middle of Washington DC, and I didn't feel like spending the whole night playing tug-o-war over two girls when there were a shitload more floating around out there. My buddy and I collected our uniform items back from the girls and headed for the door to go out on the town. Chalk one up for Pep and his boys.

Finally Somehow Home

The next time I ran into Pep was during the invasion of Iraq where we were both attached to 1st Force. His platoon ended up getting into some good shit on their extended deployment over there, so I'm happy for them. I never thought I'd run into him again.

Pep was deeply involved in the Force Recon Association even back when I had first met him, but after the desert wars kicked off there was a need for an organization that supported the entire Recon community and the boys in the fight as well as their families. The Marine Reconnaissance Foundation (MRF) had been started years before in 2013. Pep got involved in 2018 and was immediately voted in as a Vice President. After a year they made him President and he's been running ragged to this day in support of Recon Marines, Special Amphibious Reconnaissance Corpsmen (SARC), and their families.

The MRF's Mission is to provide recurring and emergency assistance to the men of the Marine Reconnaissance community and their families and perpetuate the storied history and lineage of the Reconnaissance community since the community's inception. This is accomplished by an entirely volunteer staff to ensure that all support and donations directly benefit those to whom they provide such critical support. MRF programs include but are not limited to the following:

-Annual Recurring Programs:
- Recon Gold Star Family Retreat (these retreats are for the parents and families of Recon Marines and SARCs killed in combat and training)
- Wounded Teammate & Family Retreat
- Recon Gold Star Children's Retreat
- Recon Owned Business Grant Program
- Financial Support to the Annual Recon Challenge

-Emergency Support Programs:
Identify gaps in support/coverage to support our teammates and our families such as...
- On site/in person support (e.g. disaster clean up, medical support coordination)
- Medical devices not covered by insurance/TRICARE
- Financial support (not provided by traditional means, on hand resources etc. that are approved by the BOD)
- Donated goods/services

Finally Somehow Home

-Support Active Duty/Reserve Forces:
- Providing goods/services to units, schools, houses, deployed forces
- Support to personnel wounded/injured or personnel killed in action or training
- Mentorship program
- Unit events (e.g. memorials, warrior night)
- Unit historical programs
- Command support

-Preservation of Reconnaissance History Programs:
- Unit history
- Significant Recon Teammate highlights (photo, video, narrative history)
- Significant operations & individuals in Recon history (photo, video, narrative history)

They do a lot of shit, and usually under the radar. Every day. The things you don't hear about. Like setting up college funds for the kids of suicides. Messy stuff. But it's not all gloom and doom. They recently helped a Sergeant get into MIT. He has since graduated and is now running a profitable tech startup. They had never assisted in the publishing of a book before. I hoped to be the first.

Finally Somehow Home

I called Pep out of the blue, told him what I was trying to accomplish, and crossed my fingers. He invited me to an upcoming Wounded Teammate and Family Retreat in Whitefish, Montana. Lila's Dental office was going to be on a vacation trip together during that time, so Ryker and I packed our bags and headed to Montana afew weeks later.

Chapter 40

The Lodge at Whitefish Lake was amazing. Montana was beautiful, but the most memorable part of that trip was the people. To once again, after almost 20 years find myself sitting around a fire drinking, talking shit, and laughing with my Recon Brothers. It was like getting a shot of adrenaline to the soul. Dormant parts of who I am awoke and emerged that I had forgotten were there. It was like meeting an old unrecognizable acquaintance, vaguely familiar at first, then suddenly recognizing him as my old self, and being there with those mighty men and sharing their company forced me to remember my own great strength of times past. And it brought me great peace, and joy, and rest in the presence of my Brothers.

All of the attendees of the retreat were wounded in some way. I had gotten off the lightest with some PTSD, but

Finally Somehow Home

others there were missing limbs, or hands, or otherwise bore the physical scars of battle on top of their PTS.

Jonathan was a handsome fucker. He looked like a young Mel Gibson with better hair. He had stepped on an IED in Afghanistan that had taken both his legs and sent hundreds of shards of his bone and frag into the back of Adam, his teammate. Jonathan had a tattoo on his forearm that said "Stay Dangerous." And he was. He is now a poster child and representative of the Black Rifle Coffee company whose Founder and CEO, Evan used to attend "The Church of Elvis" back in my Jerusalem days. Adam is a backcountry guide of all things outdoors in Moab, Utah.

Eddie was a mountain of a man. The only thing bigger than his smile was his persona. He was a force of nature, like an Irish tornado in a hurricane over an erupting volcano in the sunshine. The first thing you noticed about him was his booming voice and the shit eating Irish grin that followed it. The second thing you noticed about him was that he didn't have any hands. In Eddie's own words, here's how that happened:

Finally Somehow Home

The Ambush

by Eddie Wright

7 April 2004

1st Reconnaissance Battalion, Bravo Co. 2nd Plt

This was the second time in less than a mile that we halted our convoy. We were the lead vehicle in the Company movement. We tried to move as if we were walking point whenever possible. We were in column formation, same as if on foot. This was route Boston, a good place to get in a fight and something was up. It was startlingly obvious the Iraqi's were anticipating our arrival. This suburb of Fallujah usually had a steady flow of vehicle traffic, and the local residents were always outside in small groups, milling about or working. It was around noon and the day was sunny, not too hot. The gas station usually had a congregation of serious looking men out front, jaw-jackin' the day away. Today the place was eerily quiet, the gas station deserted. In the distance up ahead I saw a cluster of people dart behind a building. At the same time a lone car that was heading towards us suddenly busted a u-turn and took off in the opposite direction.

I relayed over the radio what I was observing. All I got for an answer was "Solid copy, pick up speed to 25kph." I

Finally Somehow Home

thought to myself, "Roger. Mother-fuckers." Marines, Recon Marines especially, hated operating with officers who never trained with the men they lead. I silently swore at the 119 Foxtrot (radio). I assumed this was Captain Brad's call to disregard our observations. He was the Company Commander, normally nowhere near us when we worked but today he accompanied us. We all had opinions regarding his capabilities, I didn't think too highly of him. He was untested in combat and had yet to prove himself to us. Today he would get his chance. Most of our battalion were combat veterans of the 2003 invasion and OIF I. Bravo Company 2nd Plt. Had busted our asses getting ready for this deployment. We spent nearly every waking hour training and rehearsing our Standard Operational Procedures (S.O.P's). We were some bad mothers and we knew it. We had our shit together. We resented what we considered a POG (Person Other than a Grunt) calling the shots once the boots hit the deck. I thought to myself Capt. Brad must have made that call. In two seconds, our company commander was able to assess the situation and make a command decision from his perch, a quarter mile back in the formation. It pissed me off. Now years later I have moved the finger and pointed it at myself. I could have taken a few seconds to reiterate my

Finally Somehow Home

sitrep to paint the battlespace in a way he could have conceptualized in his lofty warehouse of intelligence hidden under his "brain bucket." Nevertheless, it was Aye-Aye Sir! Off we went.

I could "what if" that following hour of my life a million times over, but it wouldn't change a thing. We knew that we were heading into an ambush. I relayed the news to the team, and we started moving again. Everyone was silent, every weapon pointed outboard. "Well here we go," I thought. I dismounted my SAW from its swing-arm mount and rested its folded bi-pod on the duct tape covered windowsill of my door, the barrel casually surveying our 3 O'clock. When the shit went down, I wanted to be mobile if needed. As we started picking up speed, I made the conscious decision to spit out my dip, just in case I got hit. I didn't want to accidentally swallow it. After all, who wants to be puking their guts out while leaking all over the place from a gunshot? This was about the point I felt my mind go to a familiar place. As I readied myself for battle, I turned off all of my emotions. I was used to combat. Fear could only hint at manifesting itself. I'd catch it and put it in check as soon as it started creeping in at the fringes of my mind. It was time for us to focus on work.

Finally Somehow Home

We were traveling at about 25kph when I heard the first shots. It was a short burst of machine gun fire from our right flank. Whoever initiated the ambush must have jumped the gun. Within a split second his buddies joined in on the action, as if they were late to the party. It was an incredible amount of gunfire, and it seemed to be concentrated entirely upon our vehicle. I hastily squeezed my radio handset and called out "Contact right!" I dropped the handset and brought my gun up as fast as I could. Immediately we executed our SOP for this type of ambush. We stopped our vehicle and started laying down a base of fire along with the rest of the Alpha element of our platoon. Meanwhile I trusted that the Bravo element, led by Gunny Griego, would be executing their Immediate Action Drills and maneuvering to flank the enemy.

We had stopped our vehicle right in the middle of the kill zone. There wasn't much of a choice. The enemy had picked a good spot. They blocked the road ahead of us, confining our vehicle to the narrow, one lane road. The rounds came in on us so thick they prevented us from dismounting from our vehicle. The only option for us was to assault through by fire and maneuver. Any inaction or hesitation could and would have killed us. The rounds

Finally Somehow Home

shredding apart our vehicle were so many I knew it was only a matter of time before I got shot in the face.

I assumed our Radio Operator, LCpl. Mazon was already dead, shot in the face by one of the many rounds that snapped by so close it's a wonder they didn't pierce him. I didn't have time to dwell on the issue. I had some work to do. In true Marine Corps fashion, I thought, "If I'm going out, I'm going out fighting."

This was a textbook close ambush, and we were fighting our way through it. I squeezed out long bursts from my saw. I remember once being told by an instructor at SOI that 5-8 round bursts was the optimal rate of fire in a firefight, so as not to get a "hot barrel." Well, not in this fight. Any grunt will tell you SAWs could be finicky, prone to jams and miss-feeds. I took pride in keeping my weapon pristine. I knew just how to keep her rocking and rolling in this type of environment. I dumped rounds down range right back at them. I employed a few really longs bursts of grazing fire just inches over the top of the berm to our 3 O'clock the enemy was using for cover. The enemy was firing from behind until they got a taste of their own medicine.

Finally Somehow Home

It did the trick; they couldn't peek over the top of their hiding places unless they wanted to catch one in the grape. They knew it too and kept their heads down. I paused in firing to move to suppress the fire that was coming from our 1 o'clock. Bullets were still raining down on us at an insane rate. They were firing at us from behind the berms and from positions scattered out across the small fields. I could also see the muzzle flashes winking at us from the dark places in the nearby buildings. They were unloading on us with at least four belt fed machine guns, or PKM's. One of the insurgents had a bead on us from our 1 o'clock. Luckily the angle of our vehicle related to his position gave us some protection as long as we didn't lean too far out of the doors to return fire. I swung my barrel to the left and was about to start suppressing that machine gun at our 1 o'clock, but I changed my mind and went back to suppressing our right flank.

Sergeant Kocher was selectively engaging individual targets, and I didn't want to shoot his M4 out of his hands. I wasn't worried about my aim, but with my gun firing across the top of his barrel from a foot away all it would take was him lifting his barrel an inch. I knew Kocher would soon pick that guy off, and I didn't want the enemy I had pinned behind the berm to get cocky and decide to

Finally Somehow Home

join the party again either. Anyways, I assumed Talbert would bring the 50 cal up in the turret rocking and rolling. "What's the hold up?" I wondered fleetingly. Making assumptions is a good way to get yourself killed. Try learning that lesson the hard way.

As the fighting had been going on I kept hearing explosions behind us. The enemy was "volley firing" RPGs at us. I assumed that the enemy was firing at the vehicles behind us. I never saw the telltale smoke trailing bottle rocket whiz by like I had in earlier engagements. I've heard people say that you never see the one that gets you. Well, that saying held true in my case.

I felt a tremendous boom. I can't adequately describe being hit by a Rocket Propelled Grenade. Take my word when I say words fall short of truly conveying it. If you can imagine, it was as if the greatest thunderclap you've ever felt in your lifetime was magnified a million times over and originated from inside your head. Everything went silent, but I was very aware. I knew I had finally been shot in the face or head. I was cognizant of everything. Time stopped. I remember screaming out at the top of my lungs, "Ahh, I'm hit!" But my voice as powerful as it is, fell on deaf ears, including mine. I knew I had yelled out loud that I

Finally Somehow Home

was hit, and I immediately felt stupid for doing it. It was so cliché, and I was irritated with myself for almost allowing myself to freak out. I shut up and told myself to relax. I knew that shock could set in and could kill me if I allowed myself to go down that road. It worked. As I took control of myself it was as if I had flipped on a light switch to the world. My senses flooded back to me.

From the moment of impact to this point seemed like a good five minutes had passed. In real time I'd say 5 seconds would be a more correct estimation. So many different thoughts had crossed my mind. In those few seconds I remember thinking I had been shot in the face. I thought to myself, "I guess I'll see what it's like to die now," and "I wonder if I'll be retarded because of a gunshot to the brain?" I thought to myself "Well, how would I even know if I'm brain damaged if I'm brain damaged?" It may sound surprising to say, but I felt peaceful. Even though I expected that I was dying, I wasn't afraid. I knew that everything would be okay, better than okay. I remember thinking how much I wished I could somehow give that peace to those I would leave behind. They would be sad, but I knew they didn't have to be. I remember seeing my time on earth as merely a fraction of my life, as if in death I was being awakened.

Finally Somehow Home

I opened my eyes. I knew I wasn't dead, not yet anyway. The world came into view. For a second I thought the enemy had stopped firing at us. They hadn't. We were all deaf from the RPG blast. It had detonated two feet from my face. My left arm was burning. I looked down and saw what was left of it. It was blown off about mid forearm. I could see my jagged, splintered bones jutting out from a bloody, scorched, flayed open stump. I knew I had lost my left hand. My right hand was killing me. I raised it up in front of my face to get a good look at it. It was blown off at the base of my hand. There were a few uneven bone fragments sticking out where my palm used to be. It looked as if some of the skin that used to be my hand was dangling, shredded to pieces like someone removed all the bone and flesh from inside. It hung like and empty glove that went a few rounds with a garbage disposal. I thought, "Fuck, both of them!" I wasn't done assessing the situation though. I looked down and saw my left leg was blown wide open, my femur split in half like a jagged splintered water hose. It pumped out huge amounts of blood with every heartbeat. Imagine a coffee cup full of blood, hot blood. Now imagine that every time your heart beats, you tossed about that much blood out of your cup and down your thigh. The coffee cup would fill up again in between heart beats. I

Finally Somehow Home

knew I only had so many cups of coffee left in me. My leg had almost been blown in half. I took one look at the gleaming white bone sticking out of a sea of red, and I knew I was dead if I didn't stop that bleeding. How was I going to get a tourniquet on my leg and both arms when I didn't have hands? The fight wasn't over yet. I knew I needed to use my head.

I understood just how grave my situation was. I was losing blood very rapidly. Everyone in the team was wounded, some worse than others. I needed a tourniquet, and I needed it fast. My leg was the main priority. My hands could wait. I turned and saw that Mazon was not dead. Surprisingly he had escaped major injury and sustained a good peppering of shrapnel. Talbert was laid out on the roof, his legs curled up along with himself behind the gun shield. He was unresponsive, maybe dead. Music, our driver, was dazed behind the wheel. He had caught a lot of shrapnel from head to shoulder, down his back and on his right side. You could tell his bell was rung. He had checked on Talbert our gunner and he kept telling us that Talbert wasn't responding. As bad as it sounds, all I could think was, "If he's dead, he's dead. Let's focus on saving the rest of our asses." It's just the nature of combat, now was not the time to slow down to mourn.

Finally Somehow Home

My attention moved to Sgt. Kocher who was quietly putting a tourniquet on his right arm with his left hand. His right arm flapped around useless from a hole the size of a silver dollar just above his elbow on his tricep, his bones shattered. I told Kocher I was hit. He responded, "I know brother. I can't help you until I get this tourniquet on." I knew that, but I guess in the moment it was something I felt I should tell my team leader. I wasn't taking any chances. I wasn't assuming anything, not anymore. My attention went back to Mazon. He was visibly shaken at the sight of me. He kept repeating, "Oh shit! Oh fuck! Oh shit! Oh fuck Corporal!" I'm sure I was quite a sight to see, but I knew I couldn't afford to let him go down that road to panic, fear and shock. I needed him to focus, slow down, take his time, and move with a purpose.

In boot camp our drill instructors would hammer that into us whenever they had us complete complicated tasks under extreme duress. The ditty they used is cemented into my mind and soul. "Slow is smooth. Smooth is fast." It works. I told Cpl. Mazon in the calmest, most authoritative voice I could muster, "Mazon, calm down. I'll be all right. Get the blow-out kit." The "blow-out" kit was our field expedient medical kit that we kept in the vehicle. The contents would vary slightly from time to time based on what we could acquire. We wanted it all. If push came to shove and we couldn't get medical support, we had to be prepared to help ourselves.

The one thing that is always in that medical kit is tourniquets. It was Cpl. Mazon's job to load it into the vehicle before we stepped off anywhere. He had done that, but the kit wasn't secured well enough to withstand the impact of an RPG. When the RPG hit us, it blew all kinds of shit all over the place. It looked like the six foot pile of footlocker guts that my drill instructors affectionately called Mt. Suribachi. "Where's my mountain?" they would shout, and ninety Charlie Company Platoon 1119 wannabe Marines would immediately and without hesitation dump our shit out of our footlockers into one single pile in the middle of the squad bay. Then the next step was for each and every one of us to retrieve a certain item, seemingly random like our "moonbeams" (flashlights) or our "go fasters" (running shoes) and get back "online" (at the position of attention) with our gear in under ten seconds. Except 10 seconds of DI time went something like "10, 9, 8, 3, 2, 1, ZERO! It was chaotic. Everyone would be knees and elbows akimbo as we converged on our footlocker guts as fast as we could. It was

Finally Somehow Home

an exercise in futility, designed to teach us to slow down, focus and utilize economy of movement and time.

So here I was watching Mazon frantically sort through our Mt. Suribachi for the blow out kit. I didn't have time for this. None of us did. I was bleeding out, and the enemy was still trying to kill us. I told him, "Fuck it, Mazon. Grab my tourniquet." Our team had spent time rehearsing our IA drills for self-aid/buddy-aid. Each of us had two tourniquets on us at all times, one in each of our Cammie blouse shoulder pockets. This was before there were enough actual tourniquets to issue, so we had come up with our own solution. We found that small six-inch bungee cords worked fantastically on both legs and arms, and they were easy to apply to yourself one handed in just seconds. I still have one of 3 the blood-stained tourniquets that were used on me that day. The docs at TQ thought so much of it they saved it and sent it home with me. That bungee cord helped save my life, and it's one of my most prized souvenirs from the war.

Almost as soon as I met Eddie, Ryker walked directly up to him and smacked him right in the balls. Ryker was right about that height where the little guy would flail his arms around and shit like that would happen. Eddie

Finally Somehow Home

grimaced in pain and brought his hook down to cover his junk in case of follow-on strikes. "Are you a robot?" Ryker asked in his toddler voice. "Ryker, that's Mr. Robot to you buddy." I corrected. And since then, Eddie has been Mr. Robot to Ryker and to no one else in this world. Because as fun loving and cheerful as Eddie is, in spite of having only a hook and a nub to work with, he'll still head-but you and beat the shit out of you in true Irish fashion. He's done it before. Eddie is like a brother to me now. He's what it means to persevere. Eddie wakes up every morning and makes life work with no fucking hands. And he's always smiling. I know it's a lot harder on him than he lets on, and he knows the cost of liberty, but he sees it for what it is and he faces it head on and wears it like a fucking badge of honor because that's exactly what it is.

Remember when I talked about Moshpit asking me to put a bullet in him if he ever got burnt up real bad? I understand where he was coming from when he asked me that because I asked the same of him for me. But now that I've grown alittle wiser in life I think we were underestimating ourselves and each other. Watching guys like Jonathan and Adam and Eddie overcome their shit was like watching a human become a fucking demi

Finally Somehow Home

god. These guys had been through hell and made it and still bore the scars that none of us who are whole can begin to imagine the pain of, let alone the daily struggle of a life without legs, or hands, or incessant pain. And I think at the end of the day, Eden overcame his obstacles as well. If there was anyone I know that was strong enough to do it, it was Eden. It hurt seeing him crippled up, a quad amputee, and incoherent due to several strokes he'd suffered as a result of his countless surgeries. But somehow, I know he was strong enough in his own mind to overcome it all. So, I'm glad I wasn't there the night he got hit. I know that in the end he was even stronger than he thought he was.

It was humbling as fuck being around so many guys who'd sacrificed so much more than I had. I think the gift in getting older and the slow acquiescence of our youth serves to show us that we are spiritual beings, because as our body declines, our soul is strengthened and comes alive. Notice how seldom you'll hear complaining in a nursing home? That's the evidence of a strong soul. Well, these guys were cut down in their prime and forced to deal with pains and limitations of their bodies so suddenly that there is a power in them beyond their years and a tenacity for life that puts the lukewarm everyday nature of the rest of us to shame. Not because they were able to circumvent their pain, but because they were able to bear it all. I learned this while I was there with them: **The only way to heal all the pain is to feel all the pain.**

The MRF ran like a well-oiled machine. Pep led the charge and with compass in hand, still the quintessential Recon Team Leader, his wife, Charity, and the many other volunteers made it into a really impressive, pleasant, and enjoyable experience. But there was one person in particular, always on the periphery, always attentive and preemptive in solving would-be issues, always working 24/7 and never dropping the ball. That was Bonnie. Sweet, brilliantly intellectual, and brimming with elegance and propriety which belied her 30+ years of Diplomatic, Philanthropic, and "Other" experience. "Other" being the type of shit that could only be written down in a book that had -TOP SECRET- stamped across the top of the page. She had grown up traveling the world as the child of Diplomats, and at a very young age was cruising around Europe on international flights with just her little sister and no adult supervision. Since then, her career had taken her to 87 different countries on all 7 continents. Yes, all

Finally Somehow Home

seven, because in addition to circumnavigating the globe three times in a fucking boat, she spent a season as an expedition guide in Antarctica, and in so doing, was part of the first team to navigate the ice fields of Lamaire Sound by kayak.

Among many, many other things, she's also the Ambassador to End Child Soldiering through a joint initiative with the Lobo Institute, wherein she brings awareness to the atrocities of human trafficking and child soldiering in such countries as Uganda, Rwanda, Syria, Sudan, Somalia, Philippines, Palestine, Afghanistan, Pakistan, Iran, Iraq, Nigeria, Central African Republic, DRC, Mali, Yemen, Russia, Ukraine, Mozambique, and Colombia.

In spite of the many different irons in her many different fires, she had a most ardent love and devotion to her Recon boys. She watched over each of us like a mother hen, ready at a moment's notice to help in any way she could, and equally poised to strike and destroy, should anyone fuck with any of us in any way. She was unassuming and pleasant to the casual observer, but it soon dawned on me that her mild manners were an obfuscation of the great power and respect she held and

Finally Somehow Home

wielded daily in other contexts. Many at the highest levels of US and foreign International Diplomacy, National Governance, Military, Intelligence, Corporate entities, and other people of great power and influence deferred to her and shut the fuck up when she spoke. And she wouldn't hesitate to call in a favor across her vast network if it would help a Recon Marine in any way, or inversely fuck someone's life up who was fucking with one of her boys. And we all knew it and wouldn't, and still won't hesitate to bust kneecaps if anyone were ever foolish enough to make the mistake of fucking with our Bonnie.

It was great to see Pep again. We gave each other a big hug and were able to catch up over drinks and throughout the following days during the many events that were planned for us, but we still hadn't really discussed anything with regard to *The Perfect Fucking Life*. Finally, on a whitewater rafting trip, we had time to talk about it. I had already sent him a copy which he had looked over, and we discussed the purpose behind the whole thing as one of shining a light back on the path for those behind us who may be dealing with things that we have dealt with in life, especially with regard to combat and Post Traumatic Stress. At the end of the day, after conferring with the Board of Directors, the Marine Reconnaissance Foundation agreed to assist in raising money and awareness for the publishing of my first book. A few short months later, on January 4, 2022, *The Perfect Fucking Life* was released to the world. After nearly six years, I had finally become a published author. I sent this to the MRF staff shortly thereafter:

ALCON:

It's been a long ten years. About this time of the year in 2013 my marriage fell apart. I had to move away from my kids. They were 5 and 3. They still don't know who I am. I haven't seen them since March 2017.

It's the hardest part of my life, and one that I don't know how to fix. I wrote this book so that maybe someday they would pick it up and read it and understand who their dad really is, despite what they may have been led to believe. The good, the bad, and the ugly, but the god damn truth and nothing but. That book was a letter to my kids. All the shit that I really thought they need to know about life because I knew I couldn't be there to teach them in person as they grew older and confronted the harshness and uncertainty of a life for someone who is truthful to

Finally Somehow Home

themselves right in the god damn shit of the depths of whatever hell they may have to face.

You have given me something I may have otherwise never had. This was my Message to Garcia. To my kids. And you delivered it.

Thank you from the bottom of my heart.

I love you all.

Fuckers.

-MO(SOC)

It was a delicious feeling. As if some of my time in the pit had been redeemed. As if suddenly, some of the most painful parts of my life became beautiful. The seeds of perseverance had taken root in the compost and waste and shit of the past and had begun to bud, and as more and more people began to read my work and relate to it and see some things that maybe they hadn't seen before that way, and maybe life made just alittle bit more sense now, those little seedlings began to bear fruit and to feed the souls of many. A lot of what this book and the *Perfect Fucking Life* really are, is this: you know when you're having a good conversation and someone maybe asks

Finally Somehow Home

you a really good question, but you're stumped at the moment, and don't really know what to say? Then afew days later you're thinking about it, and hot damn! You stumble onto the right response? You realize that you could have possibly really made an impact in someone's life if only you'd thought of it when you needed it. Fuck! Well, alot of this is that. A lot of this is those things I've come to learn or discover after the fact. Things I wish I'd known to tell some of my dearest friends. Hell, the very last time I saw Bushhog before he died, he asked me what the fuck the deal was with Abraham sacrificing Isaac. I had no answer for him. And he died without one. And it still kills me because the answer is a beautiful one. That conversation with Bushhog is what led me to discover and explore and codify the line of reasoning I mentioned when I was on the streets in DC about the Bible and child sacrifice. So, in a small way, all those missed opportunities when I didn't have an answer, have been redeemed as well. Redeemed, meaning they once more belong to me and are valuable to me. It was like getting back lost time. And it gave me peace.

Chapter 41

Two months later Russia invaded Ukraine. I didn't really think much of it at the time. It was far away and I had neither the desire nor the ability to do anything about it because the State Department had pulled my Passport due to my situation with Child Support, so I figured this was one war they'd just have to figure out without me. Around that time, I got a phone call from a phone number I didn't recognize and for some reason I answered it.

"Hi, is this Jason Morrison?"

"Yes. Who's this?"

"My name is Matt. Your old roommate Steve said we should talk." Steve had been working at DARPA when I had been at CTTSO, and he still dabbled in the Science and Technology space. No telling how Matt had met Steve, but after a conversation with him, Steve had

Finally Somehow Home

indeed passed along my contact information and recommended we chat. I was impressed with Matt right away. He was sharp as a tack when it came to getting down into the technological weeds, yet he had an acute knack for common sense and spoke as if he knew his way around a battlefield. About three weeks later I was to find out that he had been a Navy SEAL, which impressed me even more, because it's a running joke in the Special Operations Community, and if any of you have ever had the pleasure of meeting a SEAL, you'll certainly remember this experience, that the fact that they are a SEAL is the very first thing they will tell you about themselves. Matt definitely broke the mold as a no-nonsense technological genius who cared more about getting the right things done fast, than about how cool everyone thought he was... which made him pretty damn cool. We also found ourselves discussing the philosophical aspects of the war and the technological implications thereof. We immediately became fast friends. Less than a week after our first phone conversation, Matt left for Ukraine to see what he could do to help. I stayed in touch with him and became his reachback source and administrative coordinator, as well as his emergency backstop. It was the least I could

Finally Somehow Home

do to help a good man on a noble mission. Whatever you may think of that war, Matt was driven by the belief that free men who have the knowledge, understanding, and experience to defend the liberties of other free men are duty bound to do so. And he acted on those beliefs.

He soon made inroads and established relationships all throughout the country, and drawing from his experiences as a SEAL and as a technologist, having written patents and undertaken groundbreaking work in acoustic array of arrays, signal analysis, through-wall high-frequency bioluminescent radar with DARPA, low-cost intensity differential spectrometry, passive multipath 3D RF rendering and sensor fusion, among many other technologies in his area of expertise, he set out to help the people of Ukraine in any way he could. He established a strong reputation and worked closely with Aerorozvidka, the premier and most cutting-edge drone technology organization at the time, learning from them while advising the organization in the development of Techniques, Tactics, and Procedures (TTPs), drone applications, radio systems, and other areas from his experience with radars, signal processing, antenna arrays, spectrometry, electronic fingerprinting and other technologies. Several weeks later Matt invited me

Finally Somehow Home

to support him full time as co-founder of a small company.

Low-Cost Disruptive, Multi-use Technologies (LCDM Tech Inc) was officially born in June 2022 and has since grown to include a deep network of partner companies and organizations all over the world. Matt has been on the ground in Ukraine working with various Ukrainian organizations almost constantly since the war started. He is a bona fide member of an active Ukrainian military unit with the mandate to develop drone technologies. He was in Bakhmut before it fell working with Ukrainian forces on the front line as well as in the Tactical Operations Center advising and assisting with drone deployment, communications systems, and witnessing the challenges of organizing a military in the middle of a war while suffering heavy attritive losses of their most experienced forces. He has first-hand experience on both sides of drone warfare, including avoidance of tracking drones and direct attack types such as the Orlan and Shaheed. His on-the-ground experience also encompasses launching and operations in Electronic Warfare (EW) contested zones, all while dealing with enemy artillery, ATGMs, mine fields, and other battlefield threats. This breadth of experience under

Finally Somehow Home

battlefield conditions has endowed LCDM Tech with a keen understanding of the true Operational context of modern peer-to-peer conflict, and what is required to succeed therein.

In his words: "The biggest need on the battlefield is the concentration, organization, and cohesion of technologies such as drones and the personnel to operate, and command and control them to overmatch the enemy's local defenses, create breakthroughs in enemy lines, and push the Operational initiative to Strategic tipping points and ultimately Strategic gains." Matt has since worked with many Ukrainian startup companies on such technologies and has been a judge and advisor to Ukrainian hackathons to develop these types of systems. He has worked with US and Ukrainian Special Operations Forces on Operations, been offered multiple jobs in Ukrainian organizations and business, and holds a very strong reputation in the country to all who meet him. This is absolutely critical to navigating the deployment and implementation of any kind of system on the ground.

The first-hand experience in Ukraine coupled with continuous exploration of the most rapidly relevant

Finally Somehow Home

technologies in US and NATO countries to bring to the fight, led us to the formation of a concept that can generate the Operational momentum necessary to trigger Strategic tipping points though the assembly and deployment of a critical mass of drones capable of systematic destruction of the enemy's Operational Center of Gravity followed by a persistent, pervasive, domination of the battlespace over Armor and ground forces using low cost, AI enabled drones equipped to bypass and/or destroy Electronic Warfare (EW) jamming systems. The name of this system is: JUGGERNAUT.

Below is a brief summary of LCDM Tech's JUGGERNAUT Concept of Operations:

Drones have changed how modern war is fought. But they have not yet been deployed in a manner that exploits their fullest and most deadly potential – massed and coordinated. The ability to suddenly and without warning, amass overwhelming force on the battlefield in a coordinated manner at the enemy's most vulnerable points and times is the key ingredient to achieving Operational overmatch and subsequent Strategic

Finally Somehow Home

breakthroughs. Russia is clearly learning this. Whoever gets there first, wins.

JUGGERNAUT provides an immediately executable roadmap to get there first, beginning with scalable drone swarms and supporting systems that can operate in EW environments that can be deployed into battle within weeks, then immediately expanding into assembly of a Common, Combined-Arms-Integrated System of Systems. The JUGGERNAUT Concept of Operations is composed primarily of assets which have already been purchased by, and/or are presently on the ground in, or built in Ukraine and is augmented with readily and rapidly available US/NATO Commercial Off the Shelf (COTS) technologies. This will ultimately give Ukraine an intrinsic, self-sustainable, regenerative capability, impervious to political and other uncertainties that influence its warfighting capacity.

So, all that muckity-muck is saying is this: Drones are great for uses in ones and twos, but when you build a system out of many different kinds of them – mostly cheap ones, each with different capabilities and missions, and you deploy them in such a way as to systematically dismantle the enemy's defenses... now

Finally Somehow Home

you're starting to get somewhere. For instance, first you launch high quantities of drones (many of them decoys), and within that first wave are drones specifically designed to find and destroy EW systems which jam the entire battlefield while your decoy drones make the enemy use up all of their Anti-Air missiles to shoot them down. The second wave is scouting and finding and destroying remaining air defenses and command centers and identifying follow-on targets for the next wave which destroys the enemy's artillery, then armor, then troops. Within minutes and hours an entire 60km section of the battlespace has been gutted and is primed for follow-on ground and armor assault. Rinse and repeat.

The key ingredient to making this happen is a broad network of organizations, manufacturers, and other cats and dogs with the ready-made required components. There's no point in going to one drone company and telling them to create an AI enabled swarm to JUGGERNAUT specifications when all the components already exist. One component in a small company in Utah, another component created by a software company in Tampa, another manufactured in Ukraine or Poland. LCDM Tech has become the connecting tissue between hundreds of disparate organizations, each with their own components. This modular approach allows the system it comprises to morph and change rapidly to counter or stay ahead of the enemies defenses against it, as any component can be upgraded, tuned, or replaced by its supplier and simply plugged back into the system. This networked catalytic business model produces a much more agile battle system because of its decentralized approach. The entirety of JUGGERNAUT and indeed LCDM Tech is predicated on a network of strong relationships wherein each member's contribution, once systematized, renders an impact far greater than the sum of the parts of the whole.

After nearly two years of working for Matt as LCDM Tech's Director Future Operations, then as the Managing Director, I knew somehow that I needed to take a step back and finish this book. It had been 3½ years since I'd worked on *Finally Somehow Home*. I had changed in that span of time. I had healed. It wasn't from counseling or from closure or even from spending long hours trying to figure it all out. What had healed my soul was the love of my wife, Lila. When I was a younger man most of my mentors and those who helped me along through life were men. As I have grown older it is impossible to

Finally Somehow Home

ignore both the increase in the number of powerful women in my life, as well as the unique and tremendous impact they have had in it. It is a delightful departure from my own ignorance. It's not that I misogynistically expected less from women. Hell, I didn't know what to expect at all from them. Honestly, I didn't really know what the fuck I was doing when I got married. I didn't know shit about women. I didn't have a sister. I grew up in boys" dorms, surrounded by only other guys. Recon was exclusively a male unit, we didn't even have any support personnel that were women. Same with the work I did overseas after the Marine Corps. So, I was well into my late 20's and still didn't know shit about girls. By the time I got married I had only ever had a handful of girlfriends, none of whom lasted longer than a couple of months. I was never in one place long enough to get to know anyone, let alone to learn much about women, and all the married guys, or the very large majority anyway, only ever bitched about their wives, so I honestly kinda thought marriage was supposed to suck, and that's just how it was. But aside from that even, I just hadn't been around many of them until I hung up my gunbelt. There were strong and intelligent women at COIC and very notably at CTTSO as well. Denise, one of the CEOs from

Finally Somehow Home

my New York days was my first exposure to one of the modern-day Amazons. Her manner was unapologetically feminine and unflappably competent as if it never even occurred to her that she could be discriminated against except maybe in the sidelong glance in the rearview mirror at whatever small creature had been so stupid as to underestimate her. It seemed as though she had long ago realized the fact that in many cases it would be more difficult for her than for many of the men in her chosen career path, turned it up to 11 to offset the difference, and never looked back. For some reason during this season in my life, these Amazons started coming out of the woodwork to help me. There was Denise, Chris who had introduced me to Adria – yet another one, and then of course Bonnie as well. I don't know if the future is female, but it sure as shit is up for grabs, and there's just no way to stop someone who is unwilling to give themselves excuses, no matter how justly entitled to them they may be.

I first noticed this incredible strength of women in my ex-wife when David was born. Although now that I think about it, I don't know if I'd call it strength. I'd call it power. Strength is the wherewithal to move heavy shit

Finally Somehow Home

easily. Power is the wherewithal to move heavy shit even though you have no strength left in you.

And Lila loves with all her power. On our second date I had tried to break up with her. I had nothing to offer her. No way to take care of her. I still thought I was worthless. She interrupted me and said: "We've just found each other. Do you really want to give up so soon?" She might as well have asked me to marry her. Because that's when I knew she was the one. When she fought for me. For us. And I have no fucking clue how, but that love healed me. It made me whole again.

So, I started the arduous task of reliving my greatest pain. And in going back and watching myself re-feel and re-live the darkest parts of my past, I started learning things about myself that I'd have never otherwise learned. Things that I can't describe but that I know are there. What do you think you get from being a student of your own life? Whatever it is, that's it. I know myself more. And it did bring closure and peace about things I haven't had peace about in a long time. And the best part of it was I was writing again.

Chapter 42

On occasion, I'd take a break from writing and go to the range. Vale is a city in and the county seat of Malheur County, Oregon, about 12 miles west of the Idaho border. It is at the intersection of U.S. Routes 20 and 26, on the Malheur River at its confluence with Bully Creek. The little town sits smack dab on the Oregon Trail, the wagon wheel ruts still frozen in time in the dried mud of the high desert. The Old West isn't really that old in Vale and the small community that supports the farms and ranches in the area like to keep it that way. Hell, Vale should be one of the biggest towns in Eastern Oregon, but when the freeway was being built through the area back in the 1950s, the people refused to have their town so soiled, so now the freeway runs through Ontario instead, which, not surprisingly became the economic center of gravity for the county leaving Vale to languish well off the beaten path. But they still don't want their town to change. It's the kind of town where you know the people are the salt of the earth, yet at the same time you question whether you should bring your pistol or not when you go to the bar. There have been gunfights.

Just outside of Vale, heading South on Lytle Blvd, and just past the old Oregon Trail wagon ruts is an unmarked gravel road that turns off to the right. Over the cattle grate and a left turn onto another smaller gravel road leads one down a bumpy ¾ of a mile to a locked cattle gate. If you know the combination, another ¼ mile opens up into a beautiful and spacious bowl in the earth wherein some of the farmers in the area had pooled their resources and earth moving equipment and created a world class range complex. There was a 50 yard standard pistol pit off to the right. The main rifle range had steel targets out to 800 yards and a pit for long range paper targets with firing berms reaching back to 1000 yards. Two adjacent 200 and 300 yard ranges catered to smaller calibers and rimfire rifles, and a "Cowboy" range of various steel targets scattered about provided a good area for plinking – shooting pop cans, shotgun shells and multiple targets at unknown distances. This was the main range complex for the Snake River Sportsmen's Club. I loved it because there was seldom if ever anyone else out there. It was my little place of zen. That day I was out with a buddy giving my Springfield Armory M1A Loaded Precision .308 rifle a workout on the steel targets ranging from 200 to 800. An older fella had pulled up to the benchrest firing line in his pickup and eventually ambled over in true Western fashion for a neighborly handshake and to say hello.

We bullshat for awhile about shooting. He asked me some questions about my pistol belt and body armor that I had happened to bring with me that day and eventually revealed that he was the President of the Snake River Sportsmen's Club. I was intrigued. Only a couple months before I had posted ads on various internet platforms offering coaching in tactical shooting in an attempt to scrape up afew extra bucks every month. "Does anyone offer any tactical training out here?" I asked. "I'm a Department of State certified Firearms Instructor Trainer, and I've got some tactical experience."

"No, but if you wanted to do something like that, I'd be happy to bring it up to our Board of Directors."

"Really!? That would be great. I'm definitely interested. Thank you."

Finally Somehow Home

"Our next board meeting is Wednesday after next at 6 PM at the Plaza Inn Restaurant. Come by and tell the board what you're thinking and let's see what they say. It would be great to get some more people out here."

"I'll be there. Thanks, Bill."

I had about a week and a half to put something together, so I started toying around with some ideas. I might as well start a little side hustle for some extra scratch. Pickins are slim when you're just writing every day, and I'd shot so damn much over the years of my life that it really did come to me like breathing. Might as well put those skills to good use. It would be great if my students could get discounts on guns and equipment, I thought. Hell, a lot of what keeps you alive in a shitstorm is proper selection and rigging of gear, plus, just like a ghee in most Martial Arts, there is certain equipment besides just a pistol or AR that you're gonna need to learn right, so I might as well help my students with identifying and purchasing what they're going to need up front. I knew a few people in the industry, so I picked up the phone and started making calls.

Bryce, from Vortex Optics was on board from the get-go and in addition to setting up a discount through me told

Finally Somehow Home

me to send him a wish list of optics that I'd need to get things off the ground. It was a godsend. And a hell of an advertising platform for Vortex as well. Think about it, if you're a novice shooter and you see your instructor using Vortex optics every day on his own guns, you're going to learn to trust that brand, especially if you get the chance to get your hands on it and finger fuck it before you decide to make the purchase, and even more so if you get a massive discount on the shit. With this business model in mind, I got ahold of several different equipment and firearms companies and brokered agreements with them for either direct discounts to my students if they purchased with my discount code, or direct discounts to me that I could pass through to my students.

Jason had reached out to me several months before on LinkedIn. He was a former Recon Marine from 1st Recon Company, having left around the same time I got there in 1996. He'd been reading some of the excerpts from this very book that I had posted on there and got in touch to let me know he appreciated my writing. It was great to hear that the stories had resonated with him and it's always good to meet other Recondos after they've moved onto their next chapters in life and watch them continue

Finally Somehow Home

to kick ass. Jason had been working for major defense contractors such as Raytheon and was at the highest echelons of their organization when he got sick of all the stupid woke bullshit and limp dick fuckerey getting shoved into every nook and cranny of their operation and impeding support to the American Warfighter. So, he decided to pull chalks and do something else. He had grown up in Louisiana as a poor kid scrubbing shitters and doing grunt work and making it somehow all the way up to a highly compensated business executive, so he didn't really get the whole white privilege thing. Furthermore, he had grown up hunting and fishing and realized, hell if you're gonna do anything in life, do something you love, so before departing the military industrial complex he started some due diligence on prospective firearms companies he could work for. First, he looked into Winchester and discovered they were no longer American owned. Same with Browning, Colt, and Barrett who have all sold out to European conglomerates and Remington doesn't even own the rights to their name anymore and have been in chapter 11 bankruptcy no less than three times. After a little bit of discovery he realized that there were really no great American firearms companies left in the world. Most of

Finally Somehow Home

them were owned by European conglomerates. And guess where all that money that Americans pay for their American guns goes? It goes straight back to fucking Europe. Including, of course, Sig Sauer, who has somehow created the illusion that they are now an American company. The fact of the matter is that all the profits earned by these companies go back to Europe. To countries that have no say in and no support of our Second Amendment. Jason decided he was gonna change that.

And while we're on the subject of the Second Amendment, let's talk about it for a little bit. The Second Amendment has nothing to do with hunting. This question of "What do you really need an assault rifle for?" speaks to it exactly. If you want to be stupid about shit, you can put an end to hunting, but the Second Amendment was written about combat weapons. Why? Because an armed citizenry in the United States is the world's last stand against tyranny. The buck stops with this country. Do you really think that all the special interest groups who have so much power would get anywhere at all if it weren't for the United States backing their play? Do you think the leaders of the Chinese Communist Party give a good god damn about the

Finally Somehow Home

environment, or minority rights, or freedom of religion? Fuck no. Those guys are Mob thugs - made men - who happen to be in a position of government. The real question is this: "Is all the gun violence in America really worth the right to bear arms?" It's a legitimate question. Let me relay something I wrote to Bushhog awhile back that might help you put this into context.

God Damn it. Fucking Memorial Day.

Let's dredge up a shitload of the heavy stuff Day.

I always forget.

I guess I think I've gotten over it somehow.

Or past it.

I'm not even sure what "it" is.

It's not fucking pity for you. Fuck no. Only the limp dick civilians do that.

It's not mourning. You'd call me a pussy and tell me to quit bitchin'. You always hated bitchin'. It pissed you the fuck off.

Finally Somehow Home

I'm not feeling sorry for myself. Fuck no. You'd swing on me for that, for sure.

Dude, I was at a Chiropractor's office in Snohomish, Washington a few years back, and mentioned the Marine Corps and falling out of airplanes etc. as a cause of my back issues. "Was it worth it?" he asked. I still hate that fuck and hope he dies a horrible fucking death soon for it.

Was it fucking worth it?

As if we went in expecting a fucking treat after?

I wanted to kill him with my bare hands.

Was your violent fucking death worth what, exactly, Johnny?

The values of what is at stake in that question are so high as to be almost incomprehensible.

Was your death worth the chance to kill the people who would be standing in your fucking Chiropractor office laughing as you watched them in the mirror slowly saw your fucking head off? You fucking piece of shit, fuck?

Yes.

Finally Somehow Home

It was.

It was worth it.

How much is it worth to kill those who would violently kill my kids and yours and our families if they had the slightest chance?

It's worth your life, brother.

I didn't have to pay that. You did.

I know you'd be ok with that.

It will never sit right with me that you gave so much.

And I didn't have to.

That's what the "it" is.

And I miss the fuck out of you, motherfucker.

I hope I'm making you proud somehow.

   Bullshit'n with Johnny - Memorial Day 2023

So, let's ask the question again. It is not an easy one at all to answer. "Is all the gun violence in America really worth the right to bear arms?" Remember, the rights and

Finally Somehow Home

freedom of the people of the world are at stake, for if the United States should fall, either from without or from within, all the dominoes will follow after. That's the question. You decide for yourself. As much as it pains me to say it... I think it is.

Within 9 months of founding Watchtower Firearms (named after Operation Watchtower – the invasion of Guadalcanal and the turning point of WWII in the Pacific), the Watchtower Firearms Apache, a double-stacked 1911 in 9mm, and aptly named after Operation Apache Snow – Hamburger Hill in Vietnam, was on the cover of Guns and Ammo. Jason didn't fuck around, he was out to create the next great American firearms company, and by the looks of it, he's going to pull it off.

I shot him a paragraph on LinkedIn letting him know what I was trying to accomplish and got this back afew days later: "Jason, apologies for not responding sooner. I have been underwater this week. The short answer is yes, I am interested and will give you a call Monday afternoon if you have some time? How many AR platforms do you believe you would need?"

Afew months before, my good buddy Ben from my days in Israel, got me a gig in LA training stunt men in basic

Finally Somehow Home

tactics so they didn't look like dorks when it came to handling weapons. We were putting together a pitch for a potential video game of a popular action movie for Netflix. It was a great experience and got me thinking further about starting a training company. I had to have a corporation in place to get paid for the stunt work, so I created SPADILLE LLC. The Spadille is the name for the Ace of Spades card which I adopted as the logo for the company. So, I already had a corporate entity in place for it, I just had to flesh it out.

About ten days after I'd met Bill on the range, I showed up to the Board of Directors meeting thinking I'd knock it out of the park. Not so. Just like the rest of Vale, there were afew on the board that didn't like the idea of their range becoming anything different than it was. They decided to deliberate on it. I went home and kept making phone calls. I was already committed.

Afew days later a Watchtower 9mm AR pistol with a brace, a .223 Wilde AR, and an AR 10 in .308 showed up at my gunsmith's shop with my name on them. They were beautifully crafted deadly works of art. I could swear Jason had Elves in a sweatshop cranking these things out but come to find out he had abunch of Combat Veterans

Finally Somehow Home

in there instead. And these guys knew a hell of a lot more about gunfighting than Elves. I really wanted an Apache too, but the waitlist was off the chain, especially after that Guns & Ammo cover, so I'm saving up for that, or maybe for their newest pistol as of right now, the Demolitia. When Jesus comes riding back down on his white horse from heaven, I wouldn't be surprised if his first stop is Texas so he can trade in his flaming sword for a Watchtower Demolitia and a Type 15. I've made afew minor modifications to mine just to tune it, but Watchtower guns are the best bang for your buck you'll find anywhere in the world. They are premium firearms made by combat veterans sold at reasonable prices and all the parts and pieces are made and assembled in the USA by Americans, unlike all the other "American firearms companies" whose parts are made in fucking South Korea, or Japan, or fuckin Spain who haven't been in a war in almost a century and haven't won one by themselves in a millennia. Holy Shit. What a concept. Watchtower was doing it right. One of my former snuffie Lance Coconuts had retired as a fucking First Sergeant, and a combat decorated Vet at that, Eric, was now the COO at Longhorn Ammunition, and set me up with 7000 rounds of quality 9mm ammo to get me back on my game

Finally Somehow Home

and resell what I could. And that was all I had, but that was a fucking lot considering only a couple weeks' work.

Shadow Systems was another such company. Basically, an American remake of GLOCK. Henry, one of the execs there sent me an XR920P – a delicious wicked little fucker and about the best shooting you'll find in a GLOCK type frame, especially if you drop a RAMM trigger into it. Wilder Tactical, maker of the finest gun belts I've ever used, and owned by a former Ranger, set me up with a brokerage agreement. X2 Development Group, out of Boise, Idaho gave me one of their TRIDENT barrels which I promptly slapped onto my Watchtower Type 15 which gave me another 250 yards of range on that rifle, and Genesis Arms agreed to kick in one of their semi-auto 12 gauge AR based shotguns once I got up and running.

Then the questions set in. "What the fuck am I doing? I'm supposed to be writing this book and I'm fucking around with this training company that I didn't even mean to start." It conflicted me for a long time. I was spending all of my time with this new thing and it seemed to be undermining my writing and I didn't know what to do about it. Fuck.

Finally Somehow Home

Then I thought of Hemingway and how he used to have to write as a reporter to make ends meet. Well hell, I thought, I can just do both. So, I spent most of my time for a couple of months building up SPADILLE. Even though the Snake River's Sportsmen's Club declined to let me use their range I was able to make agreements with the Parma Rod and Gun Club in Parma, ID and began making agreements with other ranges in the area. I even got flood lights so we could train at night after people got off work during the week. What I was trying to set up was a martial arts program in the art of practical tactical shooting. Shooting is a martial art. You don't see Delta Force guys walking around with Samurai swords. They use fucking guns. Because guns work best. I'm not taking anything away from traditional martial arts, that is an important skill to be sure. However, you can wrestle around all day if you want but I'm just gonna shoot your dumb ass. And that's how it works. You need to know a little bit of everything. I started writing a business plan for SPADILLE, here's the Executive Summary:

Since the Chinese invented gunpowder, the most effective Martial Art in the world is that of the Gunfighter. That is why our mark is the SPADILLE. The Ace of Spades. The highest card in the deck. Mike Tyson didn't just take a

Finally Somehow Home

boxing class. He made a commitment to himself and to his discipline in the pursuit of its mastery. SPADILLE adopts the Martial Arts mentorship and proficiency model in the form of a tiered subscription-based membership which disciples the student over the course of their tutelage in the Art of Practical Tactical Shooting and recognizes demonstrated proficiency much like the administration of colored belts in most Martial Arts disciplines, with the purpose of instilling a fierce and compelling sense of personal accountability and moral responsibility in the practice of their Art.

SPADILLE's corpus of instructors will continue to grow over time as the enterprise spreads geographically. This Cadre will be entirely comprised, without exception, of Special Operations Forces (SOF) Combat Veterans such as Army Rangers, Special Forces, Delta Force, Navy SEALs, Marine Corps Force Recon, Scout Snipers, and Raiders. SPADILLE provides the unique opportunity to America's greatest and truest Heroes, who have sacrificed most of their lives for the sake of the priceless Liberty we each enjoy, to establish and operate their own business in a discipline they have already mastered, as a SPADILLE Chapter, in a location of their own choosing, within a community of their peers and brethren, from which they can derive a prosperous living, mission, and sense of purpose previously only afforded to them in the context of the intensity of their great sacrifice in war.

SPADILLE leverages a hybrid of cutting edge and highly successful business models derived from companies and industries such as Uber, CrossFit, Walmart, Airbnb, Martial Arts, Physical Fitness, and others to create an Enterprise of Goal-aligned, mutually supporting Networks in the field and Discipline of Practical Tactical Shooting.

Partnerships with manufacturers of ammunition, firearms, clothing, and equipment relevant to Practical Tactical Shooting facilitate direct access of the enterprise to the best of breed products and tools of the trade enabling students to observe daily instructor use and application of these products, handle and train with them, and ultimately purchase the very products they have trained with and/or otherwise trust at highly discounted rates. This relationship benefits Industry Partners with opportunities to showcase their products directly to their target demographic, introduce new products for test and evaluation by combat experienced Subject Matter Experts, receive product-tuning feedback, and even provide

Finally Somehow Home

hands-on training modules to SPADILLE instructors and students, facilitating immediate bulk orders and subsequent intense proliferation of their products throughout the enterprise and beyond as SPADILLE shooters rub shoulders with others in the communities of relevance across the nation.

Eventually I want to take SPADILLE national and maybe even international. Build it into a global community like CrossFit. But for now, I'm doing something I've never done before – I'm taking it one step at a time - building it from the ground up and sinking my own roots into a local community so I can finally begin to belong somewhere. We'll always be vagabonds that don't quite fit in, but that's ok. It's a tough spot, but not impossible. I've learned something important in the course of studying my life to write it down. The story is about the relationships. All of them. The good and the bad. The story is about that invisible sinue that makes us all one thing. That makes us humanity.

This is something that I struggled with throughout the writing of this book. It seemed to me there needed to be a big slam bang finish. One where I was happy and rich and had all that most people ever dream of. Well, I'm not rich. But I do have joy in my life. Within my very self exists love, joy, peace, patience, kindness, goodness, faithfulness, gentleness, and even sometimes some self-control. Of course, I do hope someday to get all of the gravy. But I already have the steak.

I'd still like to build all the things I've designed or at least some of them if I can find the funding, and after this book is finished I'll return to work for LCDM Tech creating systems for next generation warfare, but if I do nothing else in this life, at least I've written parts of it down, so maybe it won't take others so long to get through some of the shit I've had to figure out.

There is a tremendous temptation for a writer to make it look like he's got his shit together, or at least that he's not a total fucking fool. This has been a very difficult book to write, for to write it you must relive it, and in reliving it I've been forced to watch myself through many times being a fool at best and a fucking god damn bastard at worst. It's not lost on me that in years passed I'd have been stoned to death or otherwise gotten rid of by the rest of humanity for my actions. This exercise has made me understand what a truly despicable motherfucker I really am, and you can say all you want about life lessons

Finally Somehow Home

but maybe it would have been better for humanity had I been ground up slowly in a wood chipper for my sins. Others have suffered worse for simply slipping. I've somehow evaded it in spite of all my flagrant transgressions. So far anyway. The purpose of this book is not to tell a wild story that sells, but rather to face down some of the things in life that many contend with in the lonesome shameful silence of themselves, where none else may enter, because even to seek help is to expose your most vulnerable and wicked self. Few books are written for those who struggle with the deep depravities that ensnare and rape your soul while you watch, frozen in horror of yourself, because everything you've tried, to overcome it doesn't work. What help is there for the 21-year-old Tranny living in hotel rooms hookin' for the rest of their abysmal life because somehow their entire life and identity became only and all about sensation, or the pedophile trapped alone in their depravity and self-loathing with no known way of escape? Where's the book on how to get out of homelessness or finally be free of incessant suicidal ideations? There isn't one. But maybe this one comes close. Am I trying for attention by baring my soul and wretchedness to the whole world? I'm not. So why have I

Finally Somehow Home

done it? Because there is great power in bleeding, and if even only one person is ever helped in some small way by mine, that's the redemption of the blood. See it? My bleeding will be made worthy by what it can accomplish in the lives of others. See how that works? This, but infinitely more is the significance of the blood of Christ. His real blood was worth what it accomplished in this world and beyond it. Listen, God is not what you want Him to be. That's bullshit wishful thinking. If you believe that, you are creating a fantasy and then believing in it. He is only who he truly is or he is nothing at all. Those are your only choices. Relationship is discovery of another. And this exploration of what and who the fuck that nebulous triune force of essence is, who asks us to call it God, discovery of that thing is the ultimate adventure and purpose in life. And maybe there's some redemption in it. Maybe even a sliver of vindication. That's what's in it for me.

Finally Somehow Home

Chapter 43

I heard about a big meeting of the minds at Oxford University that took place over several days. The topic of discussion was something along the lines of "What makes Jesus Christ different from all other religions?" A few days into the meeting, CS Lewis walked by in the hall, and one of the other professors hailed him and told him what they were discussing. "Oh, that's easy," said Lewis, "the difference is grace." After a couple more days of deliberation, as the story went, the council decided that, Grace was indeed the one thing that set Jesus Christ apart from all other religions. Many of them have the same tenants, in fact, for a belief system to survive it must have merit, thus the alignment of desired and productive traits across belief systems. Self-destructive traits tend to kill off the belief systems that promote them. But the only way to actually produce those traits authentically is through the mechanism of grace. Beating and flogging and thrashing yourself until you manifest love, joy, peace, patience, kindness, goodness, faithfulness, gentleness, and self-control within yourself, for yourself, and unto yourself simply doesn't fucking work. It works great if the mandate is only to spread those traits around to others. Anyone can manufacture and act in love, joy, peace, patience, kindness, goodness, faithfulness, gentleness, and self-control, but only by grace, the grace of the author of all these things, in fact, can you "produce" the real thing. And the real thing is for you to experience, not for you to hand out. You can't hand out self-control. You can only experience it in and of yourself. And there's the difference. Religion mandates that everyone get their shit together. Jesus changes you into someone who has their shit together. Religion can only produce fake fruit. It looks like fruit to everyone else. But at the end of the day, the poor bastard handing out all his fruit is starving, because he's fucking empty inside. And religion tells him to keep lying to himself about how empty he really is and keep flogging himself so that he never catches on. It's fucking sick and twisted, but it's the god damn truth.

Finally Somehow Home

The substance, however, of a pure, authentic and incomprehensible relationship with the even more incomprehensible entity from which one derives these fruits, the natural byproduct of a person who truly possesses those things for and unto themselves, not for anyone else, that shit will spill over into the people and world around them completely uncontrived, unforced, unmanufactured, like a light bulb deriving the energy of its purpose from a source foreign and incomprehensible to it, and as a natural byproduct of a connection with this source, pure light emanates from it in the way that it was made to function - a blueprint that it had no knowledge of or influence of authorship, resulting in a natural emanation over which it has no control. That's the point of God in Man. That's the way it works, all else is artificial, self-contrived, and sourced from guilt, shame, obligation, or otherwise derived from that which smothers a human soul - a soul which has no intrinsic love, joy, peace, patience, kindness, goodness, faithfulness, gentleness, and self-control, but only puts on the facade of them and demands this artifice from all others. Religion is a living hell of fake for its most ardent followers that demands the visage of Right-ness and light from a vessel disconnected from any source but the

Finally Somehow Home

powerful potent angst of its own secret knowledge and shame of its emptiness and commensurate ineptitude to authentically experience these truly good things within and for its own self. Religion is slavery to guilt. It's a sick, disgusting, subversive, insidious counterfeit of the most authentic and thrivent fulfillment of purpose that a human being can experience for its own sake which brings forth as a matter of course the greatest and most potent beauty and purpose of the organism of humanity.

We never really officially dated, but Noel was the first person in my life anywhere close to a girlfriend in the post-high school sense. We met when I was at 1st Recon about six months before I left to Okinawa. She was a short little firecracker of a girl. 5'3" with dirty blonde hair just past her shoulders and enormous blue green eyes that looked like the ocean where it's really fucking deep. Her body was perfect. She was Italian but her ass was black, and her breasts bounced softly and perfectly above a toned midsection. We didn't have much time together, but we sure got a lot done. She'd call me all upset about school – she was going to San Diego State at the time - or some other such shit in the middle of the night and my dumb ass would drive 100 mph through El Nino's shitty-ass wind and rain on my buddy's Honda

Finally Somehow Home

CBR650 with tires so bald that you could see the white threads sticking out, just to bring her ice cream and sing Disney songs to her. We never really dated because she was with a SEAL who was deployed at the time, and she didn't want to break up with him while he was overseas. There's a kind of kinship between Special Operations dudes, so I felt kinda bad about it at first. But hey, fuck the SEALs. I got over it.

I had only limited and severely fucked up experience sexually until I met her. There was a strict no-touchy of the opposite sex rule at the missionary boarding schools. Hell, I hadn't even seen porn until I was 18. That shit was hard to come by for a missionary kid in Indonesia. The closest I could get to porn was spanking it to the lingerie section of the cumbersome 12lb annual SEARS catalogue.

I was six or seven years old. Me and my brothers and a friend of ours, who was probably 12 or so, were all having a sleepover out on the deck one night. I awoke to the strange and foreign sensation of someone doing things to my body that were beyond my sanction, control, or comprehension. If you've ever felt it, you know. It was the older boy. He wasn't violent or forceful.

Finally Somehow Home

He did certain things to me and asked me to do certain things to him. I felt no sexual sensation because at that young age I had no concept of it nor understanding of what was happening to my body, or my soul, or why, but he was the older kid. The cool kid. I was the chubby kid. I went along. Passing subtly, as I did, into a deep and crushing darkness that I did not understand.

I think it was two weeks before I told anyone about it. I had planned to just pretend it never happened, but I couldn't. From that moment on, all of my life that was before was gone. My new chief sensation, more intense than any other, was the fierce and vicious hatred of myself. I had no idea what had happened to me. I just knew beyond a doubt that I was a horrible person for it and at seven years old I used to look at the sharp kitchen knives and wonder if it wouldn't just be better if I used one on myself. Anything to get away from the overwhelming hatred of myself. I think it opened a Pandora's box that I wasn't ready to deal with at the time. Whatever the reason, and I suspect this is a big part of why I have always been so hypersexual, the switch got flipped far before my mind or body knew what the fuck was going on, not to mention a shitload of other baggage

Finally Somehow Home

that I didn't know how to deal with until much, much later in life.

I've heard that a very high percentage of Special Operations types experienced severe childhood trauma. Very fucking high, like in the 80-90 percentile. I think that's how we can deal with pretty much anything and go on as if nothing happened. You learn to just not think about certain things. Just bury it in the secret furnace of self-loathing of your innermost soul. No one on this earth will ever hate me as much as I have hated myself. It made everything else very easy. I deserved everything bad that ever happened to me, and much worse than that, I thought, so in my mind I was getting off easy anyway... bring on the pain, motherfuckers! It won't suck much worse than it already does, and I deserve it anyway, so hit me with your best fuckin shot! I wasn't an adrenaline junkie at all. I wasn't in it for the rush. I fucking hated the adrenaline. It made my hands shake, and my vision blur, and my throat dry. It pissed me off because it made it look like shit scared me, and I was already pissed off because it did scare me. It scared the shit out of me. I think most of us just flogged our will along at breakneck speed with guilt and pain and anything else we could get ahold of because the worst possible outcome, for me

Finally Somehow Home

anyway, wasn't death. Not even close. The worst possible outcome was that others would find out what a pathetic, weak-ass pussy I really was deep down at the core of my being. I fucking hated that pathetic welp. NOT ENOUGH, that's who I really am, I thought. I hated that motherfucker so intensely that I would endure anything, to never let anyone find out the truth about me. It was my own dark secret. I was an imposter. Death. Ha! Whatever. Death just meant the shitty movie was over sooner. Big fucking deal. Fucking up, though. Fucking up was worse than death. Fucking up was eternal hell, because it exposed the real me, the weakling who wasn't good enough, and that's all anyone would ever remember of me.

I blocked it all out eventually. When I was a kid, I mean. After awhile, I forgot why I hated myself, I just did. And maybe that's why shit was so brutal with my ex-wife. She claimed to see in me what I had been hiding from everyone else. That deep down I was pathetic. NOT ENOUGH. Maybe that's why it hurt so fucking bad. Because she actually agreed with me about who I thought I was, and she believed that about me just as much as I did. And still does. And now so do my kids. And that's why it's my own eternal hell.

Finally Somehow Home

There is an Upshot to PTSD. The Upshot is that when you finally begin to deal with it. When you finally begin to unpack the "Don't think about it bucket" that you've shoved all of your war bullshit into... Well, you can't just dump out half the bucket. You have to dump all of it out. And when I finally did, there was a huge pile of bullshit in there that had been in there for many years before I ever put on a uniform. I was confronted with a snarl of shit from my childhood that I hadn't even thought of in many years. But just because I hadn't been thinking about it doesn't mean it wasn't having a huge effect on my life. Quite the contrary. Because I had learned to cope with those things in a certain way, I had not experienced peace or happiness since I was a little kid. And I didn't know why until then. You can't flog yourself into happiness. And bludgeoning myself thus was how I'd always gotten results. It's how I'd been able to perform as good or better than many of the most elite Special Operators in the world. It worked great for that. But it precluded any chance at enjoying any of life. You can't beat someone into loving you and making you happy, including yourself. And you will always despise the person you're beating, especially if it's you. You see, that's religion. You may perform according to the

Finally Somehow Home

standard. But it's a bullshit standard. The real standard is the measure of your love, your joy, your peace, your patience, your kindness, your goodness, your faithfulness, your gentleness, and your self-control. If you don't have these things for you, you're missing the point, or you're talking to the wrong guy, or both.

Anyway, I'm not there anymore. I don't live my life under the whip any longer. But I'll be honest, I have never really put it all together in my mind until right now. I didn't realize that my self-loathing and insecurity made me such a juicy target. I made it easy for them. The most hurtful thing they could ever do to me was reinforce my own false beliefs of who I was. All they had to do was agree with me and it destroyed me. And if there is a God and a Devil, you can bet your sweet ass the Devil does the same damn thing. All he has to do is agree with you and he's got you drowning in shame. I have never seen this before now for what it is. The only way to remove their levers was to change the way I saw myself. And it occurred to me, that if that nebulous fucking triune thing claims to like me, and thinks I'm cool, and gives me grace when I fuck up, and the only one who could remove my shame sees me as Justified (Just-as-if-I'd never fucked up), and wants me to know Him because

Finally Somehow Home

He fucking loves me, because He made me exquisitely unique and razor sharp and beautiful, like no other creature in eternity, then I was lost, then He sacrificed the life of His own Son for me, so I didn't have to pay that price. Maybe it's not too far of a stretch to do the unthinkable and love myself. I used to really not care if I died. I still have some lingering hopeful anticipation that death will bring rest, but I really want to live now. When I finally turned that corner, I found that for the first time since I was seven years old, I want to live. There is a HUGE Upshot to PTSD. I'm much more fulfilled now than I have ever been. I have found peace and rest in this life. And only in the rich and fertile soil of peace will you find your joy begin to grow. Everyone wants to be happy. Fuck happy. Happy is a buzz, a line of blow, a cigarette, an orgasm. Happy is a diversion. All that keeps you from all you want most, is all you want less. Happy is all you want less, and it stands directly between you and your joy because it is not deep enough or strong enough to sustain peace.

It's interesting that all that we know of that all of us know – the only experiences to which every single living being in this universe can relate, including God, are the experiences of beauty and of pain. That's it. Those are

Finally Somehow Home

the only things that everyone can relate to. But what's really amazing about it is how it actually works – it's the pain that wrings the beauty out of it all. It took three wars, the greatest pain I've ever felt from the person who professed to love me most, separation from my own children, and utter humiliation in the eyes of everyone I've ever known, but I would have never otherwise begun to unpack the burden of shit that I'd been carrying with me since I was a little boy who hated himself and didn't know why he thought he was dirty inside and stared at the kitchen knives wondering how bad it would hurt to not feel the incessant roaring unbearable shame that I could not comprehend. When finally, I saw it all laid out at once before me, it became a beaconed pathway. And now I lift my head to see where it has brought me and find that I have been here once before, many years ago. I would have never made it back if it wasn't for the pain. Back to peace and rest and joy again. And following its harsh and jagged pathway back from the far-flung corners of this world and mind where I have dwelt and roamed, it dawns suddenly upon me where I am again, I am finally somehow home.

-THE END-

Finally Somehow Home

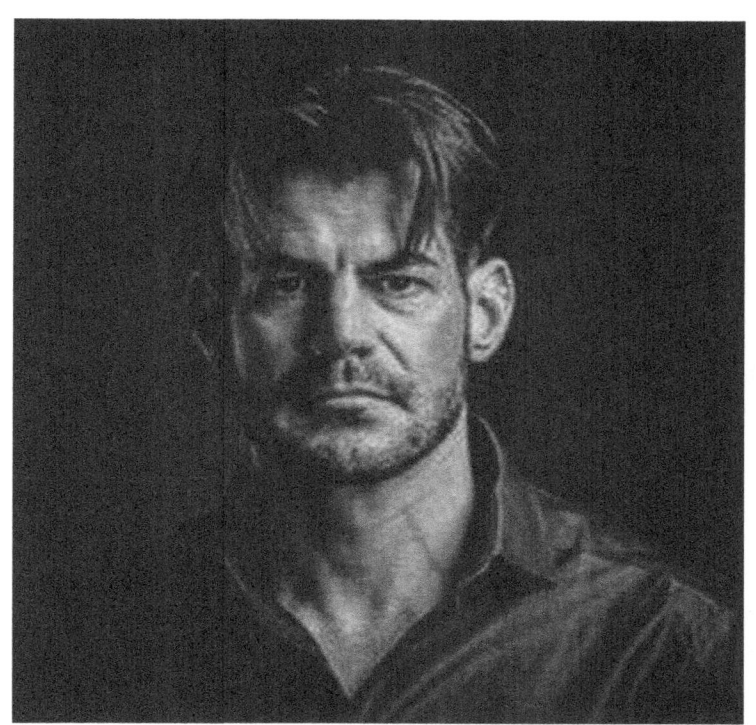

Jason Lee Morrison

FOR MORE BY JASON LEE MORRISON GO TO:

www.theperfectfuckinglife.com

Made in the USA
Las Vegas, NV
24 November 2024